INTRODUCTION TO PHARMACOLOGY

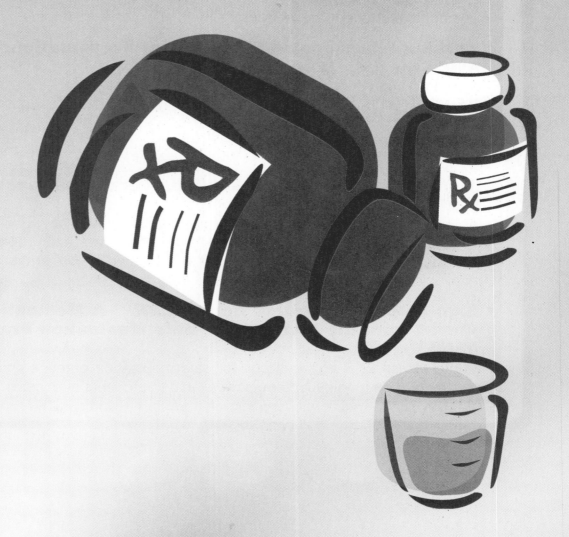

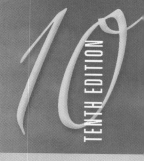

INTRODUCTION TO PHARMACOLOGY

Mary Kaye Asperheim, MD

Staff Physician
Smith Medical Clinic
Pawleys Island, South Carolina;
Formerly, Instructor of Pharmacology
St. Louis University School of Nursing and Health Services
St. Louis, Missouri

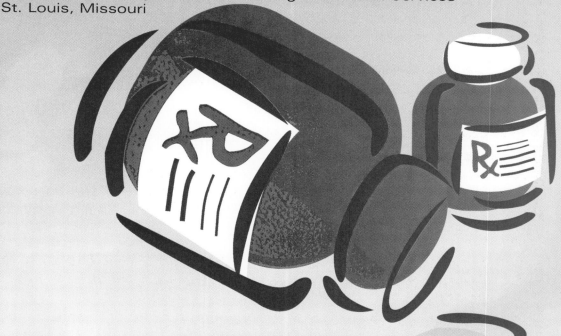

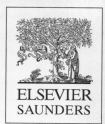

ELSEVIER
SAUNDERS

ELSEVIER
SAUNDERS

11830 Westline Industrial Drive
St. Louis, Missouri 63146

INTRODUCTION TO PHARMACOLOGY
Copyright © 2005, Elsevier Inc.

ISBN 1-4160-0189-1

NOTICE

Previous editions copyrighted 2002, 1996, 1992, 1987, 1981, 1975, 1971, 1967, 1963

International Standard Book Number 1-4160-0189-1

Editor: Lee Henderson
Senior Developmental Editor: Maureen Iannuzzi
Publishing Services Manager: Catherine Jackson
Senior Project Manager: Jeff Patterson
Designer: Bill Drone

Printed in the United States of America

Last digit is the print number: 9 8 7 6 5 4 3 2 1

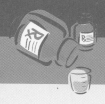

To the Instructor

Introduction to Pharmacology, 10th edition, welcomes the beginning student in practical nursing and other allied health fields to the study of pharmacology. After providing the student with a thorough grounding in mathematics and dosage calculation, *Introduction to Pharmacology* presents basic pharmacology principles and monographs on the major drugs in a concise, understandable, and straightforward manner. The many features included here make the text both a learning tool and a quick reference for current drug information and other issues involved in health care.

As in previous editions, the text is divided into four units: Mathematics of Drug Dosage, Principles of Pharmacology, Drug Classifications (categorized by anatomic systems), and Special Situations in Pharmacology.

New to this edition are two chapters: Chapter 22, Pain Medications, discusses the sensible, patient-centered use of narcotic and nonnarcotic analgesics in the treatment of chronic, nonfatal conditions. Chapter 31, Innovations: Gene Therapy, explains the principles and uses of medications resulting from the emerging fields of gene therapy and molecular medicine.

Additionally, Key Terms are now listed at the beginning of each chapter. Their in-context use is highlighted within the text, and a definition for every Key Term is included in the Glossary. New drugs have been added throughout, especially new antineoplastics and antivirals. There is increased information in the area of drug interactions, and some new methods of drug administration are included as well.

Returning from previous editions are the Lifespan Considerations and Herb Alert boxes appearing throughout the text and the Clinical Implications feature in each chapter. The Considerations boxes, Considerations for Children, Considerations for Pregnant and Nursing Women, and Considerations for Older Adults, highlight important drug considerations for each of these critical developmental stages. Herb Alert boxes highlight herb–drug interactions and contraindications—important information for a population that uses complementary and alternative therapies at an ever-increasing rate. The Clinical Implications feature offers valuable information for safe and effective drug administration and patient teaching for each drug category.

The online *Evolve Learning Resources to Accompany Introduction to Pharmacology*, 10th edition, are available free of charge with the text and offer the student a collection of Web Activities keyed to each chapter. These activities reinforce the student's understanding of important concepts presented in the text. Also on Evolve, students can sign up to receive the *Mosby/Saunders ePharmacology Update* newsletter and the *Nurse Advise-ERR*, a Medication Safety Alert from the Institute for Safe Medication Practices.

Instructors may choose the ancillary format with which they are most comfortable. A printed *Instructor's Manual to Accompany Introduction to Pharmacology* includes Tips for Teaching English as a Second Language (ESL) students, Answers to Review and Critical Thinking Questions, Web Activities, and Open-Book Quizzes. The *Instructor's Resource CD-ROM* offers both the complete Instructor's Manual and a Test Bank with approximately 400 NCLEX® Examination–style questions. The *Evolve* website offers the instructor the Student Resources mentioned previously, as well as the complete Instructor's Manual and Test Bank, Mosby's Nursing Pharmacology PowerPoint Collection, and Mosby's Electronic Image Collection for Pharmacology.

I would like to thank many who worked on this edition, particularly Linda Kerby of Mastery Educational Consultations for her accuracy review and the Test Bank. Lisa Hernandez, copy editor, Jeff Patterson, Senior Project Manager, and David Rushing, the Multimedia Producer of the Evolve website, gave helpful and skilled assistance wherever needed. I would also like to thank Alfred J. Rémillard for supplying the Canadian Drug Information for this edition.

The ongoing support and help of Editor Lee Henderson and Senior Developmental Editor Maureen Iannuzzi are greatly appreciated. The editors are present from the first conception of the edition and are involved with determining the needs of the students so that the text can respond satisfactorily.

As it has for the past nine editions, I trust that this text will continue to serve as a helpful, understandable introduction to pharmacology for beginning students.

MARY KAYE ASPERHEIM FAVARO, MD

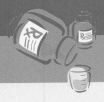

Content Threads

Introduction to Pharmacology, 10th edition, shares some features and design elements with other LPN titles on the Elsevier list. The purpose of these Content Threads is to make it easier for students and instructors to use the variety of books required by the relatively brief and demanding LPN curriculum.

The shared features in *Introduction to Pharmacology,* 10th edition, include the following:

- A **reading level evaluation** performed on every manuscript chapter during the book's development. The purpose is to increase the consistency among chapters and to make the text easy to understand.

- Cover and internal **design similarities.** The colorful, student-friendly design encourages the reading and learning of the core content.

- Numbered lists of **Objectives** that begin each chapter.

- **Key Terms** with phonetic pronunciations and page number references at the beginning of each chapter. The key terms are in color the first time they appear in the chapter.

- **Critical Thinking questions** at the end of most chapters.

- A **Glossary** at the end of the text.

And for instructors:

- A **Computerized Test Bank** with the following categories of information: Topic, Step of the Nursing Process, Objective, Cognitive Level, NCLEX® Category of Client Need, Correct Answer, Rationale, and Text Page Reference.

- A **PowerPoint slide presentation** in the Instructor's Resource CD-ROM.

- **Open-Book Quizzes** in the Instructor's Manual.

- **Tips for teaching English as a Second Language (ESL) students** in the Instructor's Manual.

In addition to content and design threads, these LPN textbooks benefit from the advice and input of the Elsevier Advisory Board.

Advisory Board

SHIRLEY ANDERSON, MSN
Kirkwood Community College
Cedar Rapids, Iowa

MARY BROTHERS, MED, RN
Coordinator, Garnet Career Center
  School of Practical Nursing
Charleston, West Virginia

**PATRICIA A. CASTALDI, RN,
BSN, MSN**
Union County College
Plainfield, New Jersey

**DOLORES ANN COTTON, RN,
BSN, MS**
Meridian Technology Center
Stillwater, Oklahoma

**LORA LEE CRAWFORD, RN,
BSN**
Emanuel Turlock Vocational Nursing
  Program
Turlock, California

**RUTH ANN ECKENSTEIN, RN,
BS, MED**
Oklahoma Department of Career and
  Technology Education
Stillwater, Oklahoma

PAM HINCKLEY, RN, MSN
Redlands Adult School
Redlands, California

**DEBORAH W. KELLER, RN,
BSN, MSN**
Erie Huron Ottawa Vocational
  Education School of Practical
  Nursing
Milan, Ohio

PATTY KNECHT, MSN, RN
Nursing Program Director
Center for Arts & Technology
Brandywine Campus
Coatesville, Pennsylvania

**SHEILA LASSITER, MSN, RN,
CRNP**
Director, Practical Nursing Program
Breslin Learning Center
District 1199 Training
Philadelphia, Pennsylvania

**FRANCES NEU SHULL, MS,
BSN, RN**
Miami Valley Career Technology
  Center
Clayton, Ohio

BEVERLEY TURNER, MA, RN
Director, Vocational Nursing
  Department
Maric College, San Diego Campus
San Diego, California

**SISTER ANN WIESEN, RN,
MRA**
Erwin Technical Center
Tampa, Florida

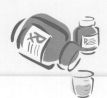

To the Student

Designed with the student in mind, this textbook will introduce you to the world of pharmacology. To guide your way, look for the following signposts.

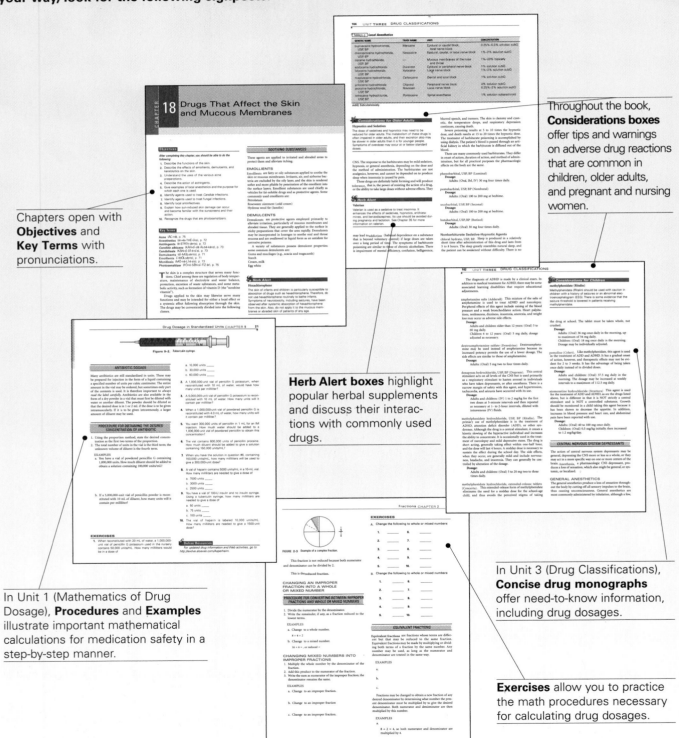

Chapters open with **Objectives** and **Key Terms** with pronunciations.

Herb Alert boxes highlight popular herbal supplements and discuss their interactions with commonly used drugs.

In Unit 1 (Mathematics of Drug Dosage), **Procedures** and **Examples** illustrate important mathematical calculations for medication safety in a step-by-step manner.

Throughout the book, **Considerations boxes** offer tips and warnings on adverse drug reactions that are common in children, older adults, and pregnant and nursing women.

In Unit 3 (Drug Classifications), **Concise drug monographs** offer need-to-know information, including drug dosages.

Exercises allow you to practice the math procedures necessary for calculating drug dosages.

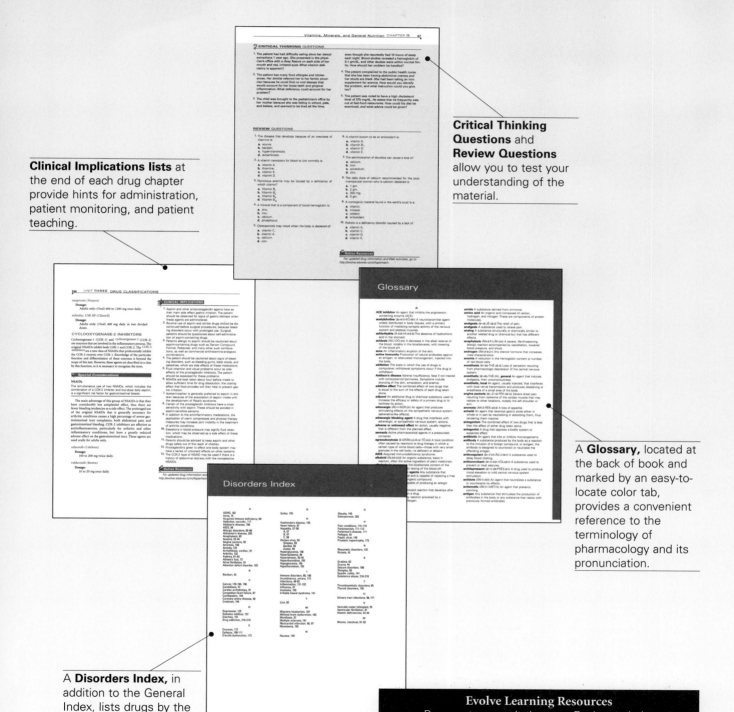

Clinical Implications lists at the end of each drug chapter provide hints for administration, patient monitoring, and patient teaching.

Critical Thinking Questions and **Review Questions** allow you to test your understanding of the material.

A **Glossary,** located at the back of book and marked by an easy-to-locate color tab, provides a convenient reference to the terminology of pharmacology and its pronunciation.

A **Disorders Index,** in addition to the General Index, lists drugs by the disorders for which they are used.

Evolve Learning Resources
Be sure to consult the new Evolve website
(http://evolve.elsevier.com/Asperheim/pharmacology/)
for web activities and signup pages for the
Mosby/Saunders ePharmacology Update newsletter and
the *Nurse Alert-ERR*™ newsletter.

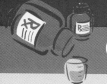

Contents

CHAPTER 1

Roman Numerals

Objectives

After completing this chapter, you should be able to do the following:

1. Write the basic Roman numerals for their Arabic equivalents.
2. Read and write Roman numerals with 100 percent accuracy.

Key Terms

Arabic (ĂR-é-bîk) **numeral system,** p. 1
Roman numeral system, p. 1

Unlike the **Arabic numeral system,** which uses symbols and decimal places to express numbers, the **Roman numeral system** uses letters to designate numbers. Their use is obviously restricted because mathematical procedures would become extremely complicated if the attempt were made to use these numerals in calculations. Lower case Roman numerals are occasionally used in prescriptions (see Chapter 13).

Basic Roman numerals are expressed as follows:

Roman Numeral	Arabic Number
I	1
V	5
X	10
L	50
C	100
D	500
M	1000

PROCEDURE FOR READING AND WRITING ROMAN NUMERALS

1. When a Roman numeral precedes one of larger value, its value is subtracted from the larger. When a numeral follows one of larger value, its value is added to the larger.

   EXAMPLES
   a. IV = (5 − 1) = 4
   b. XI = (10 + 1) = 11
   c. LXI = (50 + 10 + 1) = 61

2. When two numerals of identical value are reported in sequence, their values are added. (Numerals may never be repeated more than three times in sequence.)

   EXAMPLES
   a. XXX = 30
   b. MMXXVIII = 2028

3. When a numeral is placed between two numerals of greater value, the lesser is subtracted from the numeral following it.

   EXAMPLES
   a. XIV = (10 + 5 − 1) = 14
   b. XIX = (10 + 10 − 1) = 19
   c. CXLIX = (100 + 50 − 10 + 10 − 1) = 149

EXERCISES

A. Express the following in Roman numerals:

1. 35 _____
2. 89 _____
3. 72 _____
4. 55 _____
5. 101 _____
6. 92 _____
7. 135 _____
8. 1580 _____
9. 341 _____
10. 729 _____

B. Express the following in Arabic numbers:

1. MCCXI _____
2. DCCXX _____
3. CLXVI _____
4. DXXIX _____
5. MMMVI _____
6. DCCC _____
7. LVI _____
8. LXXV _____
9. MMDCLXXIII _____
10. LXI _____

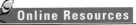
Online Resources

For updated drug information and Web activities, go to http://evolve.elsevier.com/Asperheim.

Objectives

After completing this chapter, you should be able to do the following:

1. Explain the meaning of a fraction and give an example of each type of fraction.
2. Convert between improper fractions and whole or mixed numbers.
3. Give the fundamental principles used in computing with fractions and give an example of each.
4. Demonstrate accurately the addition, subtraction, multiplication, and division of fractions and mixed numbers.

Key Terms

Complex fraction, p. 2
Equivalent (ĭ-kwĬV-ĕ-lĕnt) fraction, p. 3
Fraction, p. 2
Improper fraction, p. 2
Lowest common denominator, p. 4
Mixed number, p. 2
Proper fraction, p. 2
Reduced fraction, p. 3

A **fraction** indicates division and expresses the number of equal parts into which a whole is divided. If a whole is divided into equal parts, then one or more of this number of equal parts is called a fraction.

EXAMPLE
The fraction ⅜ means 3 of 8 equal parts (Figure 2–1). This could also be written 3 ÷ 8 because it indicates division into 8 equal parts.

In the example above, the numbers 3 and 8 are called the "terms of the fraction." The lower number of a fraction is called the *denominator*, or the divisor, and tells into how many parts the unit is divided. The upper number of the fraction is called the *numerator*, or the dividend, and tells how many parts of the unit are taken.

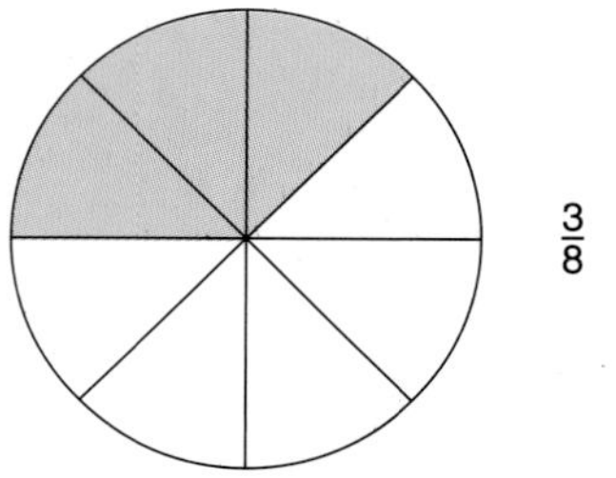

KINDS OF FRACTIONS

Proper fraction. Sometimes called a common fraction, or just "fraction," a **proper fraction** has a numerator that is smaller than the denominator and designates less than one whole unit.

EXAMPLES
$$\frac{1}{3}, \quad \frac{2}{5}, \quad \frac{3}{17}$$

Improper fraction. An **improper fraction** is one in which the numerator is larger than the denominator and designates more than one unit (Figure 2–2).

EXAMPLE
$$\frac{5}{4} \quad \text{or} \quad 1\frac{1}{4}$$

Mixed number. A mixed number consists of a whole number and a fraction.

EXAMPLES
$$3\frac{3}{7}, \quad 4\frac{2}{3}$$

Complex fraction. When both the numerator and the denominator (or just one of these) is in fraction form, we refer to the term as a **complex fraction.**

EXAMPLES
$$\frac{\frac{2}{3}}{\frac{3}{8}}, \quad \frac{\frac{4}{3}}{7}$$

Reduced fraction. A fraction is said to be reduced to its lowest terms when the numerator and denominator cannot be divided exactly by the same number (except 1).

$$\frac{3}{8}$$

FIGURE 2-1 The fraction 3/8 means 3 of 8 equal parts.

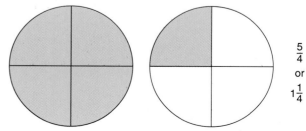

$$\frac{5}{4}$$
or
$$1\frac{1}{4}$$

FIGURE 2-2 Example of an improper fraction.

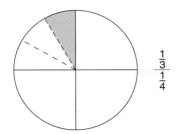

$$\frac{1}{3}$$
$$\frac{1}{4}$$

FIGURE 2-3 Example of a complex fraction.

EXAMPLE

$\frac{6}{8}$ This fraction is not reduced because both numerator and denominator can be divided by 2.

$\frac{6\,(\div 2)}{8\,(\div 2)} = \frac{3}{4}$ This is the **reduced fraction.**

PROCEDURE FOR CONVERTING BETWEEN IMPROPER FRACTIONS AND WHOLE OR MIXED NUMBERS

CHANGING AN IMPROPER FRACTION INTO A WHOLE OR MIXED NUMBER

1. Divide the numerator by the denominator.
2. Write the remainder, if any, as a fraction reduced to the lowest terms.

EXAMPLES

a. Change $\frac{8}{4}$ to a whole number.

   $8 \div 4 = 2$

b. Change $\frac{16}{6}$ to a mixed number.

   $16 \div 6 = 2\frac{4}{6}$, or reduced $= 2\frac{2}{3}$

CHANGING MIXED NUMBERS INTO IMPROPER FRACTIONS

1. Multiply the whole number by the denominator of the fraction.
2. Add this product to the numerator of the fraction.
3. Write the sum as numerator of the improper fraction; the denominator remains the same.

EXAMPLES

a. Change $2\frac{3}{8}$ to an improper fraction.

   $2 \times 8 = 16, 16 + 3 = 19 \therefore \frac{19}{8}$

b. Change $4\frac{2}{5}$ to an improper fraction

   $4 \times 5 = 20, 20 + 2 = 22$

c. Change $9\frac{1}{6}$ to an improper fraction.

   $9 \times 6 = 54, 54 + 1 = 55 \therefore \frac{55}{6}$

EXERCISES

A. Change the following to whole or mixed numbers:

1. $\frac{12}{8}$ _____		**6.** $\frac{25}{8}$ _____
2. $\frac{7}{5}$ _____		**7.** $\frac{79}{5}$ _____
3. $\frac{20}{10}$ _____		**8.** $\frac{64}{9}$ _____
4. $\frac{12}{4}$ _____		**9.** $\frac{26}{3}$ _____
5. $\frac{17}{9}$ _____		**10.** $\frac{410}{100}$ _____

B. Change the following to whole or mixed numbers:

1. $1\frac{1}{3}$ _____		**6.** $6\frac{4}{5}$ _____
2. $4\frac{1}{2}$ _____		**7.** $2\frac{1}{8}$ _____
3. $100\frac{3}{7}$ _____		**8.** $17\frac{1}{4}$ _____
4. $9\frac{1}{8}$ _____		**9.** $80\frac{5}{12}$ _____
5. $10\frac{4}{5}$ _____		**10.** $110\frac{1}{4}$ _____

EQUIVALENT FRACTIONS

Equivalent fractions are fractions whose terms are different but that may be reduced to the same fraction. Equivalent fractions may be made by multiplying or dividing both terms of a fraction by the same number. Any number may be used, as long as the numerator and denominator are treated in the same way.

EXAMPLES

a. $\frac{1\,(\times 2)}{8\,(\times 2)} = \frac{2}{16}$

b. $\frac{2\,(\times 32)}{3\,(\times 32)} = \frac{64}{96}$

c. $\frac{4\,(\div 2)}{6\,(\div 2)} = \frac{2}{3}$

Fractions may be changed to obtain a new fraction of any desired denominator by determining what number the present denominator must be multiplied by to give the desired denominator. Both numerator and denominator are then multiplied by this number.

EXAMPLES

a. $\frac{1}{2} = \frac{?}{8}$

   $8 \div 2 = 4$, so both numerator and denominator are multiplied by 4.

$$\frac{1}{2}\frac{(\times 4)}{(\times 4)} = \frac{4}{8}$$

b. $\frac{5}{9} = \frac{?}{72}$

$72 \div 9 = 8$, so both numerator and denominator are multiplied by 8.

$$\frac{5}{9}\frac{(\times 8)}{(\times 8)} = \frac{40}{72}$$

EXERCISES

Change the following fractions to equivalent fractions having the specified denominator:

1. $\frac{1}{4} = \frac{?}{20}$ _____   6. $\frac{8}{17} = \frac{?}{51}$ _____

2. $\frac{6}{13} = \frac{?}{39}$ _____   7. $\frac{7}{9} = \frac{?}{63}$ _____

3. $\frac{6}{15} = \frac{?}{60}$ _____   8. $\frac{9}{8} = \frac{?}{16}$ _____

4. $\frac{7}{18} = \frac{?}{36}$ _____   9. $\frac{6}{7} = \frac{?}{21}$ _____

5. $\frac{5}{4} = \frac{?}{32}$ _____   10. $\frac{63}{30} = \frac{?}{10}$ _____

PROCEDURE FOR FINDING THE LOWEST COMMON DENOMINATOR

1. Find the lowest possible number that is divisible by all the denominators, that is, the **lowest common denominator.**
2. Change the fractions to equivalent fractions using this denominator.

   EXAMPLE
   Find the lowest common denominator for the following:

   a. $\frac{1}{3}$ and $\frac{2}{5}$

   The lowest number divisible by 3 and 5 is 15, so this will be the new denominator.

   $$\frac{1}{3} = \frac{?}{15} = \frac{5}{15}$$
   $$\frac{2}{5} = \frac{?}{15} = \frac{6}{15}$$

   b. $\frac{2}{3}, \frac{7}{8}$, and $\frac{1}{6}$
   The lowest number divisible by 3, 8, and 6 is 24.

   $$\frac{2}{3} = \frac{?}{24} = \frac{16}{24}$$
   $$\frac{7}{8} = \frac{?}{24} = \frac{21}{24}$$
   $$\frac{1}{6} = \frac{?}{24} = \frac{4}{24}$$

   c. $\frac{2}{4}$ and $\frac{6}{8}$

The lowest common denominator is 8, so only the $\frac{2}{4}$ must be changed.

$$\frac{2}{4} = \frac{4}{8}$$
$$\frac{6}{8} = \frac{6}{8}$$

EXERCISES

Change the following to fractions having the lowest common denominator:

1. $\frac{7}{12}$ and $\frac{3}{6}$ _____   7. $\frac{2}{3}, \frac{1}{2}$, and $\frac{3}{4}$ _____

2. $\frac{6}{7}$ and $\frac{2}{3}$ _____   8. $\frac{3}{4}, \frac{5}{6}$, and $\frac{7}{8}$ _____

3. $\frac{1}{3}$ and $\frac{2}{9}$ _____   9. $\frac{8}{9}, \frac{9}{10}$, and $\frac{1}{3}$ _____

4. $\frac{2}{5}$ and $\frac{8}{20}$ _____   10. $\frac{4}{15}, \frac{3}{5}$, and $\frac{4}{25}$ _____

5. $\frac{1}{8}$ and $\frac{8}{24}$ _____   11. $1\frac{1}{3}, \frac{3}{6}$, and $\frac{1}{4}$ _____

6. $\frac{1}{4}, \frac{1}{5}$, and $\frac{1}{6}$ _____   12. $\frac{3}{5}, \frac{4}{6}$, and $\frac{4}{10}$ _____

PROCEDURE FOR ADDITION OF FRACTIONS AND MIXED NUMBERS

1. If the fractions have the same denominator, add the numerators and write the sum over the common denominator and reduce to the lowest terms.
2. If the fractions have unlike denominators, first find their lowest common denominator; then add the numerators as in step 1.
3. To add mixed numbers, first add the fractions as mentioned and then add this to the sum of the whole numbers.

EXAMPLES

a. $\frac{1}{5}$ b. $\frac{3}{5} = \frac{9}{15}$ c. $6\frac{1}{6} = 6\frac{8}{48}$

  $+\frac{2}{5}$ $+\frac{2}{3} = +\frac{10}{15}$ $+9\frac{5}{8} = +9\frac{30}{48}$

  $\frac{3}{5}$ $\frac{19}{15} = 1\frac{4}{15}$ $15\frac{38}{48} = 15\frac{19}{24}$

d. $1\frac{3}{8} = 1\frac{15}{40}$

  $+9\frac{9}{10} = +9\frac{36}{40}$

  $10\frac{51}{40}$ $\left(\frac{51}{40} = 1\frac{11}{40}\right) = 11\frac{11}{40}$

EXERCISES

Add the following numbers:

1. $\frac{1}{12}, \frac{2}{3}$, and $\frac{4}{9}$ _____

2. $\frac{3}{5}, \frac{2}{3},$ and $\frac{4}{10}$ _____

3. $2\frac{1}{3}$ and $4\frac{1}{8}$ _____

4. $7\frac{1}{4}, 6\frac{2}{8},$ and $4\frac{5}{6}$ _____

5. $\frac{2}{3}, \frac{1}{2},$ and $\frac{1}{4}$ _____

6. $3\frac{1}{2}, 2\frac{3}{10},$ and $5\frac{2}{5}$ _____

7. 5 and $\frac{7}{12}$ _____

8. $2, 1\frac{4}{4},$ and $2\frac{5}{6}$ _____

9. $24\frac{3}{8}, 12\frac{6}{7},$ and $\frac{5}{14}$ _____

10. $4\frac{1}{2}, 2\frac{3}{8},$ and $3\frac{1}{4}$ _____

PROCEDURE FOR SUBTRACTION OF FRACTIONS AND MIXED NUMBERS

1. If the fractions have the same denominator, find the difference between the numerators and write it over the common denominator. Reduce to the lowest terms.
2. If the fractions have unlike denominators, first find the lowest common denominator, then proceed as in step 1.
3. To subtract mixed numbers, first subtract the fractions as mentioned and then find the difference between the whole numbers. If the fraction in the subtrahend (bottom number) is larger than the fraction in the minuend (top number), it is necessary to borrow from the whole number before subtracting the fractions.

   EXAMPLES

   a. $\begin{aligned} \frac{4}{5} &= \frac{8}{10} \\ -\frac{1}{2} &= -\frac{5}{10} \\ &\frac{3}{10} \end{aligned}$ c. $\begin{aligned} 21\frac{7}{16} &= 20\frac{16}{16} + \frac{7}{16} = 20\frac{23}{16} \\ -7\frac{12}{16} &= \phantom{20\frac{16}{16} + \frac{7}{16} =} -7\frac{12}{16} \\ &= \phantom{20\frac{16}{16} + \frac{7}{16} =} 13\frac{11}{16} \end{aligned}$

   b. $\begin{aligned} 7\frac{16}{24} &= 7\frac{16}{24} \\ -3\frac{1}{8} &= -3\frac{3}{24} \\ &4\frac{13}{24} \end{aligned}$

EXERCISES

Subtract the following:

1. $\frac{8}{18} - \frac{3}{18}$ _____

2. $\frac{5}{7} - \frac{2}{3}$ _____

3. $\frac{7}{8} - \frac{1}{4}$ _____

4. $2\frac{4}{7} - 1\frac{1}{7}$ _____

5. $4\frac{2}{8} - 2\frac{7}{8}$ _____

6. $3\frac{10}{15} - \frac{7}{15}$ _____

7. $6 - 2\frac{2}{3}$ _____

8. $25\frac{4}{5} - 11$ _____

9. $20 - 16\frac{11}{12}$ _____

10. $4\frac{2}{3} - 1\frac{1}{2}$ _____

PROCEDURE FOR MULTIPLICATION OF FRACTIONS AND MIXED NUMBERS

1. Change mixed numbers to improper fractions.
2. Cancel if possible by dividing any numerator and denominator by the largest number contained in each.
3. Multiply remaining numerators to find numerator of answer.
4. Multiply remaining denominators to find denominator of answer.

   EXAMPLES

   a. $\frac{4}{5} \times \frac{15}{16} = \frac{\overset{1}{\cancel{4}}}{\cancel{5}} \times \frac{\overset{3}{\cancel{15}}}{\cancel{16}} = \frac{3}{4}$

   b. $6 \times \frac{3}{8} = \frac{\overset{3}{\cancel{6}}}{1} \times \frac{3}{\cancel{8}} = \frac{9}{4} = 2\frac{1}{4}$

EXERCISES

Multiply the following:

1. $\frac{1}{3} \times \frac{1}{4}$ _____

2. $\frac{7}{8} \times \frac{5}{9}$ _____

3. $3\frac{1}{3} \times 1\frac{1}{5}$ _____

4. $\frac{4}{5} \times 1\frac{8}{15}$ _____

5. $1\frac{1}{2} \times 2\frac{5}{6} \times 3\frac{1}{3}$ _____

6. $12 \times 2\frac{3}{4}$ _____

7. $\frac{2}{3} \times 6$ _____

8. $\frac{4}{200} \times 1000$ _____

9. $\frac{1}{3} \times \frac{4}{12} \times \frac{4}{6}$ _____

10. $\frac{3}{4} \times \frac{2}{5} \times \frac{2}{15}$ _____

PROCEDURE FOR DIVISION OF FRACTIONS AND MIXED NUMBERS

1. Change mixed numbers to improper fractions.
2. Invert the divisor (the number after the division sign).
3. Follow the steps for multiplication of fractions.

EXAMPLES

a. $\frac{2}{5} \div \frac{5}{8} = \frac{2}{5} \times \frac{8}{5} = \frac{16}{25}$ b. $8\frac{3}{4} \div 15 = \frac{\overset{7}{\cancel{35}}}{4} \times \frac{1}{\underset{3}{\cancel{15}}} = \frac{7}{12}$

EXERCISES

Divide the following:

1. $\frac{3}{5} \div \frac{7}{8}$ _____

2. $\frac{1}{12} \div \frac{1}{3}$ _____

3. $\frac{4}{6} \div \frac{6}{7}$ _____

4. $\frac{2}{3} \div 4$ _____

5. $3 \div \frac{1}{2}$ _____

6. $\frac{3}{4} \div \frac{4}{6}$ _____

7. $3\frac{1}{2} \div 1\frac{3}{4}$ _____

8. $1\frac{3}{4} \div 2$ _____

9. $1\frac{1}{2} \div 1\frac{1}{4}$ _____

10. $20\frac{1}{2} \div 50$ _____

RATIO

A ratio indicates the relationship of one quantity to another. It indicates division and may be expressed in fraction form.

EXAMPLES

a. $\frac{3}{9}$ may be expressed as a ratio: 3:9

b. 1:1000 may be expressed as a fraction: $\frac{1}{1000}$

EXERCISES

Express the following ratios as fractions reduced to lowest terms:

1. 1:3 _____

2. 5:7 _____

3. 2:1000 _____

4. 7:63 _____

5. 42:83 _____

6. 2:17 _____

7. 7:56 _____

8. 1:11 _____

9. 2:150 _____

10. 4:9 _____

Online Resources

For updated drug information and Web activities, go to http://evolve.elsevier.com/Asperheim.

3 Decimals

After completing this chapter, you should be able to do the following:

1. Read and write decimals with 100 percent accuracy.

2. Add, subtract, multiply, and divide decimals with 100 percent accuracy.

3. Convert decimals to fractions with 100 percent accuracy.

4. Convert common fractions to decimals with 100 percent accuracy.

Key Terms

Decimal, p. 7
Place value, p. 7

A **decimal** is a fraction whose denominator is 10 or any multiple of 10, such as 100, 1000, 10,000, and so forth. However, it differs from a common fraction in that the denominator is not written but is expressed by the proper placement of the decimal point. Usually decimal fractions and mixed decimals are just called "decimals."

PROCEDURE FOR READING AND WRITING DECIMALS

1. Observe the following scale of place values. The **place value** of a digit is its value based on its position relative to the decimal point. All whole numbers are to the left of the decimal point; all fractions are to the right.

Hundred Thousands | Ten Thousands | Thousands | Hundreds | Tens | Units | . | Tenths | Hundredths | Thousandths | Ten Thousandths | Hundred Thousandths

2. In reading a decimal fraction, read the number to the right of the decimal point and use the name that applies to the "place value" of the last figure.

EXAMPLE

0.257 = two hundred fifty-seven thousandths

3. In reading a mixed decimal, first read the whole number, then the decimal fraction. The word "and" shows the place of the decimal point.

EXAMPLE

327.006 = three hundred twenty-seven and six thousandths

EXERCISES

A. Write the following:

1. 0.03 _____

2. 0.089 _____

3. 23.5 _____

4. 5.21 _____

5. 0.0029 _____

6. 200.09 _____

7. 37.282 _____

8. 4256.353 _____

9. 256.01 _____

10. 0.0008 _____

B. Express the following as decimal fractions:

1. Four thousandths _____

2. Twenty-six hundredths _____

3. Five and three millionths _____

4. Seven hundredths _____

5. Three and one tenth _____

6. Eighty-eight thousandths _____

7. Two hundred thirty-three and fifty-seven millionths _____

8. Two and three tenths _____

9. Eight and four hundredths _____

10. Twenty-five and three thousandths _____

PROCEDURE FOR ADDITION OF DECIMALS

1. Write the decimals in a column, placing the decimal points directly under each other.
2. Add as in the addition of whole numbers. (Zeros may be added after the decimal point as place holders to prevent errors in addition; this does not change the value of the decimal.)
3. Place the decimal point in the sum directly under the decimal points in the addends (the numbers that are being added).

EXAMPLES

a. $0.8 + 0.5 =$
$$\begin{array}{r} 0.8 \\ + 0.5 \\ \hline 1.3 \end{array}$$

b. $3.27 + 0.06 + 2 =$
$$\begin{array}{r} 3.27 \\ + 0.06 \\ + 2.00 \\ \hline 5.33 \end{array}$$

EXERCISES

Add the following:

1. $7.01 + 3.888$ _____

2. $26.78 + 6.28 + 16.53$ _____

3. $7.52 + 4.9$ _____

4. $0.72 + 0.81 + 5$ _____

5. $0.76 + 2 + 300$ _____

6. $0.81 + 0.973$ _____

7. $6 + 0.09$ _____

8. $0.8 + 6 + 0.245$ _____

9. $77.1 + 0.27 + 0.31$ _____

10. $0.3 + 0.37 + 1.8$ _____

PROCEDURE FOR SUBTRACTION OF DECIMALS

1. Write the decimals in columns, keeping the decimal points under each other.
2. Subtract as with whole numbers. (Zeros may be added after the decimal point as place holders to prevent errors in subtraction; this does not change the value of the decimal.)
3. Place the decimal point in the remainder directly under the decimal point in the subtrahend (bottom number) and minuend (top number).

EXAMPLE

$0.6 - 0.524 =$
$$\begin{array}{r} 0.600 \\ - 0.524 \\ \hline 0.076 \end{array}$$

EXERCISES

Subtract the following:

1. $1.65 - 1.004$ _____

2. $0.21 - 0.17$ _____

3. $64.28 - 23$ _____

4. $756.824 - 28.127$ _____

5. $0.07 - 0.052$ _____

6. $10 - 6.78$ _____

7. $5 - 0.3$ _____

8. $36 - 1.5$ _____

9. $3 - 0.163$ _____

10. $109 - 3.29$ _____

PROCEDURE FOR MULTIPLICATION OF DECIMALS

1. Multiply as in the multiplication of whole numbers.
2. Find the total number of decimal places in the multiplier (*bottom number*) and multiplicand (top number).
3. Starting from the right and moving left, count off in the product this total number of decimal places. Put the decimal point at the left of the last of these.
4. If the product contains fewer figures than the required decimal places, add as many zeros as necessary to the left of the product.

EXAMPLE

$2.6 \times 0.0002 =$
$$\begin{array}{r} 2.6 \\ \times 0.0002 \\ \hline 0.00052 \end{array}$$

EXERCISES

Multiply the following:

1. 4×0.8 _____

2. 0.005×2.2 _____

3. 3.15×0.03 _____

4. 200×0.7 _____

5. 59.38×0.015 _____

6. 200×0.6 _____

7. 0.003×0.03 _____

8. 26.17×3.8 _____

9. 100×1.2 _____

10. 7.302×1.54 _____

PROCEDURE FOR DIVISION OF DECIMALS

1. If the divisor is a whole number, divide as in the division of whole numbers and place the decimal point in the quotient directly above the decimal point in the dividend.
2. If the divisor is a decimal, make it a whole number by moving the decimal point to the right of the last number. Move the decimal point in the dividend the same number of places; proceed in division as in Step 1. (If the dividend contains fewer places than required, zeros may be added.)

EXAMPLE

$$15 \div 0.625 = 625 \overline{)15.000.00} = 24.00$$

$$\frac{12\ 50}{2\ 500}$$
$$\frac{2\ 500}{}$$

EXERCISES

Divide the following and carry to the third decimal place:

1. $300 \div 5.0$ _____
2. $14.03 \div 6$ _____
3. $69.4 \div 0.52$ _____
4. $24.78 \div 4$ _____
5. $48 \div 2.4$ _____
6. $0.2482 \div 0.068$ _____
7. $84 \div 4.2$ _____
8. $270.6 \div 32$ _____
9. $96.2 \div 28$ _____
10. $0.06128 \div 0.72$ _____

PROCEDURE FOR CHANGING DECIMALS TO FRACTIONS

1. Express the decimal as it is written in fraction form.
2. Reduce to lowest terms.

EXAMPLES

a. $0.375 = \frac{375}{1000} = \frac{3}{8}$ c. $0.8 = \frac{8}{10} = \frac{4}{5}$

b. $0.40 = \frac{40}{100} = \frac{2}{5}$

PROCEDURE FOR CHANGING COMMON FRACTIONS TO DECIMALS

1. Divide the numerator by the denominator.
2. Place decimal point in proper position.

EXAMPLES

a. $\frac{2}{5} = 5\overline{)2.00} = 0.04$ c. $\frac{9}{7} = 7\overline{)9.000} = 1.29$

b. $\frac{19}{100} = 100\overline{)19.00} = 0.19$

EXERCISES

A. Change the following to decimals:

1. $\frac{8}{10}$ _____
2. $\frac{1}{6}$ _____
3. $\frac{22}{100}$ _____
4. $\frac{13}{15}$ _____
5. $4\frac{2}{5}$ _____
6. $7\frac{1}{8}$ _____
7. $\frac{38}{54}$ _____
8. $\frac{6754}{10,000}$ _____
9. $4\frac{23}{32}$ _____
10. $\frac{94}{36}$ _____

B. Change the following to fractions or mixed numbers:

1. 0.28 _____
2. 5.07 _____
3. 0.0022 _____
4. 1.28 _____
5. 3.04 _____
6. 0.575 _____
7. 0.76 _____
8. 0.15325 _____
9. 6.09 _____
10. 0.01 _____

Online Resources

For updated drug information and Web activities, go to http://evolve.elsevier.com/Asperheim.

Objectives

After completing this chapter, you should be able to do the following:

1. Convert percents to decimals with 100 percent accuracy.
2. Convert fractions to percents with 100 percent accuracy.
3. Convert percents to fractions with 100 percent accuracy.
4. Convert decimals to percents with 100 percent accuracy.

Key Terms

Percent, p. 10

The term **percent,** and its symbol %, mean hundredths. A percent number is a fraction whose numerator is expressed and whose denominator is understood to be 100. It can be changed to a decimal by moving the decimal point two places to the left to signify hundredths or to a fraction by expressing the denominator as 100.

EXAMPLES

a. 5% means $\frac{5}{100}$ or 0.05

b. $\frac{1}{2}$% means $\frac{\frac{1}{2}}{100}$ or 0.0005

EXERCISES

Complete the following:

	Fraction	Decimal	Percent
1.	$\frac{1}{4}$	_____	_____
2.	_____	1.25	_____
3.	_____	_____	75%
4.	$\frac{1}{8}$	_____	_____
5.	_____	0.56	_____
6.	$\frac{6}{1000}$	_____	_____
7.	_____	_____	6%
8.	_____	0.75	_____
9.	_____	_____	20%

Fraction	Decimal	Percent

	Fraction	Decimal	Percent
10.	_____	_____	12%
11.	_____	0.05	_____
12.	_____	_____	72%

PROCEDURE FOR FINDING PERCENT OF A NUMBER

1. Change the percent to a decimal or common fraction.
2. Multiply the number by this decimal.

EXAMPLES

a. 23% of 64 = ?
$64 \times 0.23 = 14.72$
b. 114% of 240 = ?
$240 \times 1.14 = 273.6$

EXERCISES

Find the following percents:

1. 6% of 300 _____

2. $\frac{1}{2}$% of 840 _____

3. 5% of 15 _____

4. 8% of 2700 _____

5. 200% of 6.7 _____

6. 0.2% of 10 _____

7. 50% of 75 _____

8. 3% of 200 _____

9. $\frac{1}{3}$% of 360 _____

10. 15.6% of 324 _____

11. $5\frac{1}{2}$% of 2500_____

12. 35% of 9.25 _____

PROCEDURE FOR FINDING WHAT PERCENT ONE NUMBER IS OF ANOTHER

1. Make a fraction of the two numbers using the number after the word "of" as the denominator.
2. Reduce the fraction to lowest terms.
3. Change the reduced fraction to a percent.

   EXAMPLES
   a. 27 is what percent of 36?
   $\frac{27}{36} = \frac{3}{4} = 75\%$
   b. 9 is ? % of 20?
   $\frac{9}{20} = 0.45 = 45\%$

EXERCISES

Find the following percents:

1. 2 is ? % of 20? _____

2. 10 is ? % of 25? _____

3. 15 is ? % of 85? _____

4. $2\frac{1}{2}$ is ? % of 8? _____

5. What % of 25 is 15? _____

6. 45 is ? % of 80? _____

7. $1\frac{1}{2}$ is ? % of $8\frac{1}{2}$? _____

8. What % of 25 is 50? _____

9. 60 is ? % of 15? _____

10. 3 is ? % of 15? _____

11. 240 is ? % of 1200? _____

12. What % of 15 is 30? _____

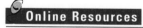 **Online Resources**

For updated drug information and Web activities, go to http://evolve.elsevier.com/Asperheim.

5 Proportion

Objectives

After completing this chapter, you should be able to use ratio-proportion technique with 100 percent accuracy.

Key Terms

Extremes, p. 12
Means, p. 12
Proportion, p. 12

A **proportion** shows the relationship between two equal ratios. A proportion may be expressed as:

$$8 : 16 :: 1 : 2$$
or
$$8 : 16 = 1 : 2$$

The first and fourth terms of a proportion are called the **extremes,** and the second and third terms are the **means.** In a proportion, the product of the means equals the product of the extremes.

It can be seen from the sample proportion above that the product of the extremes $(8 \times 2) = 16$; the product of the means $(16 \times 1) = 16$.

When one term of the proportion is unknown, it can easily be found.

PROCEDURE TO SOLVE FOR AN UNKNOWN TERM IN A PROPORTION

1. Multiply the means and the extremes, letting "x" signify the unknown term.
2. Divide the known product by the coefficient of "x" to solve for the unknown term.

EXAMPLES
a. $3 : 5 = x : 10$
$$5x = 30$$
$$x = \frac{30}{5} = 6$$

b. $\frac{1}{2} : x :: 1 : 8$
$$1x = 4 \left(8 \times \frac{1}{2} \right)$$
$$x = \frac{4}{1} = 4$$

EXERCISES

Solve the following proportions for "x":

1. $2 : x :: 10 : 20$ _____

2. $20 : x :: 30 : 600$ _____

3. $10 : 15 :: x : 30$ _____

4. $x : 300 :: 2 : 60$ _____

5. $6 : 3000 :: 10 : x$ _____

6. $8 : 24 :: 16 : x$ _____

7. $2.5 : x :: 50 : 60$ _____

8. $3.4 : x :: 17 : 25$ _____

9. $4 : 8 :: x : 72$ _____

10. $3\frac{1}{2} : 28 :: 6 : x$ _____

11. $4 : 18 :: 20 : x$ _____

12. $7 : 30 :: x : 60$ _____

13. $4 : 7 :: x : 49$ _____

14. $x : 5.2 :: 1.6 : 8$ _____

15. $20 : 100 :: 5 : x$ _____

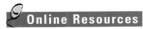

Online Resources

For updated drug information and Web activities, go to http://evolve.elsevier.com/Asperheim.

6 Fahrenheit and Celsius

Objectives

After completing this chapter, you should be able to convert temperature from the Fahrenheit scale to the Celsius scale and vice versa.

Key Terms

Fahrenheit (FĂR-ĕn-HĪT) **scale,** p. 13
Celsius (SĔL-sē-ĕs) **scale,** p. 13

Two scales are commonly used to measure temperature: the **Fahrenheit scale** and the **Celsius,** or centigrade, **scale.** The inner tube of the thermometer contains mercury, which expands and rises in the tube as the heat increases, thus showing the temperatures on the scale (Figure 6–1).

The Fahrenheit (F) scale is used on most clinical thermometers in the United States, but because some clinical thermometers do use the Celsius (C) scale, the nurse should be able to convert from one scale to the other.

Five degrees on the Celsius scale correspond to nine degrees on the Fahrenheit scale, so the ratio is 5:9. Zero degrees Celsius corresponds to 32° Fahrenheit, so 32° must be substracted from the Fahrenheit temperature in addition to considering the simple ratio.

PROCEDURE FOR CONVERTING BETWEEN FAHRENHEIT AND CELSIUS

1. Use the proportion formula $C : F - 32 :: 5 : 9$.
2. Substitute the known temperature in its proper place in the formula.
3. Solve for the unknown temperature as for the fourth term of a proportion.

EXAMPLES

a. Change 50° F to C

$$C : F - 32 :: 5 : 9$$
$$C : 50 - 32 :: 5 : 9$$
$$(18)$$
$$9 C = 18 \times 5 \ (90)$$
$$90$$
$$C = \frac{90}{9} = 10° \text{ on the Celsius scale}$$

b. Change 75° C to F

$$C : F - 32 :: 5 : 9$$
$$75 : F - 32 :: 5 : 9$$
$$5(F - 32) = 675$$
$$5 F - 160 = 675$$
$$5 F = 835$$
$$F = 167° \text{ on the Fahrenheit scale}$$

EXERCISES

Convert the following:

1. 20° C = _____ ° F

2. 60° C = _____ ° F

3. 102° C = _____ ° F

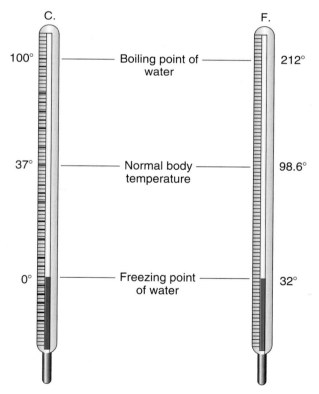

FIGURE 6-1 Celsius (*left*) and Fahrenheit (*right*) scales used to measure temperature.

4. 35° C =   _____ ° F

5. 40° C =   _____ ° F

6. 101° F =   _____ ° C

7. 70° F =   _____ ° C

8. 120° F =   _____ ° C

9. 104° F =   _____ ° C

10. 96.8° F =   _____ ° C

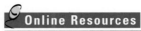 **Online Resources**

For updated drug information and Web activities, go to http://evolve.elsevier.com/Asperheim.

After completing this chapter, you should be able to do the following:

1. Convert units of measure within the metric system.
2. Convert units of measure from the Avoirdupois system to the metric system.

Avoirdupois (Ăv-ĕr-dĕ-POIZ) **system,** p. 16
Gram, p. 15
Liter, p. 15
Meter, p. 15
Metric system, p. 15

The system of weights and measures used in medicine is the **metric system.** It is essential that the health professional become familiar with this system and be able to use it accurately.

THE METRIC SYSTEM

The metric system is now being used exclusively in the *United States Pharmacopeia.* Arabic numbers and decimals are used with this system.

The units used in the metric system are

liter for volume (fluids)
gram for weight (solids)
meter for measure (length)

These basic units are multiplied and divided always by a multiple of 10 to form the entire system. There are only a few equivalents that are used in medicine, however. These are:

Volume	Weight
1000 mL = 1 liter (L)	1000 mg = 1 gram (gm)
	1000 gm = 1 kilogram (kg)

It should be noted that milliliter (mL) is the correct unit for liquid measurements. Common usage, however, interchanges the milliliter with the cubic centimer (cc) in a 1:1 ratio, with 1000 cc = 1000 mL = 1 L. The centimeter is actually a linear measurement, and the cubic centimeter is a measure of area. Therefore, milliliter and cubic centimeter should not be used interchangeably. Instead, cubic centimeters should be converted to milliliters or liters.

PROCEDURE FOR CONVERSION AMONG METRIC UNITS

1. To change milligrams to grams, to change milliliters to liters, or to change grams to kilograms, divide by 1000.
2. To change liters to milliliters, grams to milligrams, or kilograms to grams, multiply by 1000.

EXAMPLES
a. 64 mg = ? gm
$$1000 \text{ mg} : 1 \text{ gm} = 64 \text{ mg}: x \text{ gm}$$
$$1000 \, x = 64$$
$$x = \frac{64}{1000} = 0.064 \text{ gm}$$
b. 325 mL = ? L
$$1000 \text{ mL} : 1 \text{ L} = 325 \text{ mL} : x \text{ L}$$
$$1000 \, x = 325$$
$$x = \frac{325}{1000} = 0.325 \text{ L}$$

Note: These rules may be used without use of the ratio and proportion method. The use of the proportion does serve to clarify the reasoning behind multiplying or dividing, however.
c. 3.5 L = ? mL
$$1000 \text{ mL} : 1 \text{ L} = x \text{ mL} : 3.5 \text{ L}$$
$$1 \, x = 3500$$
$$x = 3500 \text{ mL}$$

EXERCISES

Change to equivalents within the metric system:

1. 1000 mg = _____ gm
2. 500 mg = _____ gm
3. 2000 mL = _____ L
4. 1500 mg = _____ gm
5. 0.1 L = _____ mL
6. 750 mg = _____ gm
7. 1 kg = _____ gm
8. 5 L = _____ mL
9. 4 mg = _____ gm
10. 100 gm = _____ kg
11. 0.25 L = _____ mL
12. 0.006 gm = _____ mg
13. 250 mg = _____ gm
14. 2.5 L = _____ mL
15. 0.05 gm = _____ mg

THE SYSTEM OF HOUSEHOLD MEASUREMENTS

The **Avoirdupois system** of common household measurements, a more familiar system in the United States, may be compared to the metric system. Household measurements include teaspoons, tablespoons, cups, pints, and quarts. These measurements, while more familiar, are not as accurate and should be avoided in the administration of medication.

The American standard teaspoon has been established by the American Standards Association as containing approximately 5 mL, and this measurement is accepted in the *United States Pharmacopeia*.

Drugs dispensed by the teaspoonful (i.e., cough syrups, antihistamines, liquid vitamins) generally do not require exactly precise measurements. It should also be noted that the household teaspoon may vary considerably in its milliliter equivalent, in some cases ranging from 3.5 to 5 mL. Exact doses for drugs such as digoxin or doses for very young children should be measured using an oral syringe, a calibrated dropper, or a pediatric dosing spoon available from pharmacies. Antibiotic suspensions may generally be administered using the teaspoon.

Some approximate equivalents to household measurements are as follows:

1 teaspoon $= \frac{1}{6}$ fluid ounce = 5 mL

1 tablespoon $= \frac{1}{2}$ fluid ounce = 15 mL
2 tablespoons $= 1$ fluid ounce = 30 mL
1 cup $= 8$ ounces = 240 mL
1 pint $= 500$ mL
1 quart $= 1000$ mL = 1 L
1 ounce $= 30$ gm
2.2 pounds (lb) $= 1$ kg

EXAMPLES

a. 45 gm = ? oz
   30 gm: 1 oz = 45 gm: x oz
   $30x = 45 \times 1$
   $x = \frac{45}{30} = 1\frac{1}{2}$ oz

b. 150 lb = ? kg
   2.2 lb: 1 kg = 150 lb: x kg
   $2.2x = 150 \times 1$
   $x = \frac{150}{2.2} = 68.2$ lb

EXERCISES

A. Change to approximate equivalents in household measurements:

1. 10 mL = _____ teaspoons

2. 2 cups = _____ ounces

3. 10 lb = _____ kg

4. 60 mL = _____ ounces

5. 22 pounds = _____ kg

6. 3 ounces = _____ gm

7. 60 mL = _____ teaspoons

8. 6 teaspoons = _____ fluid ounces

9. 3 ounces = _____ teaspoons

10. 70 kg = _____ lb

B. Convert the following:

1. 0.5 L = _____ mL

2. 4 mL = _____ cc

3. $\frac{1}{2}$ ounce = _____ mg

4. 0.1 gm = _____ mg

5. 500 mL = _____ pint

6. $\frac{1}{2}$ ounce = _____ mL

7. 30 lb = _____ kg

8. 30 mL = _____ teaspoons

9. 1500 mg = _____ gm

10. 2 ounces = _____ gm

11. 5 tablespoons = _____ mL

12. 5 tablespoons = _____ ounces

13. 1 gram = _____ mg

14. 10 mL = _____ teaspoons

15. 15 mL = _____ ounce

16. $2\frac{1}{2}$ quarts = _____ mL

17. 30 gm = _____ ounce

18. 3 kg = _____ lb

19. 165 lb = _____ kg

20. 3 pints = _____ quart

Online Resources

For updated drug information and Web activities, go to http://evolve.elsevier.com/Asperheim.

Drug Dosage for Children

Objectives

After completing this chapter, you should be able to do the following:

1. Understand the importance of referring to a drug manufacturer's recommendations on use and dosages for children.
2. Calculate a child's dose by applying the appropriate rule (Young's, Clark's, or Fried's) to the recommended adult dose.
3. Calculate a child's dose based on body surface area.

Key Terms

Clark's rule, p. 17
Fried's (FREDS) rule, p. 17
Young's rule, p. 17

Children are not able to tolerate adult doses of drugs. There are several formulas for graduating dosage according to age and weight. The recommended dosage per kilogram or pound of body weight is more accurate than calculating dosage according to age. Other factors besides age and weight enter into dosage for children. For this reason, some physicians use the "body surface area" method to estimate the dosage for children. Charts are available to determine the body surface area in square meters according to height and weight.

It is generally not the responsibility of a health care professional other than the physician to calculate the dose of a drug for children, although the following formulas give the general method used. Drug manufacturers, after considerable research, will give specific doses of drugs used for children, and these should always be carefully checked in the current drug literature or package insert. Many drugs are not advised for children because of the potential for harmful side effects on the growing child, or because they have not been sufficiently tested in children to give a recommended dosage range.

The following three formulas are useful in calculating dosage for infants and children. In **Young's rule**

$$\frac{\text{Age of child (in years)}}{\text{Age of child (in years)} + 12} \times \text{average adult dose} = \text{child's dose}$$

Young's rule is not valid after 12 years of age. If the child is small enough to warrant a reduced dose after 12 years of age,

the reduction should be calculated on the basis of **Clark's rule:**

$$\frac{\text{Weight of child (in pounds)}}{150\,\text{lb}} \times \text{average adult dose} = \text{child's dose}$$

Fried's rule, which is sometimes used in calculating dosages for infants less than 2 years old, uses the formula

$$\frac{\text{Age in months}}{150\,\text{lb}} \times \text{average adult dose} = \text{child's dose}$$

Any unit of measure may be used in these formulas. The answer will be in the same units as used. If another unit is desired, conversion may be carried out as previously illustrated.

EXAMPLES

a. Find the dose of phenobarbital for a 4-year-old child (adult dose: 30 mg).

$$\frac{4}{4+12} \times 30\,\text{mg} = 7.5\,\text{mg}$$

b. Find the dose of cortisone for a 30-pound infant (adult dose: 100 mg).

$$\frac{30}{150} \times 100\,\text{mg} = 20\,\text{mg}$$

c. If the nurse draws 2 mL of acetaminophen 120 mg/ 5 mL into an oral dosing syringe, the dose contains _____ mg of acetaminophen?

$$\frac{2}{5} \times 120\,\text{mg} = 48\,\text{mg}$$

BODY SURFACE AREA NOMOGRAM

A body surface area nomogram is used for calculating pediatric doses by square meter of body surface (Figure 8–1). The center enclosed box gives the square meters by weight in pounds only for children of normal height and weight. For children who are slender or obese, a straight line that connects the height and weight on the two outside scales can be used to read the square meters of body surface at the point where the line crosses the surface area scale in the center box.

EXERCISES

Calculate the following children's doses:

1. If the adult dose of codeine sulfate is 30 mg, what is the dose for a 3-year-old child?

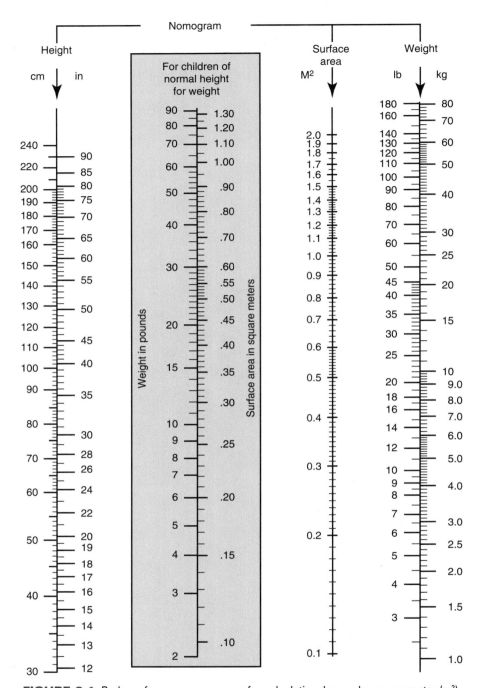

FIGURE 8-1 Body surface area nomogram for calculating dosage by square meter (m²).

2. The adult dose of Dilantin suspension is 125 mg/5 mL. How much would you use when 75 mg is ordered for a child?

3. The adult dose of Achromycin is 250 mg. What is the dose for an 8-year-old child?

4. The vial is labeled Demerol 100 mg/mL. The order is for 60 mg. How much will be given?

5. The adult dose of phenobarbital is 30 mg. How much of this drug would you administer to a 30-pound child?

6. The pediatrician has ordered Tylenol elixir 2 mL. The bottle is labeled 120 mg/5 mL. How much will be given?

7. If the adult dosage of procaine penicillin is 300,000 units once daily, calculate the dosage for a 6-year-old child using Young's rule.

8. If each milliliter of procaine penicillin supplies 300,000 units, how many milliliters would you give this 6-year-old child?

9. Gantrisin suspension is available in a dose of 500 mg/5 mL. How much is needed for a 100-mg dose?

10. The adult dose of a drug is 50 to 100 mg. What is the dose for a 6-month-old infant using the minimum dose?

11. a. Calculate the dose of Seconal for a child weighing 50 pounds. The adult dose is 100 mg.

    b. What is the metric equivalent?

12. Keflex pediatric drops are available in a dose of 100 mg/mL. The order is for 60 mg. How much will be given?

13. The adult dose of Ritalin is 15 mg. What is the dose for a 30-pound child?

14. The adult dose of paregoric is 10 mL. How much would be given to a 20-pound infant?

15. Ampicillin oral suspension 250 mg/5 mL is available. Calculate the amount to be given for the following doses:
    a. 150 mg   b. 100 mg
    c. 125 mg   d. 375 mg

16. The dose of azathioprine is 125 mg/m^2/day. Find the total daily dose for a 44-pound child of average height and weight.

17. Find the total daily dose of azathioprine for a child who is 40 inches tall and overweight at 60 pounds.

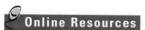
Online Resources

For updated drug information and Web activities, go to http://evolve.elsevier.com/Asperheim.

9 Drug Dosage in Standardized Units

After completing this chapter, you should be able to do the following:

1. Understand the concept of units per milliliter.
2. Accurately measure the contents of insulin and tuberculin syringes.
3. Convert insulin dosage to milliliters for injection by tuberculin syringe.
4. Calculate the desired concentration of antibiotic.

Key Terms

Insulin syringe, p. 20
Tuberculin (tū-BŭR-kyĕ-lĭn) **syringe,** p. 20
Units per milliliter, p. 20

INSULIN DOSAGE

Insulin and many other drugs that are obtained from animal sources are standardized in units based on their strengths rather than on weight measures such as milligrams and grams. The reason for this is that the strength of these animal drugs varies greatly, depending on the sources, conditions, and manner in which they are obtained. Many of the hormones (e.g., insulin) are too complex to be completely purified to obtain an exact weight of the drug per unit volume.

Insulin is supplied in 10-mL vials labeled in the number of **units per milliliter;** thus, 100-U insulin means there are 100 units per milliliter. In the past, insulin was administered in 40-U and 80-U dosage forms. Today, however, the 100-U form has almost totally replaced the weaker strengths. The smaller volume required per dose decreases local reactions at the injection site, and mathematical calculations when a fraction of a milliliter is required are obviously simplified.

The simplest and most accurate way to measure insulin is within an **insulin syringe.** The syringe is calibrated in units, and the desired dose may be read directly on the syringe. In Figure 9–1, 35 units are shown drawn up in a 100-U syringe.

If an insulin syringe is not available, a **tuberculin syringe** may be used and the unit dosage converted to the equivalent number of milliliters, using the proportion method.

EXAMPLE

Give 60 units of insulin, using 100-U insulin and a tuberculin syringe.

$$\frac{60}{100} \times 1 \text{ mL} = 0.6 \text{ mL}$$

Figure 9–2 shows a tuberculin syringe with 0.6 mL drawn up.

HEPARIN DOSAGE

Like insulin, heparin is derived from animal sources and is standardized for its activity as an anticoagulant.

Heparin is supplied in unit-dose or multiple-dose vials and in strengths ranging from 1000 to 20,000 units per milliliter. There is often no set dose for the use of heparin; the individual's requirements are obtained from blood clotting studies done initially every 4 hours. Blood clotting time is generally maintained at twice the normal clotting rate to provide a safe yet effective way to decrease the formation of blood clots in the body.

Heparin is often given intravenously to produce a rapid effect and then is given in deep subcutaneous injection in larger and more infrequent doses.

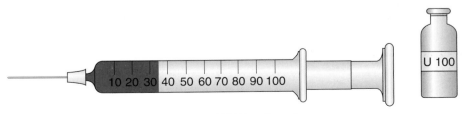

FIGURE 9-1 100-U insulin syringe.

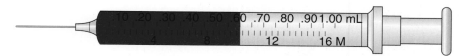

FIGURE 9-2 Tuberculin syringe.

ANTIBIOTIC DOSAGE

Many antibiotics are still standardized in units. These may be prepared for injection in the form of a liquid containing a specified number of units per cubic centimeter. The entire amount in the vial may be ordered, but sometimes only part of the contents is used. It is therefore important to *always read the label carefully*. Antibiotics are also available in the form of a dry powder in a vial that must first be diluted with water or another diluent. The powder should be diluted so that the desired dose is in 1 or 2 mL if the dose is to be given intramuscularly. If it is to be given intravenously, a larger amount of diluent may be used.

PROCEDURE FOR OBTAINING THE DESIRED CONCENTRATION OF ANTIBIOTIC

1. Using the proportion method, state the desired concentration as the first two terms of the proportion.
2. The total number of units in the vial is the third term; the unknown volume of diluent is the fourth term.

EXAMPLES

a. You have a vial of powdered penicillin G containing 1,000,000 units. How much diluent should be added to obtain a solution containing 100,000 units/mL?

$$100,000 : 1\,mL = 1,000,000 : x\,mL$$
$$100,000x = 1,000,000 \times 1$$
$$x = \frac{1,000,000}{100,000}$$
$$x = 10\,mL$$

b. If a 5,000,000-unit vial of penicillin powder is reconstituted with 10 mL of diluent, how many units will it contain per milliliter?

$$x : 1\,mL = 5,000,000 : 10\,mL$$
$$10x = 5,000,000 \times 1$$
$$x = \frac{5,000,000}{10}$$
$$x = 500,000\,units/mL$$

EXERCISES

1. When reconstituted with 20 mL of water, a 1,000,000-unit vial of penicillin G potassium used in the nursery contains 50,000 units/mL. How many milliliters would be in a dose of

   a. 10,000 units _____

   b. 30,000 units _____

   c. 60,000 units _____

2. A 1,000,000-unit vial of penicillin G potassium, when reconstituted with 10 mL of water, would have how many units per milliliter?

3. A 5,000,000-unit vial of penicillin G potassium is reconstituted with 10 mL of water. How many units will it contain per milliliter?

4. When a 1,000,000-unit vial of powdered penicillin G is reconstituted with 4.0 mL of water, how many units will it contain per milliliter?

5. You want 300,000 units of penicillin in 1 mL for an IM injection. How much water should be added to a 1,000,000-unit vial of powdered penicillin to obtain this concentration?

6. The vial contains 600,000 units of penicillin procaine. How much diluent should be added to give a solution containing 150,000 units/mL?

7. When you have the solution in question #6, containing 150,000 units/mL, how many milliliters will be used to give a 300,000-unit dose?

8. A vial of heparin contains 5000 units/mL in a 10-mL vial. How many milliliters are needed to give a dose of

   a. 7500 units _____

   b. 3000 units _____

   c. 2500 units _____

9. You have a vial of 100-U insulin and no insulin syringe. Using a tuberculin syringe, how many milliliters are needed to give a dose of

   a. 50 units _____

   b. 75 units _____

   c. 100 units _____

10. The vial of heparin is labeled 10,000 units/mL. How many milliliters are needed to give a 1500-unit dose?

Online Resources

For updated drug information and Web activities, go to http://evolve.elsevier.com/Asperheim.

10 Introduction to Pharmacology

After completing this chapter, you should be able to do the following:

1. Name four sources of drugs and give an example of each.
2. Give the definition of terms as assigned.
3. List the responsibilities of the nurse for drug administration.
4. Prepare your own objectives for this course.

The administration of medications is one of a nurse's most important responsibilities. As a member of the professional team engaged in caring for the sick, it is most important that the nurse apply him- or herself diligently in acquiring all possible knowledge of medicines, their use or abuse, correct dosage, methods of administration, symptoms of overdosage, and abnormal reactions that may arise in the treatment of various conditions. This knowledge is obviously an indispensable aid in giving the best possible patient care.

The attitude of the nurse toward drug administration is important to the effectiveness of the drug. Ideally, the body functions best when given adequate food, rest, relaxation, and freedom from undue emotional stress. However, because of physical or mental abnormalities, it is necessary at times to resort to drugs to produce a near-normal state of body function. At best, drugs are *crutches*, and undue dependence on them can be *very dangerous*. Used intelligently, they are a lifesaving boon; used unwisely, they can produce irreparable harm. The nurse who combines diligent and intelligent observation with moral integrity and plain *common sense* in administering drugs will undoubtedly make many lasting contributions to the profession and to the patients for whom she or he cares.

Pharmacology has undergone tremendous changes during the past few decades. Many new agents on the market today were totally unheard of a generation ago, and scarcely a day goes by that literature is not received on new agents or medicines and new techniques and theories of drug administration. The newest advancements are always a source of interest and intrigue to the beginning student, but it is only by applying him- or herself first of all to the task of obtaining a well-rounded background in drug therapy that the student will begin to appreciate these new "miracles of the modern age."

The information presented in this manual attempts to lay the foundation for this well-rounded background, but, as in all other areas of nursing, the responsibility for making this knowledge one's own rests with the students themselves. A true dedication to the profession only places the student in the starting position of a lifelong pursuit—a pursuit that, though admittedly arduous, promises the unfailing reward of continuous new horizons and that casts new light on the great task entrusted to the nurse in every service to the sick.

DEFINITIONS OF TERMS

GENERAL TERMINOLOGY

Pharmacology: a broad term that includes the study of drugs and their actions in the body

Pharmacy: the art of preparing, compounding, and dispensing drugs for medicinal use

Toxicology: the science that deals with poisons: their detection and the symptoms, diagnosis, and treatment of conditions caused by them

Biotechnology: the field of pharmacology that involves using living cells, usually altered cultures of *Escherichia coli*, to manufacture drugs

Drug: any substance used as medicine (e.g., used to diagnose, cure, mitigate, treat, or prevent disease). Drugs include the following:

Chemical substances: agents that may be made synthetically (e.g., sulfonamides, aspirin, sodium bicarbonate)

Plant parts or products: crude drugs that may be obtained from any part of various plants and used medicinally; leaves, bark, fruit, roots, rhizomes, resin, and other parts may be used (e.g., ergot, digitalis, opium)

Animal products: primarily glandular products that are currently obtained from animal sources (e.g., thyroid hormone, insulin)

Certain food substances: substances that under some conditions serve both as foods and as medicinal substances (i.e., vitamins and minerals in various foods)

SPECIFIC PHARMACOLOGY TERMS

Additive effect: the combined effect of two drugs that is equal to the sum of the effects of each drug taken alone

Adverse or untoward effect: an action, usually negative, that is different from the planned effect

Allergic reaction: an untoward reaction that develops after the individual has taken a drug

Analog: a chemical compound that resembles another in structure but has different effects

Antagonism: the combined effect of two drugs that is less than the effect of either drug taken alone

Biosynthesis: formation of a chemical compound by enzymes either within an organism (in vivo) or in vitro by fragments of cells

Depression: a decrease in activity of cells caused by the action of a drug

Diagnostic: pertaining to the art or act of determining the nature of a patient's disease

Idiosyncrasy (ID-e-o-SIN-kre-se): abnormal sensitivity to a drug, or a reaction not intended

Palliative: an agent or measure that relieves symptoms

Potentiation: an effect that occurs when a drug increases or prolongs the action of another drug, the total effect being greater than the sum of the effects of each used alone

Prophylactic (PRO-fi-LAK-tik): an agent or measure used to prevent disease

Side effect: an unpredictable effect that is not related to the main action of the drug

Stimulation: an increase in the activity of cells produced by drugs

Synergism: the joint action of agents in which their combined effect is more intense or longer in duration than the sum of their individual effects

Therapeutic: pertaining to treatment of disease

Tolerance: increasing resistance to the usual effects of an established dosage of a drug as a result of continued use

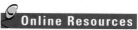

Online Resources

For updated drug information and Web activities, go to http://evolve.elsevier.com/Asperheim.

Drug Legislation and Drug Standards

After completing this chapter, you should be able to do the following:

1. Identify drugs according to the current schedule of the Controlled Substances Act.
2. List official drug standards.
3. Use the Physicians' Desk Reference to identify a selected list of drugs according to generic and proprietary names.

Key Terms

Controlled Substances Act, p. 24
Drug standards, p. 25
Schedules of controlled substances, p. 24

AMERICAN DRUG LEGISLATION

Drug legislation in the United States underwent major revisions as of May 1, 1971, when the **Controlled Substances Act** became effective. This law requires that every person who manufactures, dispenses, prescribes, or administers any controlled substance be registered annually with the Attorney General; this registration function is the responsibility of the Drug Enforcement Administration (DEA).

Legislation and controls were revised to establish a classification system that categorizes drugs by the potential for abuse, which resulted in five **schedules of controlled substances**. Drugs in the original schedules are subject to revision on an annual basis on notification by the DEA, and many changes have been made within the schedules since the legislation first went into effect.

Complete listings of the drugs in each schedule are available from district DEA offices. Only a few examples of the more well-known drugs in each schedule are included here.

SCHEDULE I

1. The drug or other substance has a high potential for abuse.
2. The drug or other substance has *no* currently accepted medicinal use in treatment in the United States.
3. There is a lack of accepted safety for use of the drug or other substance under medical supervision.

Drugs Included

1. Opioids: ketobemidone, allylprodine
2. Certain opium derivatives: heroin
3. Hallucinogens: lysergic acid diethylamide (LSD), marijuana, mescaline, peyote

SCHEDULE II

1. The drug or other substance has a high potential for abuse.
2. The drug or other substance has a currently accepted medical use in treatment in the United States or a currently accepted medical use with severe restrictions.
3. Abuse of the drug or other substance may lead to severe psychological or physical dependence.

Drugs Included

1. Many derivatives of opium (e.g., raw opium, morphine, codeine, ethylmorphine, hydrocodone, metopon, thebaine)
2. Coca leaves and derivatives (e.g., cocaine)
3. Opioids: anileridine, dihydrocodeine, diphenoxylate, levomethorphan, methadone, meperidine, oxycodone
4. Stimulants: methamphetamine, amphetamine, phenmetrazine, methylphenidate
5. Depressants: amobarbital, secobarbital, pentobarbital

SCHEDULE III

1. The drug or other substance has a potential for abuse less than the drugs in Schedule I or II.
2. The drug or other substance has a currently accepted medical use in treatment in the United States.
3. Abuse of the drug or other substance may lead to moderate or low physical dependence or high psychological dependence.

Drugs Included

1. Phendimetrazine, methyprylon, nalorphine
2. Combinations of amobarbital, secobarbital, or pentobarbital with other active ingredients
3. Compounds containing limited concentrations of codeine, dihydrocodeinone, ethylmorphine, opium, or morphine with one or more active non-narcotic ingredients in recognized therapeutic amounts

SCHEDULE IV

1. The drug or other substance has a low potential for abuse relative to the drugs or other substances in Schedule III.

2. The drug or other substance has a currently accepted medical use in treatment in the United States.
3. Abuse of the drug or other substance may lead to limited physical or psychological dependence relative to the drugs in Schedule III.

Drugs Included

Chloral hydrate, chloral betaine, ethchlorvynol, meprobamate, paraldehyde, phenobarbital, chlordiazepoxide, diazepam, propoxyphene, flurazepam, chlorazepate, pemoline, pentazocine, oxazepam

SCHEDULE V

1. The drug or other substance has a low potential for abuse relative to the drugs in Schedule IV.
2. The drug or other substance has a currently accepted medical use in treatment in the United States.
3. Abuse of the drug or other substance may lead to limited physical or psychological dependence relative to the drugs in Schedule IV.

Drugs Included

1. Compounds containing limited amounts of codeine, dihydrocodeine, ethylmorphine, opium, or diphenoxylate in combination with other non-narcotic active ingredients. (In all cases the allowable concentration of these agents is lower than those compounds included in Schedule III.)
2. Diphenoxylate and atropine preparations (e.g., Lomotil).

DRUG STANDARDS

Several organizations worldwide publish reference texts describing **drug standards** (lists of the known value, strength, quality, and ingredients of various drugs) for quality and strength. Before official standards were published, drugs, particularly those from plant sources, could vary in strength from being ineffective to providing almost a fatal dose, depending on the quality of the plant, the soil, and the growing conditions. The most prominent drug standard texts are listed below.

AMERICAN DRUG STANDARDS

The United States Pharmacopoeia/National Formulary (USP). Formerly two standards, the *Pharmacopoeia* and the *National Formulary* have been combined into one official volume. The *Pharmacopoeia* includes a list of approved drugs and defines them with respect to source, chemistry, physical properties, tests for identity, method of assay, storage, and dosage. It also provides directions for compounding and general use. It is revised periodically by an appointed committee to include new drugs and exclude those no longer in general use.

New drugs. In 1965 the American Medical Association (AMA) began publishing this annual text, which lists drugs whether or not they have been approved for official standards. It is organized according to therapeutic uses for the drugs, and the information is based on evaluation by the Council

on Drugs. The inclusion of a particular drug does not imply its acceptance by the AMA.

Additional Sources of Drug Information

Physicians' Desk Reference (PDR). Revised annually and readily supplied to all hospitals and physicians, this reference source is probably the most widely used. It is not intended as an official standard. Each manufacturer supplies information for inclusion, usually by trade name, and gives the accepted uses, side effects, and doses for commercially available pharmaceutical agents.

Drug information. This annual publication by the American Hospital Formulary Service contains useful and current information on drugs.

INTERNATIONAL DRUG STANDARDS

Pharmacopoeia Internationalis (IP). The World Health Organization was originally responsible for the publication of this text in an attempt to standardize drugs for many European nations. The names of drugs are in Latin; all doses are in the metric system.

BRITISH AND CANADIAN DRUG STANDARDS

British Pharmacopoeia (BP). Similar in content to the *United States Pharmacopoeia/National Formulary*, this text sets the standards for drugs that are official in the United Kingdom and its dominions and colonies. It is published by the British Pharmacopoeia Commission under the direction of the General Medical Council.

British Pharmaceutical Codex (BPC). A text similar to the *British Pharmacopoeia*, this is published by the Pharmaceutical Society of Great Britain and gives official drug information and standards.

Canadian Formulary (CF). Published by the Canadian Pharmaceutical Association, this text is recognized by the Canadian Food and Drug Act and contains formulas for many Canadian pharmaceutical preparations. It lists some drugs not included in the *British Pharmacopoeia*.

CANADIAN DRUG LEGISLATION

CANADIAN FOOD AND DRUG ACT

The Food and Drug Act, passed in 1941, empowers the Governor-in-Council to prescribe drug standards and limit variation in any food or drug. It contains the following schedules:

Schedule A: This schedule contains a list of diseases or disorders for which a cure may not be advertised. It includes diseases such as gangrene, influenza, and appendicitis.
Schedule B: This schedule contains lists of official drug standard texts, such as the *United States Pharmacopoeia*, the *British Pharmacopoeia*, and other previously mentioned British and Canadian volumes.

Schedule C: This schedule contains a list of drugs derived from animal tissues, such as liver extract and insulin, for which special standards of quality and purity apply.

Schedule D: This schedule contains a list of drugs obtained from microorganisms, such as antibiotics, and their requirements for manufacture.

Schedule E: This schedule contains a list of sensitivity disks or tablets and their standards.

Schedule F: Thalidomide is the only drug currently in this schedule; its sale is prohibited. Also included in this schedule is a regulation noting drugs that must be dispensed by prescription only.

Schedule G: A list of controlled drugs with strict prescribing regulations is included in this schedule. It includes amphetamines, barbiturates, benzphetamine, butorphanol, chlorphentermine, diethylpropion, methamphetamine, methaqualone, methylphenidate, pentazocine, phendimetrazine, phenmetrazine, phentermine, and thiobarbituric acid.

Schedule H: This schedule contains a list of hallucinogenic drugs that are restricted, allowing no practitioner to prescribe them, including LSD, psilocin, and harmaline.

CANADIAN NARCOTIC CONTROL ACT AND REGULATIONS

This act defines who may prescribe a narcotic drug, such as physicians, dentists, research personnel, and their agents, and places conditions on the recipient of a narcotic prescription, requiring disclosure of all previous narcotics received within the last 30 days.

In addition, the act describes procedures for record keeping and dispensing by pharmacists. Hospital regulations are also outlined.

Methadone is covered individually in this act, which sets requirements for authorized practitioners who prescribe and dispense this drug.

PROPRIETARY (TRADE) NAMES

Most pharmaceutical houses market their drugs primarily under trade names, although some are available under their generic names. Today there is a great multiplicity of trade names under which a single drug may be sold. The practice of using these brand names is often confusing to the nurse and sometimes even to the physician, to say nothing of the inconvenience to the pharmacist, who must stock four or five different brands of the same drug.

There is a trend to return to the use of official or generic names on prescriptions. In many cases this is a significant cost issue, with the price of name-brand drug being much higher compared with the less expensive generic form of the drug. Some insurance companies will pay only for the generic form of a drug if that is available, or they will only pay for the brand-name drug if the patient is responsible for a significantly higher co-payment for the prescription. Many hospital pharmacies provide their nursing divisions with a formulary that lists the official or generic names for the commercial products stocked in the pharmacy.

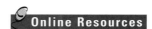 **Online Resources**

For updated drug information and Web activities, go to http://evolve.elsevier.com/Asperheim.

REVIEW QUESTIONS

1. A drug in which schedule would have the highest potential for abuse?

   a. Schedule I
   b. Schedule II
   c. Schedule III
   d. Schedule IV

2. An example of a drug in schedule III would be:

   a. nalorphine.
   b. morphine.
   c. heroin.
   d. opium.

3. The main American drug standard text is:

   a. the *Physician's Desk Reference.*
   b. the *British Pharmacopeia.*
   c. the *Merck Manual.*
   d. the *United States Pharmacopoeia.*

4. Compounds with limited amounts of codeine in a cough preparation would be in:

   a. Schedule II.
   b. Schedule III.
   c. Schedule IV.
   d. Schedule V.

5. The Canadian drug standard reference is:

   a. the *United States Pharmacopoeia.*
   b. the *British Pharmacopeia.*
   c. the *Physician's Desk Reference.*
   d. the *Canadian Formulary.*

12 Pharmaceutical Preparations

Objectives

After completing this chapter, you should be able to do the following:

1. Name all of the various pharmaceutical preparations.
2. Distinguish between an elixir and a tincture and give an example of each.
3. Discuss the advantage of administering a capsule instead of a tablet.
4. Distinguish between a lotion and a liniment and give an example of each.

Because of the various properties of the different drugs and their many uses, it is necessary to have different ways of preparing them for patient use. Listed here are the more common pharmaceutical preparations.

DEFINITIONS

Solutions: aqueous liquid preparations containing one or more substances completely dissolved. Every solution has two parts: the *solute* (the dissolved substance) and the *solvent* (the substance, usually a liquid, in which the solute is dissolved).

Waters: saturated solutions of volatile oils (e.g., peppermint water, camphor water).

Syrups: aqueous solutions of a sugar. These may or may not have medicinal substances added (e.g., simple syrup, ipecac syrup).

Spirits: alcoholic solutions of volatile substances. These are also known as essences (e.g., essence of peppermint, camphor spirit).

Elixirs: solutions containing alcohol, sugar, and water. They may or may not be aromatic and may or may not have active medicinals. Most frequently they are used as flavoring agents or solvents (e.g., terpin hydrate elixir, phenobarbital elixir).

Tinctures: alcoholic or hydroalcoholic solutions prepared from drugs (e.g., iodine tincture, digitalis tincture).

Fluid extracts: alcoholic liquid extracts of a drug made by percolation so that 1 mL of the fluid extract contains 1 gm of the drug. Only vegetable-based drugs are used (e.g., glycyrrhiza fluid extract).

Emulsions: suspensions of fat globules in water (or water globules in fat) with an emulsifying agent (e.g., Haley's MO, Petrogalar). (Homogenized milk is also an emulsion.)

Liniments: mixtures of drugs with oil, soap, water, or alcohol, intended for external application with rubbing (e.g., camphor liniment, chloroform liniment).

Lotions: aqueous preparations containing suspended materials intended for soothing, using local application. Most are patted on rather than rubbed (e.g., calamine lotion, Caladryl lotion).

Powders: single-dose quantities of a drug or mixture of drugs in powdered form wrapped separately in powder papers (e.g., Seidlitz powder).

Tablets: single-dose units made by compressing powdered drugs in a suitable mold (e.g., aspirin tablets). Special forms of tablets include *sublingual* tablets (to be held under the tongue until dissolved) and *enteric-coated* tablets (with a coating that prevents their absorption until they reach the intestinal tract).

Long-acting or sustained-release dosage forms: active pharmaceutical agents that are either layered in tablet form for release over several hours or placed in pellets within a capsule. The pellets are of varying size and disintegrate over a period of 8 to 24 hours. The sustained-release dosage forms must not be broken or crushed, because their efficacy depends on the releasing of the various layers over time.

Pills: single-dose units made by mixing the powdered drug with a liquid such as syrup and rolling it into a round or oval shape. These are largely replaced by other dosage forms today.

Capsules: powdered drugs within a gelatin container. Liquids may be placed in soft gelatin capsules (e.g., cod liver oil capsules, Benadryl capsules).

Suppositories: mixtures of drugs with some firm base such as cocoa butter, which can then be molded into shape for insertion into a body orifice. Rectal, vaginal, and urethral suppositories are the most common types (e.g., Furacin vaginal suppositories, Dulcolax suppositories), but nasal or ear (otic) suppositories may be made.

Ointments: mixtures of drugs with a fatty base for external application, usually by rubbing (e.g., zinc oxide ointment, Ben-Gay ointment).

Gels: aqueous suspensions of insoluble drugs in hydrated form. Aluminum hydroxide gel, USP, is an example.

Aerosols: active pharmaceutical agents in a pressurized container.

Troches (TRO-kes) **or lozenges:** flat, round, or rectangular preparations that are held in the mouth until dissolved.

Online Resources

For updated drug information and Web activities, go to http://evolve.elsevier.com/Asperheim.

REVIEW QUESTIONS

1. A suspension of fat globules in an aqueous preparation is called a(n):
   a. elixir.
   b. emulsion.
   c. syrup.
   d. spirit.

2. A solution containing alcohol is called a(n):
   a. syrup.
   b. solution.
   c. elixir.
   d. liniment.

3. A preparation that can be used rectally is called a(n):
   a. gel.
   b. aerosol.
   c. suppository.
   d. powder.

4. Sustained release capsules may release drug over:
   a. 30 to 60 minutes.
   b. 1 to 4 hours.
   c. 6 to 10 hours.
   d. 8 to 24 hours.

5. Which dosage form is intended to be given orally?
   a. Gel
   b. Suppository
   c. Aerosol
   d. Elixir

Special Assignment: If laboratory work is not included in the course, a visit to the hospital pharmacy to observe the various pharmaceutical preparations will enhance the learning situation at this time.

Objectives

After completing this chapter, you should be able to do the following:

1. Interpret a medication order with 100 percent accuracy.
2. Interpret a prescription with 100 percent accuracy.
3. Use accepted abbreviations with 100 percent accuracy.
4. List the factors influencing dosage.
5. Demonstrate beginning skill in transcribing orders.

Key Terms

Automatic stop policy, p. 30
Dosage, p. 29
Dose, p. 29
Drug order, p. 29
Inscription, p. 29
Prescription, p. 29
Signa (Sig), p. 29
Subscription, p. 29

Dosage is the amount of a medicine or agent prescribed for a given patient or condition. **Dose** is the measured portion of medicine to be taken at one time. Factors influencing dosage are as follows:

Age: The age of a patient will affect his or her response to drugs. Children and elderly persons require less than the usual adult dose.

Sex: The sex of a patient sometimes affects the response to drugs. Women are more susceptible to the action of certain drugs and are usually given smaller doses. The administration of medication to women in the early weeks of pregnancy may cause damage to the fetus. During the third trimester there is the possibility of premature labor caused by drugs that may stimulate muscular contractions.

Condition of the patient: Smaller doses are indicated when resistance in the patient is lowered. Impaired kidney and liver function may cause drugs to accumulate to toxic levels.

Psychological factors: A person's personality often plays an important part in his or her response to certain drugs.

Environmental factors: The setting in which drugs are given and the attitude of the nurse who is administering the medication may influence the effects of drugs.

Temperature: Heat and cold also affect the response to drugs. It may be necessary to decrease the dosage of certain drugs during hot weather.

Method of administration: Generally, larger doses are ordered when a medication is given by mouth or by rectum and smaller doses when the parenteral route is used.

Genetic factors: Drug idiosyncrasy is an abnormal susceptibility of some individuals that causes them to react differently to a drug than most people. This intolerance to small amounts of some drugs is thought to be due to genetic factors.

Body weight: The dosage of certain potent drugs is often calculated on the basis of the ratio of milligrams of the drug to pounds or kilograms of the patient's body weight. The more a person weighs the more dilute the drug will become, and a smaller amount will accumulate in the tissues. Conversely, the less a person weighs the greater the accumulation in the tissues, and a more powerful drug effect is produced.

THE PRESCRIPTION

The prescription is probably as old as the written history of humankind. The first real literature dealing with pharmacy was a scroll called the Ebers Papyrus, which included methods of conjuring away diseases as well as lists of medicinal agents and methods of compounding.

A **prescription** is an order written by a practitioner to be filled by a pharmacist indicating the medication needed by the patient and containing all the necessary directions for the pharmacist and the patient (Figure 13–1). The prescription consists of several parts:

1. The date and the patient's name and address.
2. The **inscription**, which states the name and quantities of ingredients.
3. The **subscription**, which gives directions to the pharmacist.
4. The **signa (Sig)**, which gives directions to the patient.
5. The signature, address, and registry number of the physician.

PARTS OF AN ORDER

A physician, dentist, or other qualified practitioner writes orders for the administration of drugs. A nurse who administers drugs must be familiar with the Nursing Practice Act of the state in which she or he is licensed to practice and with the policies of the employing agency.

A complete **drug order** consists of the name of the drug, the dosage, when the drug is to be given, how it is to be given,

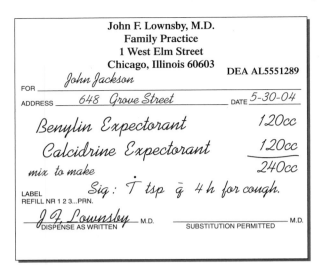

John F. Lownsby, M.D.
Family Practice
1 West Elm Street
Chicago, Illinois 60603   DEA AL5551289

FOR _John Jackson_

ADDRESS _648 Grove Street_   DATE _5-30-04_

Benylin Expectorant   _120cc_

Calcidrine Expectorant   _120cc_

mix to make   _240cc_

Sig: ꝑ tsp q̄ 4 h for cough.

LABEL
REFILL NR 1 2 3...PRN.

J. F. Lownsby M.D.   _____ M.D.
DISPENSE AS WRITTEN   SUBSTITUTION PERMITTED

FIGURE **13-1** A sample prescription.

how many times it is to be given, the date of the order, and the signature of the physician who wrote the order.

Antibiotics and narcotics are examples of drugs that have an **automatic stop policy.** A new order is required for the drug to be continued after a specified time that has been established by the institution.

PRESCRIPTION ABBREVIATIONS

To administer medications safely, it is necessary to become thoroughly familiar with accepted prescription abbreviations. The amount of a drug to be given may be written in either the metric or the apothecary system. In the metric system, the quantity of the drug is written in Arabic numbers, using decimals, before the abbreviation for the metric unit of measure. Some examples are 100 mg, 2500 mL, 0.5 gm, and 2 L. In the apothecary system both Arabic numbers and Roman numerals are used. The unit of measure is usually written before the amount of drug to be given, such as gr 10, gr 1/4, and gr IV. The abbreviation "ss" is often used to stand for 1/2, but this abbreviation should no longer be used because it can be misunderstood to mean "sliding scale," an abbreviation used with insulin, or misread as "55."

There are various ways to write drug orders using Roman numerals. Some examples are gr x, gr ix, and gr xv. When Roman numerals are used, the I is written as i. Some examples are gr ii and gr vii.

The list of abbreviations in Table 13–1 includes those most often found in prescriptions and physicians' orders.

Table 13-1 | *Common Prescription Abbreviations*

ABBREVIATION	MEANING	ABBREVIATION	MEANING
aa	of each	ou*	both eyes
ac	before meals	pc	after meals
ad lib	as much as desired	PO	by mouth
bid	twice a day	prn	as needed
c	with	q	every
caps	a capsule	qd*	every day
cc*	cubic centimeter	qh	every hour
elix	elixir	q2h	every 2 hours
et	and	q3h	every 3 hours
fldxt	fluid extract	qid	4 times a day
gm	gram	qod*	every other day
gr	grain	qs	quantity sufficient
gt	a drop	Rx	take
h	hour(s)	s	without
hs*	at bedtime	ss*	one half
HT	hypodermic tablet[M6]	SC*	subcutaneously
IM	intramuscularly	Sig	label
IV	intravenously	sp frumenti	whiskey
L	liter	stat	immediately
μg*	microgram	syr	syrup
mL	milliliter	tab	tablet
od*	once daily	tid	3 times a day
od*	left eye	tr	tincture
os*	right eye	U*	unit

*These abbreviations are considered dangerous by the Joint Commission for Accreditation of Healthcare Organizations and the Institute for Safe Medical Practice because they may be misunderstood or misread. It is recommended that these terms be written out or, in the case of "cc" and "mg," that "mL" and "mcg," respectively, be used. The complete JCAHO "Do Not Use" list of abbreviations is available at http://www.jcaho.org. See also the list of error-prone abbreviations published by the Institute for Safe Medication Practices (ISMP) at http://www.ismp.org.

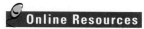
Online Resources

For updated drug information and Web activities, go to http://evolve.elsevier.com/Asperheim.

REVIEW QUESTIONS

1. Which of the following will not affect the dose of a drug given to an individual?

  a. Age

  b. Weight

  c. Impaired kidney function

  d. Time of day the medicine is administered

2. The dose of a given drug may be smaller if administered:

  a. orally.

  b. rectally.

  c. via a transdermal patch.

  d. intravenously.

3. Which part of the prescription indicates the directions to the patient?

  a. The body of the prescription

  b. The dosage form

  c. The signa

  d. The subscription

4. The measured portion of a medicine to be given to the patient is called the:

  a. mode of administration.

  b. dosage form.

  c. dose.

  d. toxic level.

5. When an individual reacts unusually to a drug, it is termed a(n):

  a. drug overdose.

  b. allergic reaction.

  c. environmental factor.

  d. idiosyncrasy.

6. Some instances of drug intolerance may be caused by:

  a. genetic factors.

  b. normalized kidney function.

  c. dosage form.

  d. dose of the drug.

7. The abbreviation for "every day" is:

  a. h.

  b. qid.

  c. qod.

  d. qd.

8. The abbreviation for "three times a day" is:

  a. bid.

  b. tid.

  c. qid.

  d. qod.

9. The abbreviation for "right eye" is:

  a. ou.

  b. od.

  c. os.

  d. PO.

10. The abbreviation for "at bedtime" is:

  a. sh.

  b. qd.

  c. hs.

  d. s.

14 Administration of Medications

Objectives

After completing this chapter, you should be able to do the following:

1. Differentiate between local and systemic effects and give four examples of each.
2. Name the four methods of administering drugs.
3. Define the term parenteral and give examples of types of parenteral methods of administering drugs.
4. List advantages and disadvantages of giving drugs by the parenteral route.
5. List guidelines for safe administration of drugs.
6. Identify reasons for errors in medication administration.
7. Use common abbreviations with 100 percent accuracy.
8. Demonstrate beginning skill in pouring medications.
9. Calibrate the rate of flow of intravenous solutions.

Key Terms

Calibration, p. 38
Dosage forms, p. 32
Local effect, p. 32
Intra-arterial injection, p. 38
Intradermal injection, p. 35
Intramuscular (IM) injection, p. 37
Intravenous (IV) injection, p. 37
Oral administration, p. 33
Parenteral administration, p. 35
Subcutaneous injection, p. 35
Sublingual administration, p. 34
Systemic effects, p. 33

GUIDELINES FOR SAFETY IN DRUG ADMINISTRATION

Safety is the paramount concern in drug administration. The following are guidelines to be used in the promotion of safe medication administration.

1. Know the policies of the hospital or agency.
2. Give only those medications for which the physician has written and signed the order.
3. Check with the head nurse or physician when in doubt about any medication.
4. Make certain that the data on the medicine card (see Fig. 14–1 below) or Kardex correspond exactly with the label on the patient's medicine.
5. Always have another person, for example, the head nurse or pharmacist, check calculations.
6. Do not converse during drug administration unless seeking help. Remember that attentiveness is the most important aspect of safety.
7. Keep the medication cabinet or drug cart locked at all times when not in use.
8. Do not give keys to the medication cabinet or drug cart to an unauthorized person.

See Box 14–1 for a summary of the "rights" of drug administration.

METHODS OF DRUG ADMINISTRATION

The methods by which drugs are administered modify their effect on the body. Certain drugs are suited to only one method of administration, whereas others may be given in a number of ways, depending on the preparation used and the reason for which the medication is given. As a general rule we are concerned with two types of drug administration: local (intended for an effect limited to the site of application) and systemic (intended for a general effect in which the drug is absorbed into the blood and carried to one or more tissues in the body).

The systems used to deliver drugs are called **dosage forms**. Drug companies package medications in certain ways to help with chemical stability and sometimes with bioavailability.

Delivery systems may also accomplish very special functions for certain drugs in certain patient populations. Patients with vomiting, seizures, asthma, or pain need quick relief. Nasal or pulmonary delivery via inhalers can achieve rapid blood levels of the required drug. Alternatively, if compliance is difficult for complicated medication routines, the patient may be better served with relatively long-acting systems such as transdermals or oral extended-release and prolonged-release injectables.

New delivery systems now being developed will include bioadhesives that allow localization in mucosal routes of administration, as well as drug carriers that will avoid removal of the drug from the body by the liver, spleen, lung, and bone.

ADMINISTRATION FOR LOCAL EFFECTS

A **local effect** is obtained when the drug is applied in the immediate area where its effect is desired. Occasionally

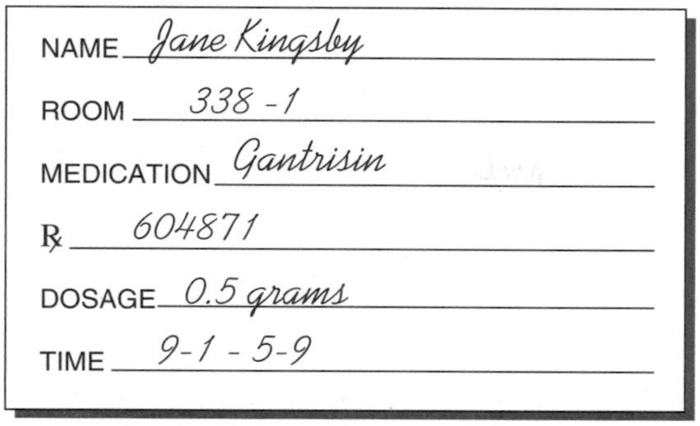

NAME *Jane Kingsley*

ROOM *338 -1*

MEDICATION *Gantrisin*

℞ *604871*

DOSAGE *0.5 grams*

TIME *9 - 1 - 5 - 9*

FIGURE 14-1 A sample medicine card.

undesired absorption may be obtained from a local site, and an untoward or toxic effect may result. Boric acid, methyl salicylate, and hexachlorophene have been shown to exert harmful effects systemically, particularly when applied to large or denuded areas.

Application to the Skin

Intact skin, with the exception of a newborn's skin, is generally impermeable to most agents. Ointments containing anti-inflammatory or antibiotic agents are useful for their local effects. Care should be taken not to apply topical agents to denuded areas without knowledge of the physician, because undesired absorption may occur.

Application to the Mucous Membrane

The application of drugs to the various mucous membranes of the body may be made for local or systemic effects. The mucous membranes in the mouth, eye, nose, vagina, and rectum are constantly bathed in watery solutions and are generally more permeable than skin.

Suppositories. Suppositories may be inserted in the rectum for local effects (e.g., Dulcolax for its local action to promote a laxative effect), or in the form of soluble bases to gain a systemic effect (i.e., antinauseants, pain-relieving agents, or drugs such as aspirin for an antipyretic effect). Vaginal suppositories are generally used for treatment of local infections, although some systemic absorption may occur.

Enemas. Enemas are most commonly used to promote a laxative effect; however, some oil-based retention enemas may contain drugs intended for systemic effects.

Intranasal preparations. Intranasal preparations may be used to treat systemic conditions such as asthma or to exert

a local effect in decreasing nasal congestion. Care should be taken that the nasal passages are free from exudate before administering a nasal preparation, and the tip of the spray bottle should be protected from contamination. Nasal spray nozzles should be cleaned after each use.

Ophthalmic preparations. Care should be taken to protect eye preparations from contamination. The eyedropper bottle or ointment tube should never touch the membranes of the eye. These preparations generally have an expiration date to guarantee their sterility; this should be checked before using any ophthalmic preparation.

Ear preparations. Absolute sterile technique is not necessary for ear preparations. With the patient lying down, the ear drops should be instilled into the ear canal after first gently pulling the external ear to straighten the ear canal. The patient should remain in a recumbent position for a few minutes after instillation of the drops to ensure their effect.

ADMINISTRATION FOR SYSTEMIC EFFECTS

To obtain **systemic effects** from a drug, it must first be absorbed into the blood and carried to the tissue or organ on which it acts. To produce these effects, drugs may be administered orally, sublingually, rectally, parenterally, by inhalation, or in some cases even by topical administration.

Oral Administration

Although it is the most popular method from the standpoint of patient acceptability and convenience, **oral administration** (i.e., allowing the drug to be swallowed) has the disadvantage of being slower in onset of action than parenteral administration; this method should not be used if a very rapid effect is desired. Some drugs, such as insulin, are not effective when given orally because they are destroyed by the juices in the gastrointestinal tract.

Drugs given orally may be administered as tablets, capsules, pills, or liquids. Taste is an important factor from the patient's viewpoint. Many drugs that have disagreeable tastes may be disguised by giving them in a large amount of fluid, such as fruit juices or effervescent drinks, or in syrups or emulsions. Fluids that have an unpleasant taste should be given cold, often with ice, and followed by a drink of water.

Food delays or reduces the absorption of many drugs, including aspirin and some forms of penicillin. Other drugs are better absorbed and less irritating to the stomach when taken with food. Examples of drugs better taken with food are iron products and some forms of erythromycin.

Reduced absorption may occur if certain drugs are given with certain food products. For example, tetracycline was given with milk for a time to reduce gastric irritation. It was later found that the tetracycline was severely disabled and rendered much less effective because the calcium, magnesium, and mineral supplements in the milk bound with the tetracycline, thus reducing the amount of the drug available to the body.

Box 14-1 *Six Rights for Correct Drug Administration*

1. Right patient
2. Right time and frequency of administration
3. Right dose
4. Right route of administration
5. Right drug
6. Right documentation

When taking oral medications, the patient should be advised as follows:

1. Read all directions, warnings, and interactions about the drug. These are generally clearly printed on the package insert that comes with the drug, or the labels of over-the-counter preparations. Over-the-counter preparations are drugs too and should not be ignored as a cause of possible side effects with prescription drugs.
2. Take medications generally with a full glass of water to enable the drug to be dissolved and begin working faster.
3. Medications should never be combined with alcohol. Some cough syrups contain alcohol in sufficient amounts to be noted.
4. Do not mix medications in hot drinks. The hot temperature can destroy some drugs, and the tannic acid in hot tea can reduce the absorption of certain medications.
5. Do not mix medications in food unless specifically ordered.
6. Vitamin, mineral, and herbal supplements have substances that can interfere with drug absorption. Information about these supplements should be noted in the same way as for over-the-counter drugs.

Procedure for pouring and administering oral medications.
Observe the following guidelines when administering oral medications:

1. Wash hands.
2. Identify the patient by checking his or her identification armband. If the armband is missing and there is any question as to the patient's ability to respond correctly to his or her name, ask a reliable staff member to identify the patient.
3. Compare the drug label with the medicine card or the Kardex when taking the container from its location, before pouring, and before returning the container to its location.
4. Pour pills, tablets, and capsules into lid of bottle before placing in medicine cup. Avoid touching them with fingers.
5. When pouring liquids, pour away from the label. Wipe neck of bottle with damp paper towel or tissue before replacing cap.
6. Hold medicine glass or graduate (see Fig. 14–2) at eye level and place thumb on glass at desired volume.
7. When giving more than one medication to a patient, the following order should be used: Give tablets and capsules followed by water or other liquid; then give liquids diluted with water as required. Cough medicine is given undiluted and is not followed by liquids. Sublingual and buccal tablets are given last.
8. Remain with patient until all medication has been swallowed.
9. Record on Kardex or medicine sheet only after medication has been given.
10. Report and record medication ordered but not given.

A medicine card similar to the one illustrated in Figure 14–1 is usually made out for each medication a patient

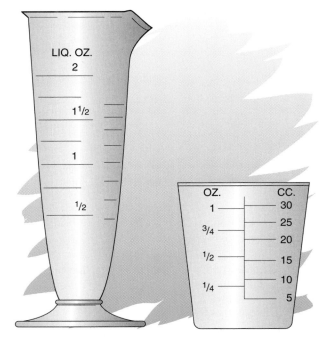

FIGURE 14-2 A graduate (*left*), a minim glass (*center*), and a medicine glass (*right*), all used to measure liquid medication.

receives. Each hospital has its own slightly modified form. Many hospitals and long-term care facilities transcribe medication orders to a Kardex.

Many commonly used drugs are available in unit-dose packages. A unit-dose package contains the amount of drug for a single dose in the proper form for administration by the prescribed route. Tablets, capsules, and liquid medications can be prepared in single-dose packages. All unit-dose packages are labeled with the generic name, trade name, precautions, expiration date if appropriate, and instructions for storing.

Packaging of drugs provides for medication safety because it is not necessary to calculate dosages. Strip packages provide for ease of counting narcotics, because all doses in the strip are numbered. This package also prevents contamination caused by pouring tablets into the hands when counting.

Liquid medications may be measured in a graduate or medicine glass, depending on the volume desired and the amount of accuracy required (Fig. 14–2). Very small or exact volumes should not be measured in a medicine glass. A syringe should be used for the measurement of volumes less than 5 mL.

Sublingual Administration

The procedure for giving sublingual medications follows that for oral administration of drugs. However, with **sublingual administration** the medication is not swallowed; it is placed under the patient's tongue, where it must be retained until it is dissolved or absorbed. The number of drugs that may be administered in this way is limited but includes nitroglycerin.

Parenteral Administration

The term *parenteral* refers to all the ways in which drugs are administered with a needle. Although **parenteral administration** is undoubtedly the most efficient method of drug administration, because it avoids all the variables of topical and gastrointestinal absorption, it can also be the most hazardous: Untoward effects may be rapid and even fatal.

Whenever the skin is punctured, it is possible for infections to develop; thus, strict aseptic technique must be used. Injections may cause nerve damage if placed incorrectly, and the accidental penetration of blood vessels may cause hematoma formation or the incorrect placement of a drug intended for intramuscular use directly into a blood vessel.

Medications intended for use by injection are supplied in the form of ampules or vials, as illustrated in Figure 14–3. Ampules are designed for use only once, and the unused portion must be discarded. Rubber-stoppered vials are used both for single-dose amounts and for multiple withdrawals of drugs. The label should be examined carefully for the strength of the drug and the intended use of that particular vial. If any sign of precipitation, color change, or cloudiness develops within the vial, it should be discarded.

Some parenteral drugs are supplied within the ampule as a powder that must first be diluted by the nurse before administration. Directions for reconstitution are enclosed with the package literature, advising dilution with sterile saline or water, and should be strictly observed.

Prefilled disposable syringes for all medications to be given subcutaneously, intramuscularly, and intravenously are available (Fig. 14–4). Some of the advantages of prefilled disposable syringes are the following:

1. Sterility is ensured.
2. Accuracy is ensured.
3. There is less trauma to tissue caused by blunt needles.
4. They are immediately available.

These unit doses of disposable syringes are the most convenient but also the most costly forms of parenteral medications.

Intradermal injection. With an **intradermal injection**, used exclusively for skin testing, the needle is inserted at an angle almost parallel to the skin surface, placing the drug within the dermis. When correctly placed, a small bubble will be raised in the skin surface where the intradermal material is deposited. The inner surface of the arm or the back is generally chosen for skin testing (Fig. 14–5).

Subcutaneous injection. In a **subcutaneous injection**, the solution is placed beneath the skin into the fat or connective tissue lying just under the dermis layer. A 25-gauge needle is generally used, with the length from 3/8 to 5/8 inch, depending on the thickness of the patient's subcutaneous tissue. A 45-degree angle is generally used, although with a short needle a 90-degree angle may be used as well (see Fig. 14–5).

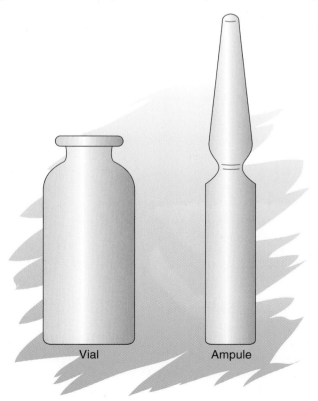

FIGURE 14-3 Injected medications are supplied in vials (*left*) and ampules (*right*).

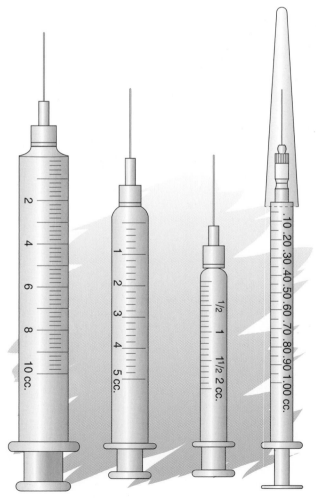

FIGURE 14-4 Prefilled disposable syringes.

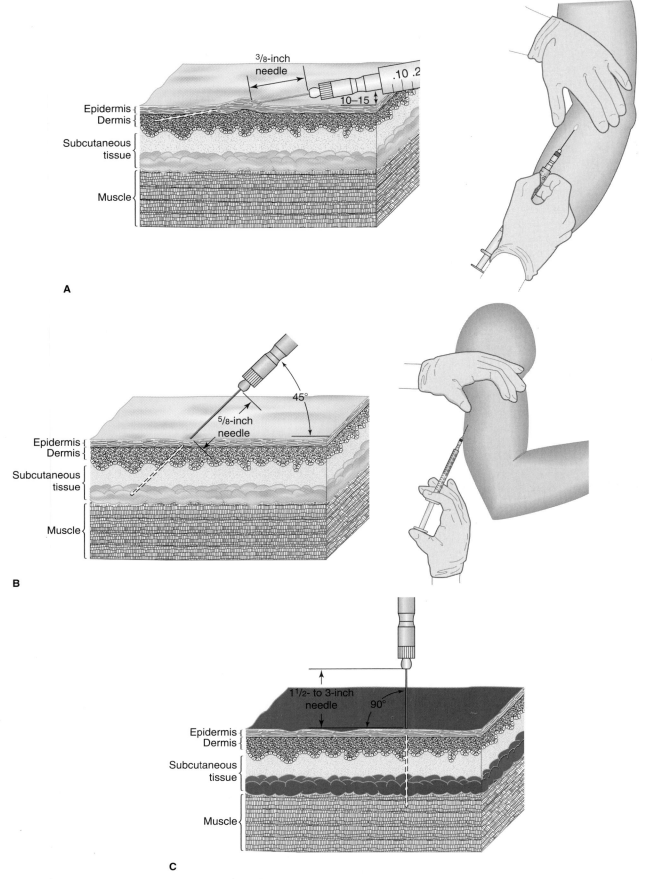

FIGURE 14-5 Three types of injections. **A,** Intradermal. **B,** Subcutaneous. **C,** Intramuscular. (From Asperheim MK: *Pharmacologic basis of patient care*, ed 5, Philadelphia, 1985, Saunders, with permission.)

After careful cleansing with alcohol or another anti-infective, the skin is gently pinched and lifted away from the muscle. The needle is inserted, and the pinched-up skin is released. Before the medication is injected, the needle is aspirated to make sure a blood vessel has not been entered, and then the material is deposited. Generally amounts injected subcutaneously are less than 2 mL.

Intramuscular injection. For **intramuscular (IM) injection** (i.e., administration directly into a muscle), a 1- to 3-inch needle is used. The gauge of the needle generally is based on the viscosity of the material injected. A 21-gauge needle is often used for penicillin injections, but a smaller gauge is chosen for solutions of other drugs.

Several sites may be used for intramuscular injections, including the deltoid muscle in the upper arm (Fig. 14–6), the vastus lateralis in the lateral thigh (Fig. 14–7), and the gluteus maximus in the buttocks (Fig. 14–8). Sites should be rotated if repeated administration of IM medications is ordered.

When giving intramuscular injections to children, a smaller length needle is chosen. With infants often a 3/8-inch needle is used. The vastus lateralis in the anterolateral thigh is the preferred site for infants and young children because the gluteal muscles are not well developed. The needle is inserted in an anteroposterior position after the muscle is firmly grasped and the child firmly restrained (Figs. 14–9 and 14–10).

Care should be taken to aspirate the syringe before the medication is delivered.

Intravenous administration. The **intravenous (IV) injection**, placing the drug directly into a vein, is used when the most rapid onset of drug action is desired. The medication is

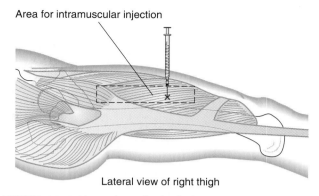

FIGURE 14-7 Vastus lateralis site for intramuscular injection in adults. (From Asperheim MK: *Pharmacologic basis of patient care*, ed 5, Philadelphia, 1985, Saunders, with permission.)

injected directly into a vein as a preparation either administered directly from an ampule especially constituted for IV use or diluted in a bottle of fluids for more gradual administration. Any surface vein may be used, or a cutdown is employed to utilize the subclavian vein or deeper extremity veins.

Just as the intended effect of the drug takes place within a few seconds in many cases, the untoward effects may occur with the same rapidity. For this reason direct supervision by a physician is often necessary.

The IV route can be used when drugs are too irritating to be injected into subcutaneous or intramuscular sites, because the intima of the blood vessels is ordinarily quite resistant to the effect of these agents. Care should be taken to prevent extravasation of these agents; sloughing of local tissues can result.

The IV route is also used to administer fluids, electrolytes, dextrose or other sugars, and proteins. Care should be taken to avoid incompatibilities when mixing drugs in various IV solutions. If cloudiness, discoloration, or precipitates occur when two drugs are mixed, the solution should not be used.

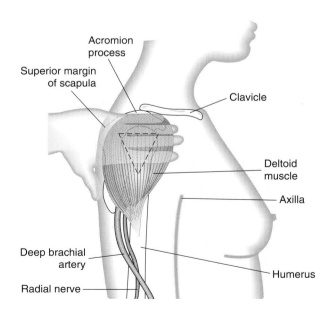

FIGURE 14-6 Two views of the deltoid site for intramuscular injection. (From Asperheim MK: *Pharmacologic basis of patient care*, ed 5, Philadelphia, 1985, Saunders, with permission.)

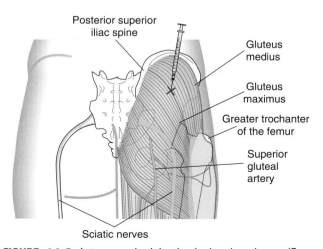

FIGURE 14-8 Intramuscular injection in the gluteal area. (From Asperheim MK: *Pharmacologic basis of patient care*, ed 5, Philadelphia, 1985, Saunders, with permission.)

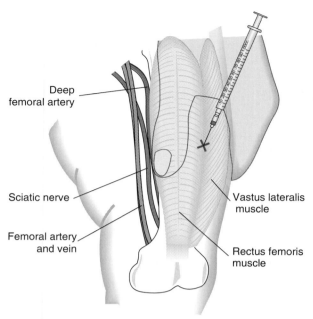

FIGURE 14-9 Vastus lateralis site for intramuscular injection in children.

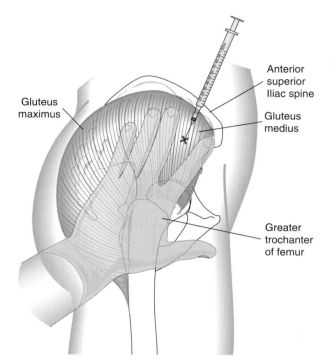

FIGURE 14-10 Ventrogluteal site. The injection is made between the index and middle fingers, which are spread apart as far as possible to form a "V." (From Asperheim MK: *Pharmacologic basis of patient care*, ed 5, Philadelphia, 1985, Saunders, with permission.)

The rate of flow of the IV solution is monitored by maintaining the proper number of drops per minute. The number of drops per minute varies with the caliber (diameter of the tubing) of the IV set used and should be carefully checked by the nurse in each instance. The **calibration**, or measurement of solution delivered "per drop," may vary from 10 to 60 drops/mL.

Calibrating the rate of intravenous solutions. IV bottles are supplied in 250-, 500-, and 1000-mL sizes. The order may read that a specified solution is to be given at stated intervals (e.g., 150 mL/hr for 8 hours), or a specified amount may be administered continuously (e.g., 500 mL is to run for a 6-hour period). In every case the proper number of drops per minute is determined by the calibration of the particular IV set used.

Example

1000 mL of 5% dextrose in water is ordered to be given over an 8-hour period. The equipment is calibrated so that 15 drops = 1 mL. What should be the rate of flow in drops per minute?

1. Determine the number of milliliters per hour.

$$\frac{1000 \text{ mL}}{8 \text{ hr}} = 125 \text{ mL/hr}$$

2. Determine the number of milliliters per minute.

$$\frac{125 \text{ mL/hr}}{60 \text{ min/hr}} = 2.1 \text{ (or 2 mL/min)}$$

3. Convert the milliliters per minute to the number of drops required.

$$1 \text{ mL} = 15 \text{ drops}$$

Therefore, 2 mL = 30 drops per minute

Example

How long will it take for 250 mL of IV solution to be delivered if it is flowing at 30 drops/minute? This set is calibrated at 60 drops/mL.

1. Convert drops to milliliters.

If 60 drops = 1 mL, 30 drops = 0.5 mL/minute

2. Determine how many minutes it will take for this amount of fluid to be absorbed.

$$\frac{250 \text{ mL}}{0.5 \text{ mL/minute}} = 500 \text{ minutes}$$

3. Convert minutes to hours.

$$\frac{500 \text{ minutes}}{60 \text{ min/hr}} = 8.3 \text{ hr}$$

Intra-arterial injection. In special cases, most notably in the administration of antineoplastic agents, an **intra-arterial injection** is used: the drug is injected directly into an artery leading to the affected tissue or organ. A special administration set is used for this purpose. Intra-arterial administration can deliver high doses of a drug to a restricted area of the body, thus eliminating some of the systemic side effects of the agent. Presently, patients can be discharged with intra-arterial medications prepared for self-administration over extended periods of time.

INNOVATIVE DRUG DELIVERY SYSTEMS

Historically, systems to deliver drugs had the primary purpose of allowing "no harm to the drug," and to deliver the drug to the intended site unaltered by body processes and defenses, so that an acceptable therapeutic blood level could be attained.

Modern drug delivery systems are intended to perform very special functions with regard to certain drugs in certain patient populations.

Patients with vomiting, seizures, migraine headaches, and breakthrough pain, for example, need quick relief. Nasal or pulmonary delivery can achieve high and rapid drug blood levels for them. In populations where compliance is an issue, such as the elderly and patients with neurologic diseases, long-acting systems such as transdermals and oral extended-release and prolonged-release injectables perform better to increase patient compliance.

New innovations in drug delivery fit into the following broad categories:

- Biocompatible subcutaneous or intramuscular injectables.
- Reticuloendothelial systems, drug carriers that avoid removal from the body by the liver, spleen, lung, and bone.
- Bioadhesives that allow localization in mucosal routes of administration.
- Systems for oral delivery of peptides and proteins, most of which are now destroyed upon oral administration.
- New polymers for tissue engineering.

- New systems to solubilize new drugs (43% of new drugs are insoluble in water.)
- Implantable polymer chips, which could replace many of the oral and injectable forms now in use. The paper-thin, dime-sized chip contains a series of tiny reservoirs. Each reservoir can store a single drug dose and is sealed with a membrane made from a second polymer. The membranes can be programmed to burst and release the reservoir's contents at specific times. Microchips now developed have up to 36 reservoirs and release their drugs over 35 to 60 days. When the chip is empty the biocompatible materials will slowly degrade. The development of and research on polymer chips continues.

Research into tissue engineering is changing many aspects of medicine. Development in this field started with artificial skin; now other engineered artificial tissues, such as cartilage, are progressing toward Food and Drug Administration approval. By designing polymers that do not fit the white blood cell receptors, it is possible to prevent white blood cells from attacking the polymers as they would foreign tissue. This will have implications in organ transplant, drug delivery, wound healing, and tissue engineering.

Online Resources

For updated drug information and Web activities, go to http://evolve.elsevier.com/Asperheim.

REVIEW QUESTIONS

1. Which preparation would not be expected to produce a systemic effect?

   a. Intranasal preparation
   b. Ear drop
   c. Rectal suppository
   d. Oral tablet

2. The most convenient systemic dosage form is:

   a. IV medication.
   b. subcutaneous injection.
   c. oral tablet.
   d. rectal suppository.

3. Which method of administration would have the most rapid systemic effect?

   a. Intravenous
   b. Subcutaneous
   c. Intramuscular
   d. Intradermal

4. An IV solution should generally not be used if it is:

   a. cloudy.
   b. discolored.
   c. noted to have 'floaters.'
   d. all of the above.

5. Parenteral administration means:

   a. local administration.
   b. administration into the parenchyma.
   c. administration by injection.
   d. topical administration.

6. The main advantage of prefilled disposable syringes is:

   a. cost.
   b. fewer side effects.
   c. accuracy.
   d. less tissue trauma.

7. Patient compliance may be increased with all except which dosage form?

   a. Transdermal patches
   b. Four-times-daily oral medication
   c. Extended-release tablets
   d. Long-acting injections

8. Preparations generally applied for local effect are:

   a. ointments.
   b. subcutaneous injections.
   c. oral tablets.
   d. transdermal patches.

Continued

REVIEW QUESTIONS—CONT'D

9. The dosage form that has been shown to avoid removal/inactivation of the drug by the liver and spleen is:
   a. extended-release tablets.
   b. intravenous administration.
   c. transdermal patches.
   d. oral short-acting tablets.

10. The hourly volume administered by an intravenous solution is calculated by:
    a. drops per minute.
    b. noting how long the IV bottle lasts.
    c. milliliters per second.
    d. urine volume of the patient.

ADDITIONAL LEARNING OPPORTUNITIES:

1. If the course in pharmacology does not correlate with the basic nursing course, it is recommended that equipment for pouring the various forms of oral medications be provided for examination.
2. Practice transcribing orders by various methods.

15 Vitamins, Minerals, and General Nutrition

Objectives

After completing this chapter, you should be able to do the following:

1. List the characteristics of vitamins.
2. State the function of vitamins in the body.
3. State the function of minerals in the body.
4. Identify fat-soluble vitamins.
5. Identify water-soluble vitamins.
6. Give an example of a source of each vitamin.
7. Identify symptoms of specific vitamin deficiencies.
8. Identify symptoms of specific mineral deficiencies.
9. Identify the components of a healthy diet.
10. Understand the significance of the food pyramid.
11. Understand the role of antioxidants in nutrition.
12. Realize that nutrition can affect various bodily functions.

Key Terms

Anemia, p. 41
Antioxidants (ĂN-tĭ-ŎK-sĭ-děnts), p. 42
Avitaminosis, p. 41
Essential fatty acids, p. 41
Fiber, p. 42
Hypervitaminosis, p. 41
Minerals, p. 41
Recommended Daily Allowance (RDA), p. 42
Vitamins, p. 41

The old adage "you are what you eat" is very true. Modern understanding of nutrition has shown us that the body needs a balance of nutrients—vitamins, minerals, protein, water, carbohydrates, fiber, and essential fatty acids—for optimum health. An improper diet has been related to increased incidences of death from heart disease, certain types of cancer, stroke, and diabetes. Nutrition can also affect various neurologic states such as depression, insomnia, migraine headaches, and mood disorders.

At the lowest scale of life, primitive microorganisms are able to synthesize most of the nutrients they need and demand few ready-made raw materials from their environment. However, some of this ability to synthesize required nutrients is lost in higher plants and animals, because they have many highly specialized cells and organs that depend entirely on other cells for their nourishment. Humans depend on other organisms to supply many vital constituents of their food; this is particularly true of one class of organic compounds that is required in minute amounts: the vitamins.

It has been known for some time that vitamin deficiencies in the diet cause diseases. A condition that develops as a result of a lack of vitamins is referred to as avitaminosis (or hypovitaminosis). For example, it was noticed by the British that sailors on long voyages, without sufficient supplies of fresh fruits and vegetables, developed a disease known as *scurvy*, which was characterized by loosening of the teeth, bleeding gums, irritability, and fatigue. It was found that, if citrus fruits were part of the diet, this disease could be prevented. (Citrus fruits are notably rich in vitamin C.) One of the fruits frequently used was the lime; hence, the word "limey" was often applied to the English sailor.

Unfavorable symptoms are also noted when an overdose of vitamins (especially the fat-soluble vitamins) is consumed—a condition known as hypervitaminosis. Actual toxicity may be produced. Polar bear liver, because of the extremely high concentration of stored fat-soluble vitamins, produces toxicity of this type if it is consumed by humans.

Minerals are nonorganic materials found in the earth's crust. Some, such as calcium, zinc, and iron, are essential components of the human body. It is now understood that the calcium you consume in your early years plays an important part in preventing osteoporosis in later years. The mineral zinc as well as vitamins A and C may help to prevent macular degeneration in the eye by blocking free radical damage to retinal blood vessels. One cause of anemia, a condition in which the number of red blood cells and/or the amount of hemoglobin in cells is less than normal, is a deficiency of iron in one's diet.

Essential fatty acids are molecules found within fats that are not produced by the body but are necessary for proper functioning. Each fatty acid molecule is composed of carbon and hydrogen. Those that contain the maximum number of hydrogen atoms for each carbon atom are called *saturated fatty acids* and can be produced by the human body. *Monounsaturated fatty acids* contain one less hydrogen atom per carbon atom; *polyunsaturated fatty acids* contain several fewer hydrogen atoms than do saturated fatty acids. Unsaturated fatty acids are found in plants and fish and cannot be produced by the human body. Excessive fat and cholesterol are harmful to the body, but the brain and nervous

Table 15-1 | *Sources of Fiber*

SOURCE	PORTION	FIBER CONTENT (GM)
Apple	Small	2.8
Banana	Medium	2.0
Beans, green	½ cup	2.1
Beans, kidney	½ cup	5.5
Beans, lima	½ cup	4.4
Bread, whole wheat	Slice	2.0
Broccoli	¾ cup	5.0
Carrots	4 sticks	1.7
Peas	½ cup	3.0
Oat bran	½ cup	3.0
Orange	Small	3.0
Peach	Medium	2.0
Pear	Small	3.0
Potato	Small	4.2
Rice, brown	½ cup	5.5
Watermelon	Thick slice	2.8

system need polyunsaturated fatty acids for proper nerve functioning. It has been found that strict limitation of all fats in infants and toddlers has delayed maturation of the nervous system. Thus moderation is in order, but fats should not be strictly limited—especially in the very young.

Antioxidants are agents that inhibit oxidation, thereby neutralizing the effects of free radicals and other substances believed to play a part in tissue damage and the aging process. The antioxidant power of certain foods, such as blueberries, and foods containing vitamins C and E is just now becoming apparent. It is thought that age-related memory impairment may be prevented and/or reversed by a diet rich in antioxidants. Vitamin C and other antioxidants such as lutein and zeaxanthin are being studied because they may help fight sunlight-induced damage to the retina and may help to prevent cataracts as well. Long-term vitamin C consumption has been shown to prevent or delay cataract formation.

Nutrition is also adversely affected by gastrointestinal conditions such as constipation, diarrhea, diverticulosis, irritable bowel syndrome, lactose intolerance, and malabsorption. **Fiber** is a food substance found only in plants that is not digested by gastrointestinal enzymes. A high-fiber diet rich in vegetables such as broccoli and cauliflower may help prevent colon cancer (Table 15–1). A diet rich in tomato products may help prevent prostate cancer because of a substance called lycopene that is present in tomatoes.

To guide us in obtaining the nutrients necessary for good health, the U.S. Department of Agriculture publishes the **Recommended Daily Allowance (RDA)** for vitamins and minerals. All RDAs in this chapter are those recommended for the adult male. The recommendations for women and children, and in some instances for the elderly, may vary.

NOMENCLATURE OF VITAMINS

The duplication and confusion apparent in the naming of vitamins are understandable only in the historical context of the development of our knowledge of vitamins. Successive letters of the alphabet were assigned to new vitamins as they were characterized and isolated, but some letters were assigned out of order. Vitamin K, for example, refers to the Swedish word *Koagulation*, because of the part this vitamin plays in the clotting mechanism of blood. Vitamin H refers to the German word *Haut*, which means skin.

It soon became evident that the original vitamin B was not a single vitamin at all but actually a group of vitamins; therefore, subscript numbers were added, giving us vitamins B_1, B_2, and others. There are currently many numbers missing in the series, because some of the subtypes that were identified during early research were later found to be identical.

CHARACTERISTICS OF VITAMINS

Vitamins are:
- Organic in nature
- Required in very small amounts
- Required preformed in the diet or synthesized by intestinal flora
- Necessary for normal growth and maintenance
- Sensitive to light, heat, and oxidation and so must be stored in a cool place in dark bottles
- Necessary for enzyme systems

General vitamin-deficiency symptoms include tiredness, aches, pains, and a general "poor feeling." The general populace has far too many symptoms of this type, however, to blame them on vitamin deficiencies exclusively. An adequate diet is the best answer for the prevention of vitamin deficiencies.

FAT-SOLUBLE VITAMINS

VITAMIN A

Source: Fish liver oils (especially cod liver), dairy products, and vegetables such as carrots and spinach

Deficiency symptoms: Night blindness, nerve degeneration of the spinal cord and peripheral nerves, skin lesions

RDA: 1000 mcg

VITAMIN D

Source: Fish liver oils (especially cod and halibut), ultraviolet radiation (sunshine), dairy products

Deficiency symptoms: If the deficiency occurs in childhood, the condition is known as *rickets* and is characterized by an abnormally large abdominal region, soft skull, and deformed arms and legs; if the deficiency occurs in later life, it is known as *osteomalacia* and is characterized by softening of the bones.

Activity: This vitamin enables the body to deposit calcium and phosphorus in the bones. An overdose leads to low calcium concentration in the blood, tetany, and eventual death.

RDA: 5 mcg

VITAMIN K

Source: Alfalfa; synthesized by intestinal flora
Deficiency symptoms: Hemorrhagic tendency
Activity: This vitamin is required for the formation of prothrombin in the liver, which is needed for blood to clot normally.
RDA: 80 mcg

VITAMIN E (ALPHA-TOCOPHEROL)

Source: Wheat germ, vegetable oils, nuts, seeds
Deficiency symptoms: No deficiency states have been identified.
Activity: Vitamin E is an antioxidant. Antioxidants have been linked with decreased atherosclerosis in experimental studies. Studies have also suggested that it may boost the immune system and ward off cataracts. There is some evidence that vitamin E may have a protective effect against coronary events by reducing the oxidation of low-density lipoprotein (LDL, or bad cholesterol) that can cause atherosclerosis. It is believed by some to have some activity in slowing down the progression of Alzheimer's disease.
Toxic effects: Vitamin E prolongs bleeding time, thus causing an increased tendency to hemorrhage. Those persons with bleeding disorders and those who take anticoagulants are generally advised not to take supplemental vitamin E.
RDA: 10 mg alpha-tocopherol equivalents

WATER-SOLUBLE VITAMINS

These vitamins may be subdivided into two general groups: those concerned with the release of energy from food (e.g., thiamine, riboflavin) and those concerned with the formation of red blood cells (e.g., folic acid, vitamin B_{12}).

THIAMINE (VITAMIN B₁)

Source: Widely distributed in nature, especially in yeast, liver, and lean meat
Deficiency symptoms: The deficiency of thiamine produces a condition is known as *beriberi*, which is characterized by inflammation of the peripheral nerves, paralysis, mixed sensations of heat and cold, congestive heart failure, and edema.
RDA: 1.2 mg

RIBOFLAVIN (VITAMIN B₂)

Source: Liver, kidney, milk
Deficiency symptoms: Vascularization of the cornea followed by ulcerations, dermatitis, and lip lesions
RDA: 1.3 mg

NICOTINAMIDE (NIACINAMIDE) AND NICOTINIC ACID (NIACIN)

Source: Liver, yeast, peanuts
Deficiency symptoms: The condition produced by deficiency of niacin is known as *pellagra*. The symptoms are insomnia, appetite loss, irritability, dizziness, and morbid fears, followed by subsequent lesions of the mucous membranes and dermatoses, especially on areas of the chest and neck exposed to the sun.
Side effect: A facial flush occurs quite often when nicotinic acid is administered, but the flush is not commonly seen when nicotinamide is used.
RDA: 16 mg

PYRIDOXINE (VITAMIN B₆)

Source: Liver, yeast, milk, meats, molasses
Deficiency symptoms: Skin lesions, hypochromic anemia, and convulsions in some instances
RDA: 1.3 mg

PANTOTHENIC ACID

Source: Meat, vegetables, cereals, legumes, eggs, milk
Deficiency symptoms: Deficiency symptoms as an isolated deficiency have not been described; occurs in overall deficiency states.
RDA: 5 mg

FOLIC ACID

Source: Green leafy vegetables, liver, yeast
Deficiency symptoms: Macrocytic anemia. The erythrocytes (red blood cells) do not mature properly and are larger than normal. This increased size reduces the amount of total surface area; consequently, less oxygen is transported to the tissues.
RDA: 0.4 mg

 Considerations for Pregnant and Nursing Women

Folic Acid

Folic acid is particularly important for pregnant women. Evidence indicates that prophylactic therapy with folic acid initiated at least 1 month before pregnancy and continued through early pregnancy can reduce the incidence of neural tube defects, including spina bifida, anencephaly, and encephalocele. Women of childbearing age should consume 0.4 mg of folic acid from fortified food or supplements in addition to that available in a balanced diet.

VITAMIN B₁₂ (CYANOCOBALAMIN)

Source: Animal tissue, especially liver
Deficiency symptoms: Pernicious anemia. Vitamin B_{12} is known as the extrinsic factor for the production of red blood cells. For effective utilization of this vitamin from the gastrointestinal system, the intrinsic factor must be present in the stomach of the individual. If it is not, the vitamin is not absorbed. In most cases of demonstrated deficiency of this vitamin, it is actually this intrinsic factor that is at fault, because vitamin B_{12} is so widely distributed in nature that it would be rather unlikely that the individual has a dietary inadequacy. In a deficiency, then, vitamin B_{12} is ordinarily administered parenterally to circumvent the lack of this intrinsic factor needed for absorption from the oral route.
RDA: 2.4 mcg

ASCORBIC ACID OR CEVITAMIC ACID (VITAMIN C)

Source: Green vegetables, berries, fruits. Because this vitamin is rapidly destroyed by air, the fruits must be fresh. Canning and cooking destroy the vitamin.

Deficiency symptoms: Scurvy, characterized by gingivitis, loose teeth, slow healing of wounds, and petechial hemorrhages.

Activity: Large doses of vitamin C—1000 mg or more daily—have been used to prevent or lessen the severity of respiratory viral illnesses, although this is controversial. At these dose levels severe abdominal cramps, nausea, vomiting, and diarrhea have occurred. The use of these megadoses is generally not recommended. Vitamin C is a popular daily supplement used for its antioxidant properties. A dose of 100 mg daily is generally recommended for a supplement. Increased vitamin C requirements may be associated with pregnancy, lactation, fever, stress, infection, smoking, and the use of certain drugs (e.g., estrogens, oral contraceptives, tetracyclines, barbiturates, and salicylates).

RDA: 60 mg

MULTIPLE VITAMIN PREPARATIONS

It is well recognized that, when one vitamin deficiency exists, there is invariably a dietary deficiency in several other vitamins as well. Thus most commonly a multiple vitamin supplement is prescribed. There are many multivitamin supplements available.

The multivitamins available for over-the-counter purchasing generally have a lower vitamin content, particularly in the fat-soluble vitamins, than those available by prescription only.

MINERALS

There are many minerals, or essential elements, necessary for normal body functions. Most of these are required in trace amounts only and are found so freely in the environment, the soil, plants used for food, and seafood that they rarely, if ever, need to be discussed in terms of a deficiency leading to ill health.

Those minerals known as trace elements are used by the body as components of enzymes and in some cases as catalysts necessary for proper enzymatic function. Copper, cobalt, fluorine, manganese, and zinc are a few of the trace elements known to be essential. Zinc is believed to help in the prevention of age-related retinal deterioration by slowing down the disease process.

Other minerals perform a more dynamic function in the body and must be ingested regularly in some form, because they either are excreted daily in urine or feces or are depleted in the process of forming or repairing body tissues.

IRON

Iron has long been known to be an essential component of blood hemoglobin. Blood is not a static tissue but is constantly being re-formed as old red blood cells are trapped and destroyed by the spleen and other organs. Iron can be stored in the body, most notably in the bone marrow, but a dietary deficiency or a malabsorption problem in the intestinal tract soon manifests itself as an iron deficiency anemia.

Iron-enriched infant formulas, such as Similac with Iron and Enfamil with Iron, have been designed to prevent this problem in very young children. Cow's milk is a very poor source of iron, and iron deficiency anemia is a very frequent finding in children ages 6 months to 3 years. The problem is compounded if the infant is allowed to stay on the bottle after 1 year of age and to satisfy most of his or her appetite with a bottle of milk between meals, thus coming to mealtime with a poor appetite for the more nutritious meats and vegetables.

Considerations for Children

Iron

Iron deficiency is a very common cause of anemia in children, resulting in developmental delays and behavioral disturbances. Childhood anemia is generally nutritional, but it may also be caused by lead poisoning. Blood tests for persistent childhood anemia will therefore usually include serum lead levels.

The teenage years are another time in life when iron deficiency anemias are common. This is primarily due to the teenager's common pattern of fad diets and generally poor eating habits.

Menstruating women lose iron in the menstrual flow each month and are much more susceptible to deficiencies than males of the same age. Pregnancy is likewise a common time for anemia, because the developing fetus takes what it needs for development and can cause alarmingly low hemoglobin values in women whose diets are nutritionally inadequate.

Sources: Meat, green vegetables, legumes, fortified cereals

RDA: 10 mg

Commercial Preparations of Iron

ferrous sulfate, USP, BP (Feosol). This preparation is the most inexpensive and most commonly used form of iron supplement. It is available in tablet and liquid forms. Occasional abdominal cramping or discomfort is noted if it is taken on an empty stomach. The patient should be advised that all iron supplements will turn the stool black.

> **Dosage:**
> (Oral) 325 mg three times daily.

ferrous gluconate, USP, BP (Fergon). Very little therapeutic difference is noted between the gluconate and sulfate salts of iron. This preparation has the advantage of being slightly less irritating to the gastric mucosa but the disadvantage of being relatively more expensive.

> **Dosage:**
> (Oral) 435 mg once daily.

iron dextran injection, USP, BP (Imferon). Designed for deep intramuscular injection, this preparation is reserved for cases of severe iron deficiency anemia and malabsorption problems. It should be administered with the Z-track technique in the upper outer quadrant of the buttock to minimize skin discoloration and irritation at the site of injection.

The primary disadvantage of this, as of any parenteral iron preparation, is the ever-present danger of iron overdosage. Hemosiderosis, fever, urticaria, and headache are among the symptoms of iron overload.

> **Dosage:**
>
> Calculated individually, based on the patient's hemoglobin level and weight. The range of dosage is generally 0.5 to 2 mL/day given IM or IV.

CALCIUM AND PHOSPHORUS

Unlike iron deficiencies, conditions arising from calcium and phosphorus deficiencies are usually due to metabolic problems rather than nutritional deficits. These elements perform a very dynamic and complex function in the body under the control of the parathyroid glands. A constant balance is maintained between levels of these minerals in the blood and levels in calcified tissues of the body, primarily bone. Serum calcium levels should vary only slightly in healthy individuals. If calcium levels are too low, tetany occurs; if they are too high, cardiac irregularities are noted.

The kidneys are primarily responsible for the excretion of calcium, and severe or prolonged kidney damage can produce calcium deficiencies unrelated to the endocrine system. This condition is termed *renal rickets.*

Vitamin D–deficient rickets, in which insufficient amounts of vitamin D limit proper calcium absorption, is extremely uncommon in the United States but may still be noted in underdeveloped countries.

Osteoporosis is a condition in which there is thinning of the calcified portions of bones owing to deficient formation of bone matrix. It may be seen in postmenopausal women as well as individuals with a severely protein-deficient diet. Osteoporosis in women may be alleviated by oral calcium supplements. It has been shown that the amount of calcium you consume in the first 3 decades of life can dramatically influence your future risk for developing osteoporosis. Osteoporosis is also discussed in Chapter 32 (Drug Therapy in Older Adults).

The RDA for elemental calcium is 1 gm. One of the best sources of calcium is nonfat milk. Besides providing calcium, milk is fortified with vitamin D, which helps the body absorb calcium.

The dosage for the treatment of calcium depletion is 2 gm of elemental calcium daily. It should be noted that certain salts of calcium contain a relatively small percentage of elemental calcium; for example, calcium lactate contains only 84.5 mg of elemental calcium per 650 mg of the salt. Thus large doses of the salt are required to obtain the desired amount of elemental calcium.

Calcium salts are used intravenously in advanced cardiac life support during cardiopulmonary resuscitation. The dose may be repeated intravenously every 10 minutes if necessary.

Commercial Preparations of Calcium

calcium lactate, USP, BP
> **Dosage:**
>
> (Oral) 23 1/2 tablets (each 650-mg tablet has 84.5 mg of elemental calcium).

calcium gluconate, USP, BP
> **Dosage:**
>
> (Oral) 34 tablets (each 650-mg tablet has 58.5 mg of elemental calcium). (IV) 10 mL of 10% solution.

calcium chloride, USP, BP
> **Dosage:**
>
> (IV) 5 to 20 mL of a 5% solution.

calcium carbonate, USP, BP (Os-Cal, Biocal)
> **Dosage:**
>
> (Oral) 8 tablets (each 625-mg tablet has 250 mg of elemental calcium).

POTASSIUM

Potassium, like sodium and chloride, has a dynamic function in the maintenance of water and electrolyte concentrations within the body tissues and cells. In addition, potassium has a unique function in the transmission of nerve impulses and the control of cardiac rhythm.

Potassium depletion results from the metabolic changes occurring in diabetic acidosis, in prolonged vomiting or diarrhea, and in the debilitation caused by surgery. It is often accidentally induced by prolonged administration of certain diuretics. Familial periodic paralysis is a hereditary disease characterized by bouts of muscular weakness and hypokalemia.

Commercial Preparations of Potassium

potassium chloride, USP, BP
> **Dosage:**
>
> (Oral) 1 to 3 gm daily in divided doses. (IV) Based on potassium depletion. Maximum rate of administration would be 20 mEq/hr; usually 40 to 80 mEq is given in a 24-hour period. Maximum daily dose by IV infusion is 200 mEq per 24 hours. CAUTION: This must be diluted before IV infusion; it may be fatal if given by IV push.

Slow-K. This coated tablet has 600 mg (8 mEq) of potassium chloride in a wax matrix to minimize gastrointestinal irritation.
> **Dosage:**
>
> (Oral) 1 tablet three or four times daily.

TEN-K. Each tablet has 10 mEq of potassium chloride.
> **Dosage:**
>
> (Oral) 1 tablet three times daily.

K-DUR 10. Each tablet has 10 mEq of potassium chloride.
> **Dosage:**
>
> (Oral) 1 tablet three times daily.

CHANGES IN NUTRITIONAL INFORMATION

For many years it was believed that proper nutrition could be achieved by eating the basic food groups: proteins (meat, fish, and eggs), breads and grains, fruits, vegetables, and dairy products.

Increased information has become available with regard to overnutrition, particularly in the red meat and fat groups, with resulting elevation of cholesterol and increased incidence of vascular diseases, cerebrovascular accidents (CVAs, or strokes), and heart attacks. It has become important to control and reduce the amount of these food items in the diet.

The Food Guide Pyramid (Figure 15–1) shows the current dietary recommendations of the U.S. Department of Health and Human Services. The pyramid emphasizes that the most nutritious and healthy diet should stress food groups in different proportions in the diet, with complex carbohydrates as the base of the pyramid and then other foods in decreasing amounts.

Some nutritionists now recommend that fish or poultry be consumed only two or three times a week, with consumption of red meat being reduced to two or three times a month. It has been recommended that no more than 30% of the calories a person consumes come from fat.

Caloric requirements vary with age and activity. Children and active teenagers and adult males may need up to 2800 calories a day. Sedentary adults may require only 1600 calories.

Food labels can often be misleading. For instance,
- "Cholesterol free" does *not* mean fat free. Cholesterol only comes from animal sources. A food that does not contain animal products may still be fatty.
- "Made with vegetable oil" may or may not be a good sign. Good oil choices are canola, olive, corn, sunflower, and soybean oils. Saturated fats are present in coconut oil, palm kernel oil, or any hydrogenated oil.

Look on the back of the package for the grams of fat or saturated fat per serving.

★ CLINICAL IMPLICATIONS

1. Discuss the patient's diet, and review the natural sources of vitamins. Be familiar with the basic food groups and the vitamins and minerals they supply.
2. In some cases, a vitamin deficiency may be caused by a self-administered medication, such as mineral oil, which prevents absorption of the fat-soluble vitamins. Patients should be questioned about self-administered medications.
3. Self-administered medications such as vitamins—most notably the fat-soluble vitamins A, D, E, and K—can produce toxic effects.
4. Patients and their families should be instructed to store all vitamins in a cool place and away from direct light and heat.
5. Individuals on a vegetarian diet should be advised of their special need for vitamin and mineral supplements.
6. Water-soluble vitamins can be destroyed by overcooking foods.
7. Certain vitamins, such as vitamin C, appear to have activities outside their "vitamin" status and may be useful in higher doses in the prevention of viral illnesses, such as the common cold.
8. Iron supplements may be used in the prevention of anemia, particularly in premenopausal women and children or adults with limited dietary preferences.
9. Calcium supplements are useful in the prevention of osteoporosis in postmenopausal women.
10. Certain minerals, such as calcium and potassium, may have cardiotoxic effects when their levels in the body are too high or too low.
11. The food pyramid describes a healthy diet and the relative proportions of foods allowed.
12. A healthy diet should contain fiber and antioxidants and limited fat content.

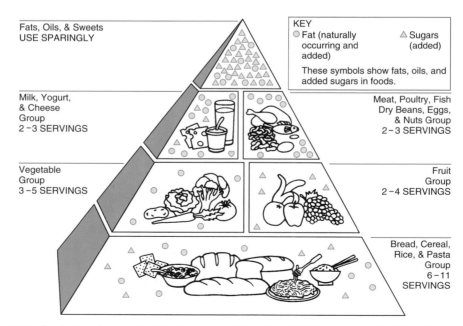

FIGURE 15-1 The food guide pyramid. (U.S. Department of Agriculture, U.S. Department of Health and Human Services.)

CRITICAL THINKING QUESTIONS

1. The patient has had difficulty eating since her dental extractions 1 year ago. She presented in the physician's office with a deep fissure on each side of her mouth and red, irritated eyes. What vitamin deficiency is apparent?

2. The patient has many food allergies and intolerances. Her dentist referred her to her family physician because he could find no oral disease that would account for her loose teeth and gingival inflammation. What deficiency could account for her problem?

3. The child was brought to the pediatrician's office by her mother because she was failing in school, pale, and listless, and seemed to be tired all the time,

even though she reportedly had 10 hours of sleep each night. Blood studies revealed a hemoglobin of 9.1 gm/dL, and other studies were within normal limits. How should her problem be handled?

4. The patient complained to the public health nurse that she has been having abdominal cramps and her stools are black. She had been taking an iron supplement for anemia. How would you identify the problem, and what instruction could you give her?

5. The patient was noted to have a high cholesterol level of 375 mg/dL. He states that he frequently eats out at fast-food restaurants. How could his diet be examined, and what advice could be given?

REVIEW QUESTIONS

1. The disease that develops because of an overdose of vitamins is:
   a. scurvy.
   b. beriberi.
   c. hypervitaminosis.
   d. avitaminosis.

2. A vitamin necessary for blood to clot normally is:
   a. vitamin A.
   b. thiamine.
   c. vitamin K.
   d. vitamin D.

3. Pernicious anemia may be caused by a deficiency of which vitamin?
   a. Vitamin B_1
   b. Vitamin B_2
   c. Vitamin B_6
   d. Vitamin B_{12}

4. A mineral that is a component of blood hemoglobin is:
   a. zinc.
   b. iron.
   c. calcium.
   d. phosphorus.

5. Osteoporosis may result when the body is depleted of:
   a. vitamin C.
   b. vitamin A.
   c. calcium.
   d. iron.

6. A vitamin known to be an antioxidant is:
   a. vitamin A.
   b. vitamin B_1.
   c. vitamin D.
   d. vitamin E.

7. The administration of diuretics can cause a loss of:
   a. calcium.
   b. iron.
   c. potassium.
   d. zinc.

8. The daily dose of calcium recommended for the postmenopausal woman who is calcium depleted is:
   a. 1 gm.
   b. 2 gm.
   c. 300 mg.
   d. 5 gm.

9. A nonorganic material found in the earth's crust is a:
   a. vitamin.
   b. mineral.
   c. oxidant.
   d. antioxidant.

10. Rickets is a deficiency disorder caused by a lack of:
    a. vitamin A.
    b. vitamin C.
    c. vitamin D.
    d. vitamin E.

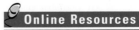

Online Resources

For updated drug information and Web activities, go to http://evolve.elsevier.com/Asperheim.

16 Antibiotics and Antifungal, Antiviral, and Antiparasitic Agents

Objectives

After completing this chapter, you should be able to do the following:

1. Identify the antibiotics and give their general uses.
2. Identify serious side effects of antibiotics.
3. Distinguish between a broad-spectrum antibiotic and a narrow-spectrum antibiotic.
4. Distinguish among first-, second-, and third-generation cephalosporins.
5. Give examples of antibiotics that are used to treat specific conditions.
6. Identify common antiparasitic agents.
7. Identify antiviral agents and their general uses.
8. List the current uses of sulfonamides.
9. List symptoms of toxic effects of sulfa drugs.

Key Terms

Antibiotics, p. 48
Broad-spectrum antibiotic, p. 48
Cephalosporins (SĔF-ĕ-lō-SPŎR-ĭns), p. 49
Fungus (pl. fungi), p. 57
Narrow-spectrum antibiotic, p. 48
Para-aminobenzoic acid (PABA), p. 53
Penicillin, p. 48
Quinolones (KWĬN-ĕ-lōns), p. 52
Sulfonamides ("sulfa drugs") (sĕl-FŌN-ĕ-mīds), p. 53
Tetracyclines (TĔT-rĕ-SĪ-klēns), p. 50
Virus, p. 57

ANTIBIOTICS

Antibiotics are substances produced by living cells (or the synthetic analog) that kill or inhibit the growth of microorganisms. The first knowledge of antibiotics was given to us by Sir Alexander Fleming in 1928, when he discovered that a product of the *Penicillium* mold had the power to destroy many disease-producing microorganisms.

Currently, we obtain many antibiotics from molds, bacteria, and yeasts, but an increasing number are now manufactured synthetically. Often only a small change in the structure of a naturally produced antibiotic can result in significant changes in the action and effect of a drug.

Each antibiotic has its own characteristic "spectrum" of activity against various microorganisms. A **broad-spectrum antibiotic** is effective against many microorganisms; a **narrow-spectrum antibiotic** is effective against only a few.

Much has been discovered in recent years about the growing resistance of many microorganisms to the action of antibiotics. It is believed that the use of antibiotics to treat many trivial infections has allowed microorganisms to develop mutant forms that are resistant to these drugs. This is particularly likely if an antibiotic is taken for only a few days instead of the generally prescribed 10-day minimum for antibiotic use. When treatment time is shortened, the organisms that are more naturally resistant to the drug are allowed to increase and multiply, and only the weaker ones are killed.

Considerations for Children

Unnecessary Antibiotics

Children do not need an antibiotic to treat every minor illness. However, busy parents often want an efficient, sure-fire cure. Teach parents that such overuse of antibiotics is producing antibiotic-resistant organisms, and reassure them when antibiotics are not necessary.

Allergic reactions to various antibiotics are also common. With repeated exposure to a drug, various defensive mechanisms of the body begin to be sensitized, and allergic reactions result. Often these reactions are mild and may produce just a rash, which is easily treated. Subsequent exposures to the drug may produce severe and even fatal reactions, however.

THE PENICILLINS

A **penicillin** is any antibiotic derived from the *Penicillium* mold. Since its discovery as the first antibiotic, there have been many alterations in the structure of penicillin to increase its usefulness.

penicillin G, USP; benzylpenicillin, BP. Utilized as either the sodium salt (given only intramuscularly [IM]) or the potassium salt (given IM or intravenously [IV]) to increase its water solubility, this early form of penicillin remains in common use for the treatment of streptococcal and pneumococcal infections, as well as gonorrhea, syphilis, meningitis, and other infections caused by penicillin-sensitive organisms. Its main disadvantage is that, in its crystalline form, it has a short duration of action and must be injected because it is destroyed by stomach acids when taken orally. Before any form of penicillin is given, the patient must be carefully questioned concerning allergic reactions to the drug.

Dosage:

Adults: (IV) 5 million to 20 million units daily in divided doses. Dosage is individualized.

Children: (IM, IV) 25,000 to 50,000 units/kg/day in divided doses four times daily. Dosage is individualized.

Neonates: (IM, IV) 25,000 units twice daily. Dosage is individualized.

Long-Acting Forms of Penicillin G

Because of the short duration of the crystalline form of penicillin G, several long-acting forms have been developed. These have the advantage of being given intramuscularly, so that a repository of the drug remains in the muscle tissue and can be absorbed slowly by the body.

These long-acting forms may be given ONLY intramuscularly. They can produce fatal embolization if incorrectly administered intravenously.

penicillin G procaine, USP, BP (Mycillin, Crysticillin, Duracillin). The addition of procaine to the penicillin molecule gives a product that provides good blood levels of penicillin for about 6 hours.

Dosage:

Adults: (IM) 600,000 to 4 million units daily in divided doses every 6 hours.

Children: (IM) 300,000 to 1.2 million units daily in divided doses every 6 hours.

Neonates: This form is not recommended.

penicillin G benzathine, USP, BP (Bicillin). By the addition of benzathine to the penicillin molecule, a very insoluble form of penicillin is formed. The drug is slowly leached from the repository in the muscle and may give prolonged but low doses of penicillin for as long as 1 month. This form is used in monthly injections for prophylaxis in patients who have had rheumatic fever and in the treatment of syphilis, as well as in other cases when prolonged action is desired.

Bicillin L-A. Pure benzathine penicillin.

Dosage:

Adults: (IM only) 1.2 million to 4.8 million units.

Children: (IM only) 600,000 to 1.2 million units.

Bicillin C-R. This drug combines equal parts of benzathine penicillin and procaine penicillin, so that a therapeutic blood level is reached sooner. Dosage range is similar to that of Bicillin L-A.

penicillin V, USP, BP (V-Cillin, Pen Vee). By changing the structure of penicillin G, a form of penicillin was developed that can be absorbed orally. It is primarily used to treat respiratory infections.

Dosage:

Adults: (Oral) 250 to 500 mg every 6 hours.

Children: (Oral) 15 to 50 mg/kg daily in four divided doses.

Semisynthetic Penicillins

Considerable research and alteration of the penicillin molecule have resulted in new forms of penicillin that have a broader spectrum of activity than the parent molecule and greater effectiveness with oral administration. Table 16–1 shows an overview of this class of antibiotics.

General Toxicity and Side Effects

Hypersensitivity to the penicillins should always be considered. In some instances, however, individuals who are sensitive to penicillin G may be able to tolerate the altered forms of penicillin. When prescribed orally, abdominal cramping or diarrhea may result. Overgrowth of nonsusceptible organisms such as *Monilia* may occur, with resultant vaginal or perineal infections.

THE BETA-LACTAM ANTIBIOTICS: THE CEPHALOSPORINS

Also derived originally from a mold, the **cephalosporins** are structurally related to the penicillins. Like penicillin, these agents exert their activity against young dividing bacterial cells by interfering with the formation of cell walls.

Because of their similarity to the penicillin molecule, there is a considerable cross sensitivity with penicillin. Although it is thought that the cross-allergic reaction occurs only about 25% of the time, all patients with a history of allergy to penicillin should be given these agents with caution.

General toxic effects of these agents include gastrointestinal distress when they are administered orally, as well as allergic skin rashes.

The cephalosporins are divided into three general groups on the basis of their spectrum of activity; because of the order in which they were developed, these groups are referred to as the first, second, and third generations.

First-Generation Cephalosporins

These agents are effective against organisms such as streptococci and some strains of staphylococci. In addition, they are effective against some organisms that invade the urinary tract. They are listed in Table 16–2.

Second-Generation Cephalosporins

In addition to activity against the same organisms as the first generation, these agents are also effective against *Haemophilus influenzae*, a common invader of the middle ear and respiratory tract. They are listed in Table 16–3.

Third-Generation Cephalosporins

This group is less effective against the streptococci and pneumococci than the early cephalosporins but more effective against the gram-negative invaders of the gastrointestinal and urinary tracts. They are generally reserved for serious

Table 16-1 | *Semisynthetic Penicillins*

GENERIC NAME	TRADE NAME	GENERAL USES	DOSAGE
amoxicillin, USP, BP	Amoxil	Same as ampicillin	Adults: (Oral) 250–500 mg q8h Children: (Oral) 20–40 mg/kg/day in divided doses q8h

amoxicillin and
  clavulanic acid
	Augmentin	Same as ampicillin, but includes
		  some ampicillin-resistant
		  organisms
			Adults: (Oral) 250–500 mg q8h
			Children: (Oral) 20 mg/kg/day in
			  divided doses q8h

ampicillin, USP, BP	Many	Otitis media, respiratory tract
		  infections, urinary tract
		  infections, meningitis (in IV form)
			Adults: (Oral, IM, IV) 1–2 gm/day in
			  divided doses
			Children: (Oral) 50–400 mg/kg/day

ampicillin sodium
  and sulbactam
  sodium
	Unasym	Severe skin, bone, abdominal
		  infections
			Adults: (IM or IV) 1.5–3 gm q6h
			Children: Not recommended under
			  40 kg; over 40 kg same as adult dose

bacampicillin hydrochloride, USP	Spectrobid	Same as ampicillin	Adults: (Oral) 400 mg q12h Children: (Oral) 12.5 mg/kg q12h

carbenicillin indanyl
  sodium
	Geocillin	Urinary tract infections	Adults: (Oral) 1–2 tablets (382 mg)
			  4 times daily
			Children: Not recommended

cloxacillin sodium,
  USP, BP
	Tegopen	Respiratory tract and soft
		  tissue infections
			Adults: (Oral) 0.25–1 gm q4–6h
			Children: (Oral) 12.5–25 mg/kg/day
			  in divided doses

dicloxacillin sodium,
  USP, BP
	Dynapen	Staphylococcal infections	Adults: (Oral, IM, IV) 250–500 mg q6h
			Children: (Oral, IM, IV)
			  12.5–50 mg/kg/day in divided doses

mezlocillin sodium,
  USP, BP
	Mezlin	Serious postsurgical abdominal,
		  GI, and soft tissue infections
			Adults: (IM, IV) 3–4 gm q4–6h
			Children: (IM, IV) 300 mg/kg/day in
			  divided doses

nafcillin sodium,
  USP, BP
	Unipen	Staphylococcal infections	Adults: (Oral, IM, IV) 250 mg–1 gm
			  4–6 times daily
			Children: (Oral, IM, IV)
			  25–50 mg/kg/day in divided doses

oxacillin sodium,
  USP, BP
	Prostaphlin,
	  Bactocill
		Staphylococcal infections	Adults: (Oral, IM, IV) 250–500 mg
			  q4–6h
			Children: (Oral, IM, IV) 50 mg/kg/day
			  in 4 divided doses

piperacillin sodium,
  USP
	Pipracil	Serious postsurgical infections,
		  some urinary tract infections
			Adults: (IV or IM) 6–18 gm/day
			  in divided doses
			Children: Not recommended
			  under 12 yr

piperacillin and
  tazobactam sodium
	Zosyn	Abdominal, skin, and respiratory
		  tract infections
			Adults: (IV) 3.375 gm q4h
			Children: Not recommended
			  under 12 yr

ticarcillin disodium,
  USP, BP
	Ticar	Urinary tract infections	Adults: (IM or IV) 1 gm q6h
			Children: (IM) 50–100 mg/kg/day
			  (IV) 150–200 mg/kg/day in 4–6
			  divided doses

ticarcillin disodium
  and clavulanate
  potassium
	Timentin	Urinary tract infections	Adults: (IM or IV) 3.1 gm q4–6h
			Children: (IM or IV) 200 mg/kg/day
			  in divided doses

GI, Gastrointestinal; IM, intramuscular; IV, intravenous.

infections that do not respond to other agents. The third-generation cephalosporins are listed in Table 16–4.

THE TETRACYCLINES

The **tetracyclines** are broad-spectrum antibiotics that are effective against many organisms, particularly those infecting the respiratory system and soft tissues. Although many can be given parenterally, they are well absorbed orally and are generally given by mouth.

Tetracyclines are used principally in the treatment of infections caused by susceptible *Rickettsia*, *Chlamydia*, and *Mycoplasma* organisms and a variety of gram-negative and gram-positive bacteria. Tetracycline is the drug of choice for Rocky Mountain spotted fever and Lyme disease.

Table 16-2 | *First-Generation Cephalosporins*

GENERIC NAME	TRADE NAME	DOSAGE
cefadroxil, USP, BP	Duricef	Adults: (Oral) 1–2 gm/day in 1–2 divided doses Children: (Oral) 10–15 mg/kg twice daily
cefazolin sodium, USP, BP	Ancef, Kefzol	Adults: (Oral, IM, IV) 250 mg–1.5 gm q6h Children: (Oral, IM, IV) 25–50 mg/kg/day in 3–4 divided doses
cephalexin, USP, BP	Keflex	Adults: (Oral) 250–500 mg q6h Children: (Oral) 25–50 mg/kg/day in divided doses
cephradine, USP, BP	Anspor, Velosef	Adults: (Oral) 250 mg q6h (IM, IV) 500 mg q12h Children: (Oral, IM, IV) 50–100 mg/kg/day in 4 divided doses

IM, Intramuscular; IV, intravenous.

Table 16-3 | *Second-Generation Cephalosporins*

GENERIC NAME	TRADE NAME	DOSAGE
cefaclor, USP, BP	Ceclor	Adults: (Oral) 250 mg q8h Children: (Oral) 20 mg/kg/day in divided doses q8h
cefamandole nafate, USP, BP	Mandol	Adults: (IM, IV) 500 mg–1 gm q4–8h Children: (IM, IV) 50–100 mg/kg/day in divided doses q4–8h
cefotetan disodium, USP, BP	Cefotan	Adults: (IM, IV) 1–2 gm q12h Children: (IM, IV) 40–60 mg/kg/day in 2 divided doses
cefoxitin sodium, USP, BP	Mefoxin	Adults: (IM, IV) 1–2 gm q6–8h Children: (IM, IV) 80–160 mg/kg/day in 4–6 divided doses
cefprozil, USP, BP	Cefzil	Adults: (Oral) 250–500 mg q12h Children 6 mo–12 yr: (Oral) 15 mg/kg q12h
cefuroxime axetil, USP	Ceftin	Adults: (Oral) 250–500 mg twice daily Children: (Oral) 125–250 mg twice daily
cefuroxime sodium, USP	Zinacef	Adults: (IM, IV) 750 mg–1.5 gm q8h Children: (IM, IV) 50–100 mg/kg/day in divided doses

IM, Intramuscular; IV, intravenous.

Table 16-4 | *Third-Generation Cephalosporins*

GENERIC NAME	TRADE NAME	DOSAGE
cefdinir, USP	Omnicef	Adults: (Oral) 600 mg daily, 1 dose or divided Children: (Oral) 14 mg/kg/day, 1 dose or divided
cefixime, USP	Suprax	Adults: (Oral) 400 mg daily in 1 or 2 doses Children: (Oral) 8 mg/kg/day in 1 or 2 doses
cefoperazone sodium, USP	Cefobid	Adults: (IV) 2–4 gm daily in divided doses q12h Children: No dose established
cefotaxime sodium, USP, BP	Claforan	Adults: (IM, IV) 1–2 gm q6–8h Children: (IM, IV) 25–180 mg/kg/day in 4–6 divided doses
cefpodoxime proxetil	Vantin	Adults: (Oral) 100–400 mg q12h Children: (Oral) 10 mg/kg/day in 2 divided doses
ceftazidime sodium, USP, BP	Tazidime, Fortaz, Ceptaz, Tazicef	Adults: (IM, IV) 1 gm q8–12h Children: (IV) 30–50 mg/kg q8h
ceftibuten, USP	Cedax	Adults: (Oral) 400 mg once daily Children: (Oral) 9 mg/kg once daily
ceftizoxime sodium, USP, BP	Cefizox	Adults: (IM, IV) 1–2 gm q8–12h Children: (IM, IV) 50 mg/kg q6–8h
ceftriaxone sodium, USP, BP	Rocephin	Adults: (IM, IV) 1–2 gm/day in 1 or 2 divided doses Children: (IM, IV) 50–75 mg/kg/day in 2 divided doses

IM, Intramuscular; IV, intravenous.

General adverse effects include gastrointestinal irritation; the overgrowth of nonsusceptible organisms, such as yeasts, which may produce diarrhea; a perineal monilial rash; and vaginal infection. The tetracyclines should not be given during pregnancy or to any child younger than 8 years, because the drug concentrates in developing tooth enamel and produces a brown or yellow stain on the teeth. The tetracyclines are described in Table 16–5. All doses given are for adults and children older than 8 years.

THE MACROLIDE ANTIBIOTICS: THE ERYTHROMYCINS

Erythromycin is a macrolide antibiotic, and this class of antibiotics, as it has become more diverse, has become known as the macrolides.

Erythromycin itself is usually only bacteriostatic and exerts its effect only against multiplying organisms. It is a relatively narrow-spectrum antibiotic, effective generally against the same organisms that penicillin affects. It is often used in penicillin-sensitive patients. Although effective par-

enterally, it is generally used orally, primarily for upper and lower respiratory tract infections. It is effective against gram-positive cocci, such as staphylococci and streptococci, and gram-positive bacilli, such as *Bacillus anthracis*, the causative agent of anthrax.

The synthetic agents in this class, such as azithromycin, clarithromycin, and dirithromycin, have expanded spectrums of activity and generally are more potent than erythromycin itself.

General untoward effects include pain and cramping after oral administration, as well as skin reactions. The macrolide antibiotics are listed in Table 16–6.

QUINOLONE ANTIMICROBIAL AGENTS

The **quinolones** are a class of orally effective antimicrobial agents that act by inhibiting the bacterial enzyme DNA gyrase. They are effective against pathogens of the respiratory, urinary, and gastrointestinal tracts and against some organisms that cause sexually transmitted diseases. They may be used in infections resistant to older antibiotics.

Table 16-5 | *Tetracyclines*

GENERIC NAME	TRADE NAME	DOSAGE*
demeclocycline hydrochloride, USP, BP	Declomycin	(Oral) 150 mg q6h
doxycycline hyclate, USP, BP	Vibramycin	(Oral) 100–200 mg initially, then 100 mg 2–3 times daily
minocycline hydrochloride, USP, BP	Minocin	(Oral, IV) 200 mg initially, then 100 mg q12h
oxytetracycline hydrochloride, USP, BP	Terramycin	Same as tetracycline
tetracycline hydrochloride, USP, BP	Achromycin	(Oral) 250–500 mg q6h
		(IM) 100 mg 2–3 times daily
		(IV) 500 mg q12h

*All dosages are for adults and children older than 8 years.

Table 16-6 | *Macrolide Antibiotics: The Erythromycins*

GENERIC NAME	TRADE NAME	DOSAGE
ERYTHROMYCINS		
erythromycin, USP, BP	Ilotycin, Erythrocin	Adults: (Oral) 250–500 mg q6h
		Children: (Oral) 7–25 mg/kg/day in 4 divided doses
erythromycin estolate, USP, BP	Ilosone	Adults: (Oral) 250–500 mg q6h
		Children: (Oral) 30–50 mg/kg/day in 4 divided doses
erythromycin ethylsuccinate, USP, BP	EES, Ery-Ped	Adults: (Oral) 400 mg twice daily
		Children: (Oral) 30–50 mg/kg/day in 2–4 divided doses
erythromycin lactobionate, USP, BP	Erythrocin lactobionate	Adults: (IV) 15–20 mg/kg/day in 4 divided doses
		Children: Same as adults
SYNTHETIC MACROLIDES		
azithromycin, USP, BP	Zithromax	Adults: (Oral, IV) 250–500 mg once daily
		Children: (Oral) 30–50 mg/kg in divided doses over 3 days
		(Oral) A single dose of 30 mg/kg for otitis media
clarithromycin, USP, BP	Biaxin	Adults: (Oral) 250–500 mg once daily
		Children: Not recommended
DERIVATIVE		
dirithromycin, USP	Dynabac	Adults: (Oral) 500 mg once daily
		Children: Not advised under 12 yr

IM, Intramuscular; IV, intravenous.

These agents are analogs of nalidixic acid, USP (covered in Chapter 28, Diuretics and Other Drugs That Affect the Urinary System). They are entirely synthetic, and they act specifically to inhibit DNA synthesis by the microorganism, causing abnormalities that result in death of the microbe.

The quinolones exhibit concentration-dependent bacterial killing. That is, bactericidal activity is more pronounced as the serum drug concentration increases. They are well absorbed orally even in the presence of food. Their slow rate of elimination allows administration every 12 to 24 hours. Because of this slow elimination, the doses may have to be adjusted for patients with renal or hepatic impairment.

Quinolone resistance has significant clinical impact. Mutations may occur rapidly during therapy and may be the most significant factor limiting the use of these antimicrobials.

Side effects are mild with these agents and usually do not cause them to be discontinued. The most common reactions are gastrointestinal (i.e., nausea and vomiting). Rashes, insomnia, irritability, and arthralgia occur less commonly. The quinolones should be administered with caution in patients taking anticoagulants, because in some cases they have prolonged the bleeding time.

The quinolones are listed in Table 16–7.

OTHER ANTIBIOTICS

Other antibiotics in common use for a variety of bacterial infections are listed in Table 16–8.

 Considerations for Children

Antibiotics and Ototoxicity (Auditory Damage)

Many antibiotics, but particularly the aminoglycosides such as gentamicin (Garamycin) and kanamycin (Kantrex), may produce auditory damage as a side effect. They are generally reserved for serious infections caused by gram-negative organisms, and the dosage must be carefully controlled. Hearing testing at an early age is beneficial when these agents have been used in the neonatal period.

SULFONAMIDE DRUGS

The **sulfonamides**, more commonly called "the sulfa drugs," combat infection in the body by checking the growth of bacteria and other microorganisms, thus enabling the body's own defenses to cope with the infection. These are synthetic drugs and are made to resemble **para-aminobenzoic acid (PABA)**, a substance that the microorganisms need

Table 16-7 | *Quinolone Antimicrobials*

GENERIC NAME	TRADE NAME	GENERAL USES	DOSAGE (ADULTS ONLY)
ciprofloxacin hydrochloride, USP	Cipro	Respiratory tract, urinary tract, bone, soft tissue infections	(Oral) 250–500 mg q12h
enoxacin	Penetrex	Sexually transmitted diseases and urinary tract infections	(Oral) 200–400 mg q12h
gatifloxacin	Tequin	Effective against a wide range of gram-positive and gram-negative organisms	(Oral, IV) 200-400 mg once daily
levofloxacin, USP	Levaquin	Sinus, respiratory tract, and soft tissue infections	(Oral or IV) 250–500 mg q24h
lomefloxacin hydrochloride	Maxaquin	Infections of respiratory and urinary tracts	(Oral) 400 mg once daily
moxifloxacin hydrochloride	Avelox	Respiratory tract infections	(Oral) 400 mg once daily
nalidixic acid, USP	NegGram	Urinary tract infections	(Oral) 1 gm 4 times daily
norfloxacin, USP	Noroxin	Urinary tract infections and sexually transmitted diseases	(Oral) 400 mg q12h
ofloxacin	Floxin	Respiratory tract, prostate, and urinary tract infections and sexually transmitted diseases	(Oral) 200–400 mg q12h
sparfloxacin	Zagam	Respiratory tract infections	(Oral) 400 mg on first day, then 200 mg once daily
trovafloxacin	Trovan	Life-threatening illnesses, generally in health care facilities	(Oral, IV) 200–300 mg once daily

IM, Intramuscular; IV, intravenous.

Table 16-8 *Other Antibiotics*

GENERIC NAME	TRADE NAME	USES	TOXIC EFFECTS	DOSAGE
amikacin sulfate, USP	Amikin	Serious infections of bone, soft tissues	Auditory and kidney damage	Adults: (IM, IV) 15 mg/kg/day in divided doses Children: Same as adults
aztreonam	Azactam	Urinary tract and lower respiratory tract infections	Anemia, diarrhea, rash	Adults (IM or IV) 500 mg–1 gm q8–12h Children: (IM or IV) up to 120 mg/kg/day in divided doses
chloramphenicol, USP, BP	Chloromycetin	Meningitis, typhoid fever	Bone marrow depression	Adults: (Oral, IV) 12.5 mg/kg 4 times daily Children: (Oral, IV) 6 mg/kg 4 times daily
clindamycin hydrochloride, USP, BP	Cleocin	Infections of respiratory tract, soft tissues	Leukopenia, vomiting, diarrhea, skin rash	Adults: (Oral) 150–300 mg twice daily (IM, IV) 600 mg q6h Children: (Oral, IM, IV) 10–40 mg/kg/day in divided doses
colistimethate sodium, USP, BP	Coly-Mycin M	Infections of urinary tract, soft tissues	Kidney damage	Adults: (Oral) 3–5 mg/kg/day in 3 divided doses
colistin sulfate, USP, BP	Coly-Mycin S	Same as Coly-Mycin M	Same as Coly-Mycin M	Adults: (IM, IV) 1.5–5.0 mg/kg/day in 2–4 divided doses (Intrathecal) 5–15 mg every other day Children: Same as adults
ethambutol hydrochloride, USP, BP	Myambutol	Tuberculosis	Optic neuritis, rash, mental changes	Adults: (Oral) 10–15 mg/kg/day Children: Same as adults
gentamicin sulfate, USP, BP	Garamycin	Serious infections of soft tissue, GU tract, respiratory tract	Auditory and kidney damage	Adults: (IM, IV) 1–2 mg/kg/day in 2–3 divided doses Children: Same as adults
imipenem and cilastatin sodium	Primaxin, ADD-Vantage	Serious infections of abdomen, respiratory tract, bone, kidneys	GI effects, seizures, bone marrow suppression	Adults: (IV) Up to 50 mg/kg/day Children: (IV) 15–25 mg/kg q6h
isoniazid, USP, BP	INH, Nydrazid	Tuberculosis	Neuritis, liver dysfunction	Adults: (Oral) 5–10 mg/kg/day Children: (Oral) 10–20 mg/kg/day
kanamycin sulfate, USP, BP	Kantrex	Infections of bone, GU tract, respiratory tract, soft tissues	Auditory damage	Adults: (Oral) 1 gm 3–4 times daily (IM, IV) 7.5 mg/kg twice daily Children: (Oral) 12.5 mg/kg 4 times daily (IM, IV) 3–7.5 mg/kg twice daily

Generic name	Trade name	Uses	Adverse reactions	Dosage
lincomycin hydrochloride, USP, BP	Lincocin	Infections of soft tissue, bone, respiratory tract	Vomiting, diarrhea, skin rashes	Adults: (Oral) 500 mg 3 times daily (IM, IV) 600 mg q12h; Children: (Oral) 30–60 mg/kg/day in 3–4 divided doses (IM, IV) 10–20 mg/kg/day in 2–3 divided doses
loracarbef, USP	Lorabid	Respiratory tract infection	Diarrhea, skin rash	Adults: (Oral) 200–400 mg q12h; Children: (Oral) 7.5 mg/kg q12h
metronidazole, USP, BP	Flagyl	Trichomoniasis	Metallic taste, giardiasis, amebiasis, diarrhea, intolerance to alcohol, rash	Adults: (Oral) Single dose of 2 gm or 250 mg 3 times daily for 7 days; Children: (Oral) 15 mg/kg/day
polymyxin B sulfate, USP, BP	Aerosporin	Serious infections of soft tissue or urinary tract	Neurologic and kidney damage	Adults: (IM) 6250–7500 units/kg 4 times daily (IV) 7500–12,500 units/kg twice daily (Intrathecal) 50,000 units once daily; Children: Same as adults
pyrazinamide, USP, BP	—	Tuberculosis	Liver toxicity, rash	Adults: (Oral) 20–35 mg/kg/day; Children: (Oral) 15–30 mg/kg/day
rifampin, USP, BP	Rifadin, Rifamate	Tuberculosis, carriers of meningitis organisms	Diarrhea, anemia, liver and kidney toxicity	Adults: (Oral) 600 mg/day; Children: (Oral) 10–15 mg/kg/day
spectinomycin hydrochloride, USP, BP	Trobicin	Gonorrhea	Chills, fever, nausea, dizziness, kidney damage	Adults only: (IM) 4 gm as a single injection
streptomycin sulfate, USP, BP	Streptomycin	Tuberculosis	Auditory damage	Adults: (IM) 0.5–1.0 gm 4 times daily; Children: (IM) 10 mg/kg 2–4 times daily
tobramycin sulfate, USP, BP	Nebcin	Serious infections of bone, soft tissue, respiratory tract	Auditory and kidney damage	Adults: (IM, IV) 1 mg/kg q8h; Children: Same as adults
troleandomycin, USP, BP	Tao	Respiratory, GI, GU tract infections	Liver damage	Adults: (Oral) 250 mg q4–6h (IM) 200 mg q6h (IV) 1–2 gm/day in divided doses; Children: (Oral IM, IV) 30–50 mg/kg/day in 2–4 divided doses
vancomycin hydrochloride, USP, BP	Vancocin	Severe septicemia, meningitis	Nausea, thrombophlebitis at IV site, skin rashes	Adults: (IV) 1 gm q12h; Children: (IV) 5–10 mg/kg 4 times daily

GI, Gastrointestinal; GU, genitourinary; IM, intramuscular; IV, intravenous.

for the synthesis of folic acid, an essential enzyme. The microorganism takes in the sulfa drug but cannot use it to make folic acid; thus it is prevented from growing and multiplying.

The sulfa drugs are less effective in the presence of a large amount of PABA because the microorganisms prefer PABA to the drug. For this reason the patient must not be taking medications containing PABA (e.g., Pabalate, an agent used for rheumatic conditions) when taking sulfa drugs.

These drugs are usually administered by mouth, the method of choice from the standpoint of convenience and because they are well absorbed from the intestinal tract.

There has been concern over the increasing frequency of bacterial resistance to the sulfonamides. In addition, the development of newer and more effective agents has sharply limited the usefulness of sulfonamides in many instances. The use of sulfonamides is recommended for the following conditions only:

1. Chancroid
2. Trachoma
3. Inclusion conjunctivitis
4. Nocardiosis
5. Uncomplicated urinary tract infections caused by susceptible organisms
6. Toxoplasmosis
7. Malaria, as adjunctive therapy in some cases
8. *Haemophilus influenzae* infections of the middle ear

Although sulfa drugs obviously aid in controlling infections, they now have been largely replaced by the antibiotics, which have faster action and fewer side effects.

It is important that a patient taking sulfa drugs maintain an adequate fluid intake. Sulfonamides have a tendency to crystallize in the urine and be deposited in the kidneys, resulting in a painful and dangerous condition. The chances of crystallization in the urine are minimized if the urine is kept dilute by a high fluid intake.

Sulfa drugs used today produce fewer symptoms of toxicity than the older compounds. However, toxic reactions may result from the use of any drugs that are absorbed and exert systemic effects. In this case toxic reactions include nausea, vomiting, cyanosis, drug fever (often confused with a recurrent fever from the infection), rash, acidosis, jaundice, blood complications, and kidney damage. In a few cases, Stevens-Johnson syndrome, which may be fatal, has occurred.

The general treatment of the toxic symptoms includes discontinuing the drug and forcing fluids. The severity of the symptoms determines whether the drug is permanently discontinued. The high incidence of toxicity associated with the sulfonamides explains why they have been largely supplanted by the antibiotics.

Drug interactions have occurred with the anticoagulants, such as coumarin. The effect of coumarin may be potentiated. The sulfonamides may also potentiate the hypoglycemic effects of the oral antidiabetic agents. Interference with the absorption/metabolism of digoxin and phenytoin has been described.

sulfamethizole combination (Urobiotic). Urobiotic is a combination of the following in each capsule:

    250 mg sulfamethizole
    250 mg oxytetracycline
    50 mg phenazopyridine

The combination is an effective remedy for urinary tract infections.

    Dosage:
        Adults only: (Oral) 1 to 2 capsules four times a day.

LONG-ACTING SULFONAMIDES

Because most of the sulfonamides are excreted fairly rapidly, until recently it has been necessary to give relatively high doses at short intervals to maintain an effective blood level of the drug. The use of the long-acting sulfonamides, however, permits lower doses to be given, because the drug remains in effective concentrations for a longer time in the blood. Often only one dose is needed daily to maintain effective blood levels. Because a lower dose may be used, side effects occur less frequently than with other sulfa drugs.

sulfasalazine, USP, BP (Azulfidine). Sulfasalazine is used orally in the treatment of ulcerative colitis and Crohn's disease. It is often used in conjunction with corticosteroid therapy.

    Dosage:
        Adults: (Oral) 2 to 4 gm daily in divided doses.
        Children: (Oral) 40 to 60 mg/kg/day in three to six divided doses.

co-trimoxazole (trimethoprim and sulfamethoxazole), USP, BP (Bactrim, Septra, Bactrim DS, Septra DS). This combination of agents blocks two successive steps in bacterial growth and has become one of the more successful antibacterial agents in the sulfonamide groups.

The regular strength of the two brands of this combination contains 80 mg of trimethoprim and 400 mg of sulfamethoxazole. The "DS" form noted for both of these signifies the double strength of the tablet. The suspension contains 40 mg of trimethoprim and 200 mg of sulfamethoxazole per teaspoonful.

In addition to considerable effectiveness in the treatment of urinary tract infections, this combination is now used successfully in the treatment of acute otitis media, particularly when routine antibiotic therapy has been ineffective. It should not be used in the treatment of streptococcal pharyngitis, because it has been shown to have little effect.

    Dosage:
        Adults: (Oral) Regular strength, 1 to 2 tablets every 12 hours; double strength, 1 tablet every 12 hours.
        Children: (Oral) 8 mg/kg of trimethoprim and 40 mg/kg of sulfamethoxazole per 24 hours in two divided doses.

ALLERGIC REACTIONS TO SULFONAMIDES AND CROSS-REACTION ALLERGIES WITH OTHER MEDICATIONS

Particularly common among the allergic reactions to sulfonamides is an extensive bright red, pruritic rash, which may occur in 3% of persons prescribed sulfonamides. Also, there is an association between hypersensitivity reactions that may develop after taking a sulfonamide and a subsequent allergic reaction after taking a drug with a similar sulfanilamide base. Cross-reaction with the related drugs then is extremely common. Of particular note are the number of thiazide diuretics and antidiabetic agents that may react with sulfonamides (Box 16–1).

ANTIFUNGAL AGENTS

Fungi are members of the plant family that are able to survive only as parasites because they contain no chlorophyll for self-nourishment. Fungal infections of humans can be as simple as tinea pedis (athlete's foot), tinea corporis (fungal rashes on the skin), or thrush (a superficial infection of the mouth often seen in infants).

When the immune system is impaired, fungal infections can become overwhelming and life threatening. Acquired immunodeficiency syndrome (AIDS) and AIDS-related complex (ARC) are both caused by the human immunodeficiency virus (HIV), and because of their severely compromised immune system, patients with these conditions are often subject to severe and life-threatening fungal infections. Cryptococcal meningitis, severe oropharyngeal candidiasis, and esophageal candidiasis can occur in these patients. Intravenous forms of the antifungal agents are generally used to treat these conditions (Table 16–9).

Box 16-1 *Related Drugs That May Cross-react with Sulfonamides*

acetazolamide	glipazide
acetohexamide	glyburide
bendroflumethiazide	hydrochlorothiazide
benzthiazide	hydroflumethiazide
bumetanide	indapamide
chlorothiazide	methyclothiazide
chlorpropamide	metolazone
chlorthalidone	piretanide
clopamide	polythiazide
cyclopenthiazide	probenecid
dapsone	quinethazone
diazoxide	sulfasalazine
dichlorphenamide	tolazamide
furosemide	tolbutamide
gliclazide	torsemide
glimepiride	

ANTIVIRAL AGENTS

A **virus** is a microscopic infectious agent that requires an intact living host cell for metabolism; when it enters this host cell, the virus is able to reproduce and mutate. Using the host cell's metabolic processes, viruses can direct the synthesis of hundreds to thousands of progeny viruses (viral copies) during a single cycle of infection. When the discovery of antibiotics began a revolution in the ability to treat bacterial infections, it was anticipated that similarly effective antiviral agents would soon be identified as well. A major problem in the development of antiviral agents has been the more intimate relationship between viral and host metabolic activities. It is this relationship that makes it nearly impossible to develop a drug to effectively kill the virus in a person's body without also causing great harm to the body's existing cells. The search for selective inhibitors of viral activity that are not too toxic to the human host has been much more difficult than first appreciated.

The primary uses of the available antiviral agents are in the treatment of influenza, hepatitis, herpesvirus infections, and AIDS. Antiviral agents commonly used for these infections are discussed below; additional antiviral agents are listed in Table 16–10.

ANTIVIRALS USED IN THE TREATMENT OF INFLUENZA

When oseltamivir (Tamiflu) and zanamivir (Relenza) (see Table 16-10) are used for the treatment of acute influenza, they have been shown to reduce the duration of the symptoms of influenza, although only by a few days. In general, the elderly and the very young are at the greatest risk from serious complications of the flu, thus these suppressants may be considered for therapy in these groups especially. They were shown not to have any prophylactic effects in preventing infection with the influenza virus.

ANTIVIRALS USED IN THE TREATMENT OF HEPATITIS AND HERPES VIRUSES

Hepatitis Viruses

Hepatitis A. This hepatitis virus is generally a short-lived virus and is not treated with antiviral agents.

Hepatitis B. Hepatitis B virus affects 5% of the worldwide population and may lead to cirrhosis and hepatocellular carcinoma. It is considered to be chronic when the surface antigen persists for more than 6 months. The chronic condition is generally treated with the following drugs.

Other forms of hepatitis up to hepatitis G are now identified but are less common than A and B.

interferon alfa-2b (Intron A). Interferon alfa, a synthetic version of the naturally occurring interferon-alpha, is composed of a family of proteins that possess antiviral, antineoplastic, and immunomodulating properties. Studies in hepatitis B patients have shown that virologic remission can occur, in which case tests for the hepatitis B surface antigen, which indicates active infection, will no longer be positive.

Table 16-9 *Antifungal Agents*

GENERIC NAME	TRADE NAME	USES	DOSAGE
amphotericin B, USP, BP	Fungizone	Serious systemic fungal infections	Adults: (IV) 0.25 mg/kg in diluted infusion every 2–4 days Children: (IV) 0.1 mg/kg in diluted infusion every 2–4 days
fluconazole	Diflucan	Vaginal candidiasis	Adults: (Oral, IV) 50–100 mg/day Children: No dose established
flucytosine, USP, BP	Ancobon	Serious systemic infections	Adults: (Oral) 50–150 mg/kg day in 4 divided doses Children: Same as adults
griseofulvin, USP, BP	Fulvicin, Grifulvin, Grisactin	Superficial fungal infections	Adults: (Oral) 250–500 mg/day Children: (Oral) 3.3 mg/kg 3 times daily
itraconazole	Sporanox	Systemic fungal infection in the immunocompromised patients	Adults: (Oral) 200 mg 2–3 times daily (IV) 200 mg 1–2 times daily Children: Not established
ketoconazole USP, BP	Nizoral	Serious systemic infections	Adults: (Oral) 200–400 mg/day as a single dose Children: (Oral) 3.3–6.6 mg/kg/day, single dose
miconazole, USP, BP	Monistat	Vaginally and topically for yeast infections Systemically for major infections	Adults: (IV) 1.2–3.6 gm/day in divided doses (Vaginal or topical) 2%-4% cream Children: (IV) 20–40 mg/day in divided doses
nystatin, USP, BP	Mycostatin	Orally for moniliasis Topically and vaginally for skin monilia	Adults: (Oral) 500,000–1,000,000 units 3 times daily (Vaginal) 100,000-unit suppository 3 times daily Children: (Oral) 100,000–200,000 units 4 times daily
terbinafine hydrochloride, USP	Lamisil	Orally for toenail and fingernail fungal infections	Adults: (Oral) 250 mg daily Children: Not recommended under age 18 yr

IV, Intravenous.

Infrequently thyroid abnormalities will occur during treatment, thus the thyroid should be evaluated before the start of therapy.

> **Dosage:**
> Adult: (subQ or IM) 30 million to 35 million International Units per week

lamivudine (Epivir, Epivir-HBV). This synthetic nucleoside analog has activity against the hepatitis B virus as well as the AIDS virus. Clinical exacerbations of hepatitis B have occurred after the drug is discontinued, as demonstrated by an increased level of alanine aminotransferase (ALT).

> **Dosage:**
> Adult: (Oral) 100 mg once daily.
> Children 2 to 17 years: (Oral) 3 mg/kg once daily.

Hepatitis C. Hepatitis C virus is the most frequent cause of end-stage liver disease in the United States, and the leading indicator for liver transplant. Treatment is indicated in patients with a detectable hepatitis C RNA viral load and a persistently elevated ALT. Nearly 85% of infected persons develop chronic hepatitis. Treatment is with the following agents.

peg-interferon (PEG-Intron). This agent is a conjugate of recombinant alfa-2b interferon. It binds to cell receptors and initiates intracellular events such as induction of certain enzymes, and suppression of cell proliferation.

> **Dosage:**
> Adult: (subQ) 1.5 mcg/kg once weekly.

ribavirin (Rebetol). This agent is not effective for the treatment of hepatitis C when used alone, but is a useful adjunct when used with peg-interferon.

> **Dosage:**
> Adult: (Oral) 600 mg twice daily.

Rebetron. This is a combination therapy product containing ribavirin capsules and interferon alfa-2b injection.

> **The dosages are as noted for the two separate drugs above.**

Herpes Viruses

Herpes viruses are DNA viruses that can lie dormant in sensory neurons after initial infection, then later reactivate and cause disease. Viruses in this family are the herpes simplex virus (HSV) and the varicella-zoster virus (VZV).

Table 16-10 *Antiviral Agents*

GENERIC NAME	TRADE NAME	USES	DOSAGE
acyclovir sodium, USP	Zovirax	Herpes simplex infections, oral or genital varicella-zoster (shingles), varicella (chickenpox) in immunocompromised patients	Adults: (Oral) 200–800 mg q4h 5 times daily (IV) 5 mg/kg Children: (IV) 5–15 mg/kg q8h (Oral) 20 mg/kg 4 times daily
amantadine hydrochloride, USP, BP	Symmetrel	Prevention and treatment of influenza A infections	Adults: (Oral) 100–200 mg/day Children: (Oral) 4.4–8.8 mg/kg/day in 1–2 doses
cidofovir didanosine (ddI), USP	Vistide, Videx	Cytomegalovirus; retinitis in AIDS Advanced HIV infection	Adults only: (Oral) 5 mg/kg weekly Adults: (Oral) 125–250 mg twice daily
famciclovir	Famvir	Herpes zoster; genital herpes	Adults only: (Oral) 500 mg 3 times daily
foscarnet sodium, USP	Foscavir	Cytomegalovirus retinitis Herpes simplex and varicella zoster	Adults: (IV) 60 mg/kg q8h for 14–21 days Adults: (IV) 40 mg/kg q8h
ganciclovir sodium, USP	Cytovene	Cytomegalovirus, retinitis in immunocompromised patients	Adults: (IV) 5 mg/kg q12h Children: Same as adults
oseltamivir	Tamiflu	Influenza A and B	Adults only: (Oral) 75 mg twice daily
palivizumab	Synagis	Respiratory syncytial virus	Adults: NA Children: (IM) 15 mg/kg once a month
ribavirin, USP	Virazole	Respiratory syncytial virus infections, adenovirus pneumonia, chronic hepatitis C	Adults: (Nasal) Aerosol mist containing 190 mg/L for 12–18 hr/day for 3–7 days Children: Same as adults
rimantadine hydrochloride, USP	Flumadine	Influenza A prophylaxis	Adults: 100 mg orally twice daily for up to 6 wk Children: 5 mg/kg/day up to 150 mg/day maximum for under age 10 yr
trifluridine, USP	Viroptic	Herpes simplex conjunctivitis, keratitis of eye	Adults: (Topical) 1% solution applied to eye for 7–14 days Children: Same as adults
valacyclovir hydrochloride	Valtrex	Herpes zoster	Adults only: (Oral) 1 gm twice daily
vidarabine, USP, BP	Vira-A	IV: herpes simplex encephalitis, neonatal herpes infections, varicella in immunocompromised patients, herpes zoster Topically to eyes for herpes simplex keratitis	Adults: (IV) 15 mg/kg/day for 5–10 days Children: Same as adults Adults: (Topical) 3% ointment applied 5 times a day Children: Same as adults
zanamivir	Relenza	Influenza A and B	Adults only: (Oral inhalation) 2 inhalations (10 mg) twice daily

AIDS, Acquired immunodeficiency syndrome; ARC, AIDS-related complex; HIV, human immunodeficiency virus; IV, intravenous.

Agents used to treat these viruses may be oral or topical.

Oral agents are:

Acyclovir (Zovirax)—see Table 16–10

Famciclovir (Famvir)—see Table 16–10

Valacyclovir (Valtrex)—see Table 16–10

Topical agents are:

Acyclovir (Zovirax). For genital herpes infection.

Dosage:

Adult: (Topical) Apply six times daily for 7 days.

Penciclovir (Denavir). For orolabial herpes.

Dosage:

(Topical) Apply every 2 hours while awake for 4 days.

Docosanol (Abreva). For orolabial herpes.

Dosage:

(Topical) Apply five times daily until healed.

ANTIVIRALS USED IN THE TREATMENT OF AIDS

The explosion of AIDS since its identification in the early 1970s has generated much research into antivirals that would be effective against this disease. AIDS is caused by HIV, a virus of the family Retroviridae. It is a ribonucleic acid (RNA) virus and has two strands of RNA as its genetic material. It is called a retrovirus because it converts genetic information "backward" from RNA to DNA. (Information generally goes from DNA to RNA. The twisted strand of DNA "unzips" itself to allow the RNA within to be copied.)

HIV fuses with a host cell's membrane and then enters the cytoplasm of the cell. Packaged within the AIDS virus is a DNA polymerase called reverse transcriptase, which transcribes single-stranded viral RNA into numerous copies of single strands of viral DNA, and then combines these into double-stranded viral DNA. The viral DNA is then transcribed in the normal way to form viral RNA. Some of these RNA copies are used to make new HIV virus, which is assembled near the surface of the host cell in a process that involves the action of the enzyme protease.

Drug development for AIDS treatment has concentrated on drugs that will interfere with the activity of the viral RNA, primarily at the point of fusion with the host cell, during the process of reverse transcription, or at the point of action of protease on the new virus. These drugs are usually given to patients in combinations because of the high likelihood that the virus will develop resistance to any one of them. This happens because HIV reverse transcriptase is prone to making errors during transcription of viral RNA into viral DNA, which can allow HIV to mutate to a drug-resistant form.

Two mechanisms are available to determine the progression of AIDS and the need to treat or to change drugs if the treatment is becoming less effective:

- *Viral load.* This is directly measured at the HIV RNA level in units indicating the number of viral copies per microliter. At a viral count of over 30,000/microliter, therapy is recommended. The goal is an undetectable viral load, or at least one under 5000 copies per microliter.
- *CD4 cell count.* CD4 cells are the subpopulation of lymphocytes referred to as the helper T cells (T4 cells). The severity of the CD4 count reduction corresponds to the severity of the AIDS disease progression. The CD4 cell count in unaffected individuals should be significantly greater than 400 cells/mL. At this time, treatment is recommended when the CD4 count falls below 350 cells/mL.

Three major categories of antiviral drugs are used in the treatment of AIDS: nucleoside reverse transcriptase inhibitors (NRTIs), nonnucleoside reverse transcriptase inhibitors (NNRTIs), and protease inhibitors. A fourth category, the fusion inhibitors, is used less often. Dosages given below are for adults only.

Nucleoside Reverse Transcriptase Inhibitors

The NRTIs exert their antiviral activity by intracellular conversion of the drug to a triphosphate metabolite. These triple-phosphated metabolites are analogs of one of the four essential components of the DNA molecule (adenine, thymine, guanine, or cytosine), and thus can fit into a DNA molecule that is being assembled. The analog slips into the viral DNA molecule during its construction and interferes with the viral RNA–directed DNA polymerase (i.e., reverse transcriptase) activity, causing the assembly of the viral DNA molecule to stop prematurely.

zidovudine (Retrovir). Zidovudine triphosphate competes with thymidine triphosphate for incorporation into the viral DNA. DNA synthesis is then prematurely terminated. Side effects include nausea and vomiting; generally there are no hematologic effects.

Dosage:

(Oral) 600 mg daily in two to three divided doses.

didanosine (Videx). Didanosine triphosphate competes with adenosine triphosphate for incorporation into the viral DNA. Antacids increase the bioavailability of this drug by preventing its breakdown in the acid pH of the stomach. Didanosine has been associated with fatal pancreatitis; thus the patient must be observed for abdominal symptoms. Patients need frequent eye examinations to assess for optic neuritis or retinal changes. This drug also has been associated with peripheral neuropathy and renal impairment.

Dosage:

(Oral) 200 mg once daily.

zalcitabine (Hivid). Zalcitabine competes with deoxycytidine triphosphate. Side effects include peripheral neuropathy, oral and esophageal ulcers, and leukopenia.

Dosage:

(Oral) 0.75 mg (750 mcg) every 8 hours.

stavudine (Zerit)

Dosage:

(Oral) 20 mg every 12 hours.

lamivudine (Epivir)

Dosage:

(Oral) 150 mg once daily.

abacavir (Ziagen)

Dosage:

(Oral) 300 mg twice daily.

Nonnucleoside Reverse Transcriptase Inhibitors

The NNRTIs interfere with the AIDS virus by binding directly to the viral reverse transcriptase and thus act as specific reverse transcriptase inhibitors. Unlike the NRTIs, they do not require conversion to a metabolite.

nevirapine (Viramune). Nevirapine is active against HIV type 1 but not HIV type 2. Resistance develops quickly unless it is used with other antiviral agents. Side effects include severe skin reactions (Stevens-Johnson syndrome type of bullous lesions) and hepatotoxicity.

Dosage:
(Oral) 200 mg once daily.

delavirdine mesylate (Rescriptor). Although delavirdine is active against HIV type 1, as with nevirapine, resistance develops quickly, so it should be used with other agents to diminish resistance. Delavirdine is ineffective against type 2 viruses. It should be taken with an acidic beverage (e.g., orange juice) to enhance absorption. Rash is the major side effect.

Dosage:
(Oral) 400 mg every 8 hours.

efavirenz (Sustiva). Efavirenz is also effective only against type 1 HIV, and should be used with other agents to diminish resistance. Side effects include central nervous system effects, abnormal dreams, vertigo, delusions, rash, nausea, and liver toxicity.

Dosage:
(Oral) 600 mg once daily.

Protease Inhibitors

These drugs directly interfere with viral protease, which plays an essential role in the replication cycle of HIV and the formation of infectious virus. The protease inhibitors act at a different stage of the HIV replication cycle than do the NRTIs or NNRTIs and may be used alone or in combination with other agents. Cross-resistance forms between drugs within this class.

saquinavir (Fortovase, Invirase). Saquinavir is active against both type 1 and type 2 HIV. Its absorption is decreased by 45% if taken with food; it should not be used alone because of resistance. Peripheral neuropathy occurs in up to 50% of the patients; hepatotoxicity and pancreatitis also may occur.

Dosage:
(Oral) 40 mg every 12 hours.

ritonavir (Norvir). This agent works against both type 1 and type 2 HIV. Side effects include nausea, vomiting, diarrhea, taste perversion, and peripheral paresthesias.

Dosage:
(Oral) 600 mg every 12 hours.

indinavir sulfate (Crixivan). Indinavir works against both type 1 and type 2 HIV. Side effects include nausea, vomiting, hyperbilirubinemia, skin rash, and anaphylaxis.

Dosage:
(Oral) 800 mg every 8 hours.

nelfinavir mesylate (Viracept). Nelfinavir is active against both types 1 and 2 HIV. Side effects include diarrhea, skin rashes, and new-onset diabetes.

Dosage:
(Oral) 750 mg three times daily.

amprenavir (Agenerase). This agent is active against both types 1 and 2 HIV. Persons taking this drug should not take supplemental vitamin E because each capsule already contains 109 units of vitamin E. The daily dosage may be as many as 16 capsules. Side effects include nausea, vomiting, skin rash, paresthesias, and new-onset diabetes.

Dosage:
(Oral) available in 150-mg capsules; dosage is up to 1200 mg (8 capsules) twice daily.

Fusion Inhibitors

The fusion inhibitor class of antiretroviral drugs is mainly used when the available combination antiretroviral regimens are no longer effective because of the development of viral resistance. These agents prevent the fusion of the HIV type 1 transmembrane glycoprotein with the CD4 receptor of the host cell. The fusion inhibitors can work synergistically with the other classes of AIDS drugs. Only one agent in this class is approved for use.

enfuvirtide (Fuzeon). This agent is useful when the patient has become resistant to the more standard combinations of AIDS drugs. However, it must be administered subcutaneously (subQ).

Dosage:
Adults: (subQ) 90 mg twice daily.
Children older than 6 years: (subQ) 2 mg/kg twice daily.

ANTIPARASITIC AGENTS

A number of parasites, including the helminths (worms), are able to invade the human body. The tropical parasites are not covered in this text.

ANTHELMINTIC DRUGS

Worm infestations appear throughout the world but are particularly prominent in the warmer climates. Cultural hygienic practices are important in the prevention of worm infestations, because in every case they are spread by a feces-to-mouth route. Day care centers, where the diaper changer is also the food handler, have been important sources for the spread of worms and other parasites.

albendazole, USP (Albenza). Albendazole is used for the treatment of active central nervous system lesions caused by

Herb Alert

Goldenseal

Goldenseal has shown some clinical effectiveness in the treatment of bacterial infections, notably infections with *Salmonella*, *Shigella*, and *Klebsiella* species, as well as in vitro activity against intestinal parasites such as *Giardia lamblia*, *Trichomonas*, and *Entamoeba histolytica*. It has been used in the past for the treatment of eye infections, notably trachoma. Prolonged use can cause digestive disorders, including constipation, as well as mucous membrane irritation and occasionally hallucinations. It reduces the anticoagulant activity of heparin and enhances the effect of antihypertensives and sedatives. Avoid the use of goldenseal in patients with glucose-6-phosphate dehydrogenase (G-6-PD) deficiency. See Chapter 35 for more information on goldenseal.

---

the larval form of *Taenia solium* (pork tapeworm), generally in combination with corticosteroids. In addition, it is used for cystic hydatid disease involving lesions in the lung, liver, and peritoneum caused by the larval form of the dog tapeworm.

> **Dosage:**
> Adults: (Oral) 400 mg twice daily for 8 to 30 days.
> Children: (Oral) 15 mg/kg divided in two doses for 8 to 30 days.

mebendazole, USP, BP (Vermox). This agent is used in the treatment of roundworm, hookworm, threadworm, pinworm, and many tropical parasites.

> **Dosage:**
> Adults and children: (Oral) One 100-mg tablet twice daily for 3 days.

piperazine citrate, USP. This agent is used to treat roundworm (*Ascaris*) and pinworm infestations.

> **Dosage:**
> Adults and children: (Oral) 65 mg/kg for 7 days.

praziquantel (Biltricide). Praziquantel has been shown to be active against many tapeworms pathogenic to humans, including fish tapeworm, dog and cat tapeworms, and beef and pork tapeworms. It is also active against all *Schistosoma* species. Generally treatment is for 1 day only.

> **Dosage:**
> Adults and children: (Oral) 60 to 75 mg/kg/day in three divided doses.

thiabendazole, USP, BP (Mintezol). This agent is used for cutaneous larva migrans (creeping eruption) and threadworm infestations.

> **Dosage:**
> Adults and children: (Oral) 25 mg/kg twice daily for 2 days. A 10% suspension of the drug may be

applied topically to cutaneous larva migrans as well.

MEDICATION FOR LICE AND SCABIES

Lice and scabies occur indiscriminately among all socioeconomic groups. Outbreaks of head lice in school systems create a public health challenge, particularly in the fall. It is often not possible to see the lice themselves, but the infestation is characterized by pruritus and the presence of nits, which are the small, silver eggs attached to the hair shaft.

Scabies is caused by a mite that burrows under the skin and causes intense body pruritus. It is often spread by shaking hands, because the thin skin between the fingers is a typical spot for infestation.

lindane, USP, BP (Kwell). This agent may be used as a shampoo for head lice or as an application to the entire body for scabies. Because of the possibility of neurotoxic effects, this prescription product should not be used unless the other over-the-counter agents have failed.

> **Dosage:**
> Adults and children: (Topical) 1% solution applied to the body or scalp once. Treatment may be repeated one more time in a week, if necessary.

permethrin cream rinse (Nix). This product is recommended as a single-dose treatment for head lice.

> **Dosage:**
> Adults and children: (Topical) After the hair has been washed, rinsed, and towel dried, the cream rinse is applied and left on the hair for 10 minutes.

permethrin topical cream (Acticin, Elimite). When applied as a skin cream, this agent is effective against scabies. It should be applied evenly to all skin surfaces and left on for 8 to 14 hours, then washed off thoroughly.

> **Dosage:**
> Adults and children: (Topical) One application of the cream; may be repeated in 2 weeks if necessary.

pyrethrins with piperonyl butoxide (R & C Lice Treatment, Blue Gel, Tisit Liquid, Licide). When used in combination, these agents are very effective as a topical treatment for head lice and pubic lice. They are supplied as a solution, shampoo, or gel containing 0.17% to 0.33% pyrethrins.

> **Dosage:**
> Adults and children: (Topical) Apply to affected body surface once, wash off after 10 minutes. May be repeated in 7 to 10 days if necessary.

CLINICAL IMPLICATIONS

1. All injectable antibiotics should be carefully checked for the expiration date before administration.
2. The patient should be carefully questioned concerning previous allergic reactions to antibiotics.
3. After administration, the patient should be checked for possible untoward effects, such as a skin rash, respiratory distress, or other allergic responses.
4. Become familiar with the special tags placed on patients' charts noting drug allergies.
5. Remember to check for MedicAlert tags that an unresponsive patient may be wearing.
6. The nurse should be aware of cross sensitivity reactions of the antibiotics, such as those between penicillin and the cephalosporins.
7. Patients should be carefully instructed to take their entire supply of antibiotics to prevent the development of resistant strains of bacteria.
8. Old antibiotic prescriptions should be discarded if they are not finished, because antibiotics quickly become outdated.
9. Aseptic technique is still the most effective way to prevent infection. Antibiotics must not be relied on to remedy infections caused by disregard for asepsis.
10. Many antibiotics are irritating when given by injection. Intramuscular injections should be given deeply in large muscles.
11. Resolution of fever is a sign used to check the early effectiveness of an antibiotic against an infection.
12. The student should be aware of possible side effects of the antibiotic agents.
13. Superinfection by organisms not susceptible to antibiotics is a common sequela to antibiotic therapy. Superinfections may occur as a rash, commonly *Monilia* in the oral or genital region, or as diarrhea.
14. Good nutrition, adequate rest, and general cleanliness are important to the overall well-being of a patient recovering from an infection.
15. Instruct patients in the importance of hygiene in preventing the spread of parasites. Short fingernails that are kept very clean, good hand-washing techniques, and the avoidance of "mouthing" of objects, such as pencils, and nail biting should be stressed.
16. Become familiar with steps used to prevent head lice cross infection. Combs, brushes, and other toilet articles should not be shared. Outer garments hung in cloakrooms can spread the infestation from garment to garment.
17. Stools should be inspected for the presence of worms. Transmission of infestations by toilet seats and bedpans should be considered and avoided.
18. Superinfections with fungal and bacterial agents are common in immunocompromised patients. These patients should be observed carefully and instructed to report changes in skin, mucous membranes, or bowel habits.
19. Infections such as chickenpox and common colds can have life-threatening implications for the immunocompromised patient. The patient and the family should be instructed to avoid infected persons.
20. The urine should remain acid for optimum effectiveness of the sulfonamides. Prunes and cranberries in any form promote an acid urine. The patient should be encouraged to drink plenty of fluids while taking sulfonamides.
21. Sulfonamides produce frequent allergic reactions, most notably a pruritic, bright red skin rash, and occasionally a drug fever.
22. Patients should be carefully questioned about former drug allergic reactions whenever they begin taking a new drug. Agents that commonly cross-react with sulfa drugs include the thiazide diuretics and antidiabetic agents.

Online Resources

For updated drug information and Web activities, go to http://evolve.elsevier.com/Asperheim.

CRITICAL THINKING QUESTIONS

1. The patient was referred by his family doctor to a local ear, nose, and throat specialist for his hearing deficit. The physician took the following case history: The patient had been well until age 35 years, when he had suffered a severe case of lobar pneumonia that did not resolve on appropriate penicillin therapy. Further studies showed that he had tuberculosis, and he was treated effectively in a sanitarium. What further inquiries might be made as to the cause of his deafness?

2. The patient was treated for recurrent and persistent sinusitis with tetracycline and the decongestant Ornade. On the eighth day of medication her condition improved, but she presented with complaints of diarrhea and abdominal gripping discomfort. What recommendations should be made?

3. A mother brought her 2-month-old infant in for a routine well-baby examination. The infant's height and weight had increased normally. The baby appeared healthy except for a yellowish-white plaque that covered most of her tongue, and a few spots that were noted on the buccal mucous membranes. What is this? How is it treated? Is it serious?

CRITICAL THINKING QUESTIONS—cont'd

4. A patient, age 3 years, was placed on ampicillin 3 days ago for otitis media. Today his mother called to report that she noted a pale-pink flat rash on his chest when she bathed him. The rash did not appear to itch. She also reported that his fever was gone now, and he did not complain of his earache anymore. Should the medication be discontinued? What precautions should be taken?

5. An elderly woman, 76 years old, presented with a new rash that was quite pruritic. She had formerly been in good health, but recently had been placed on Verapamil and hydrochlorothiazide for her hypertension. What questions may be included in the evaluation?

REVIEW QUESTIONS

1. The term used for an antibiotic that is effective against many different types of bacteria is:
   a. broad spectrum.
   b. narrow spectrum.
   c. fungicide.
   d. anthelmintic.

2. Penicillin may be used prophylactically (without evidence of an acute infection) in the management of:
   a. sinusitis.
   b. allergies to penicillin.
   c. rheumatic fever.
   d. tuberculosis.

3. Amoxicillin is superior to oral penicillin V in every respect except:
   a. it has increased absorption after oral administration.
   b. it is less likely to be broken down in the stomach.
   c. it needs to be taken more frequently during the day.
   d. it has a broader spectrum of activity.

4. A cross sensitivity may occur between penicillin and:
   a. tetracycline.
   b. erythromycin.
   c. cephalexin.
   d. zidovudine.

5. Another name for the macrolide antibiotics is:
   a. the penicillins.
   b. the tetracyclines.
   c. the fungicides.
   d. the erythromycins.

6. Viruses differ from other microorganisms in that they:
   a. are less likely to cause severe illnesses.
   b. are more easily treated.
   c. require an intact cell to replicate.
   d. reproduce slowly.

7. Interferon alfa is used in the treatment of:
   a. the common cold.
   b. hepatitis A.
   c. hepatitis B.
   d. AIDS.

8. An agent often used in the treatment of AIDS is:
   a. zidovudine.
   b. Zithromax.
   c. Zelnorm.
   d. Xanax.

9. A common use for the sulfonamides is for:
   a. drug allergies.
   b. urinary tract infections.
   c. strep throat.
   d. respiratory tract infections.

10. Drugs that may cross-react with a sulfonamide to cause an allergic reaction include all of the following except:
    a. hydrochlorothiazide.
    b. tolazamide.
    c. dapsone.
    d. penicillin.

17 Antihistamines

Objectives

After completing this chapter, you should be able to do the following:

1. Identify the symptoms of an allergic reaction.
2. Understand the role of histamine in allergic reactions.
3. Understand the antigen-antibody reaction and how it may cause allergic reactions.
4. Help detect the various environmental causes of allergic reactions.
5. Discuss information the health care professional should give to a patient taking antihistamines.
6. Describe the symptoms of anaphylaxis.
7. Understand drug allergies and their importance in drug therapy.

Key Terms

Allergen, p. 65
Allergy, p. 65
Anaphylaxis (ĂN-ĕ-fĭ-LĂK-sĭs), p. 65
Antibody, p. 65
Antigen, p. 65
Antihistamines (ĂN-tĭ-HĬS-ta-mēns), p. 66
Drug allergies, p. 66
Histamine (HĬS-tă-mēn), p. 65
Immunotherapy (IM-yĕ-nō-THĔR-ĕ-pē), p. 68

Early in the 20th century it was discovered that the release of histamine from body tissues was in large part responsible for symptoms that occurred after certain viral infections or the introduction of sensitizing foreign substances into the body. **Histamine** is an amino acid that is released from body tissues in response to an allergic reaction. It is found in many plant and animal tissues. Under normal circumstances it is probably bound to an intracellular protein. It is the histamine, then, that evokes the symptoms, more commonly known as the "allergic reaction," which may be manifested by red watery eyes, urticaria, sneezing, coryza, rash, the bronchiolar constriction of asthma, and so forth.

ALLERGIC REACTIONS

When an **antigen** (the general term for a foreign substance capable of inducing sensitivity and causing an allergic reac-

tion) is introduced into the body, it evokes a tissue response in the form of a substance called an **antibody,** which is synthesized specifically to combat the particular antigen. When the tissue response is a hypersensitive reaction, known as an **allergy,** the antigen is referred to as an **allergen.** It is believed that the complex reactions and interactions that follow cause the release of histamine.

Anaphylaxis is a severe, life-threatening allergic reaction, marked by an extreme drop in blood pressure and body temperature, a decrease in the circulating blood volume, and cardiac abnormalities. If emergency measures are not taken immediately (e.g., administration of epinephrine or corticosteroids and the rapid administration of intravenous fluids), death may occur.

The emotional component of allergic reactions is less well understood. It is a well-established fact that certain persons can experience urticaria, or hives, after severe emotional stress. It has likewise been observed that asthmatic children and occasionally adults develop severe and even life-threatening attacks of asthma in times of emotional upheaval and stress, when no precipitating antigen can be demonstrated.

Allergic rhinitis is characterized by nasal itching, sneezing, watery rhinorrhea, and nasal congestion. It also may cause a variety of nonnasal physical symptoms that include headache, sore throat, postnasal drip, plugged or itchy ears, chronic cough, and ocular symptoms such as itching, tearing, and swelling. It has been estimated that allergic rhinitis may affect 30% of adults and at least 40% of children. The symptoms may exert a significant negative impact on the quality of life.

A wide variety of complications may affect patients with chronic congestion caused by allergic rhinitis, including sinusitis, halitosis, sleep disturbances (including apnea and frequent arousals), allergic "shiners" (dark coloring under eyes from venous congestion), and exacerbations of asthma. Up to 38% of patients with rhinitis have also received a diagnosis of asthma. In many cases the diagnosis of allergic rhinitis precedes the diagnosis of asthma, but the two disorders may present simultaneously as well.

The prevalence of allergic rhinitis over the past 4 decades has increased dramatically. This is believed to be due to the increasing concentrations of airborne pollutants, growing dust-mite populations, and poor ventilation in buildings.

DETERMINING THE CAUSE OF THE ALLERGY

In some cases the source of the allergy can be determined by a little investigation or attention to circumstances prevailing when allergic symptoms appear. For instance, persons allergic to certain animal dander often determine this fact for themselves, noting that symptoms arise shortly after contacting dogs, cats, or other animals. Likewise, an individual who sneezes uncontrollably after contact with a certain flower is likely to remember the circumstances and avoid the allergen in the future.

Food allergies are somewhat more difficult to determine in some instances, but if suspected, they can often be discovered if the individual keeps a careful record of all food eaten. Allergic reactions to a food may occur within a 3-day period after the offending food is eaten; thus the meals of this time span should be investigated. Fish, chocolate, wheat, milk, eggs, and nuts are common offenders, but any food may be involved. Peanut allergies are relatively common and often severe enough to be life-threatening.

Skin tests may be used to determine the offending allergen, but these are often disappointing. Obviously, it is impossible to prepare testing solutions of every existing antigen. It is also rare to have one or even two allergens defined as the offending substance even under optimum conditions. Many persons react to multiple allergens with wheals of varying size. At best, a probable diagnosis can be obtained, and some improvement in severe allergic reactions can be achieved following regular injection of desensitizing vaccine.

ADVERSE DRUG REACTIONS (DRUG ALLERGIES)

Adverse drug reactions, or **drug allergies,** are common, but identifying a true drug allergy is often difficult. The over-diagnosing of drug allergies is common because they can be confused with a viral rash or other unusual or unwanted symptom that may have appeared as part of an illness. In addition, there are very few laboratory tests available for drug allergy, thus the diagnosis is dependent on clinical findings.

Drug reactions can be classified into immunologic, or immune-mediated, and nonimmunologic causes. *Idiosyncratic reactions* are abnormal reactions not related to the known pharmacologic action of the drug, and occur in only a small percentage of the population. An idiosyncratic reaction would be the hemolysis that occurs when a person with glucose-6-phosphate dehydrogenase (G-6-PD) deficiency takes a drug such as a sulfonamide. *Drug intolerance* would be defined as a lower threshold to the normal action of a drug, such as experiencing tinnitus after a single tablet of aspirin, or abdominal pain after a single dose of erythromycin.

In some cases an adverse effect may be tolerated if it is minimal and not too disruptive. The signs of a generalized allergic reaction are more alarming. Warning signs of impending cardiovascular collapse include urticaria, laryn-geal or upper airway edema, wheezing, and hypotension. The presence of fever, mucous membrane lesions, lymphadenopathy, joint tenderness or swelling, and a generalized skin rash are also suggestive of more serious reactions.

The most important therapeutic measure is the discontinuation of the drug. In a majority of patients the symptoms will resolve within 2 weeks. Antihistamines and corticosteroids may be given to lessen symptoms and hasten recovery.

General criteria for drug hypersensitivity reactions are as follows:

1. The patient's symptoms are consistent with a drug reaction.
2. The patient was administered a drug known to cause such symptoms.
3. The timing of the appearance of symptoms is consistent with a drug reaction.
4. Other causes of the symptoms are excluded.

THE TREATMENT OF ALLERGIES

Environmental controls should not be overlooked in the management of allergies. Encasing the mattress and pillow in plastic covers, replacing woolen blankets with cotton, replacing carpeting with hardwood flooring, replacing fabric curtains with plastic or wooden blinds, vacuuming with a system that filters through water, avoiding humidifiers, and freezing soft toys in a plastic bag for 24 hours may all be used to minimize the exposure to allergens.

When it is necessary to use drug therapy, **antihistamines** (drugs that combat the symptoms generated by histamine in an allergic reaction) are the mainstay of treatment for allergic reactions. The older antihistamines, although effective in treating the symptoms of allergic symptoms, have been implicated in actually worsening the quality of life by causing drowsiness and exacerbating the fatigue, depression, and other effects of disturbed sleep. For this reason they should not be taken when working around machinery, when driving, or at any other time when drowsiness could be hazardous. The sedative effect of these agents is greatly increased when combined with another depressant such as alcohol, tranquilizers, sleeping pills, and many of the antihypertensive agents. Thus the combination of these agents is to be avoided.

 Considerations for Older Adults

Antihistamines

The elderly are much more susceptible to the sedating effects of antihistamines than are younger people. Before administering antihistamines, ask about other prescriptions for any other sedating drugs, such as sedatives, hypnotics, and tranquilizers.

These agents are also associated with anticholinergic effects, such as dry mouth, dry eyes, and urinary retention.

TRADITIONAL (SEDATING) ANTIHISTAMINES

diphenhydramine hydrochloride, USP, BP (Benadryl). This agent is useful both orally and intravenously (IV) or intramuscularly (IM) to control moderately severe allergic reactions, such as those occurring in serum sickness, urticaria, and drug reactions. In addition, it is used occasionally as a mild sedative, particularly in the elderly, in whom more potent agents are not advisable.

Dosage:
Adults: (Oral) 50 mg three to four times daily. (IV or IM) 10 to 50 mg three times daily. Dosage not to exceed 300 mg orally in 24 hours, or 400 mg IV or IM per 24 hours.
Children weighing more than 20 lb: (Oral) 12.5 to 25 mg three to four times daily.

chlorpheniramine maleate, USP, BP (Chlor-Trimeton, Teldrin). This agent is available in both tablet form and delayed-action preparations, which allow effective release of the antihistamine for up to 8 hours. As a general rule, drowsiness is more troublesome in the delayed-release forms.

Dosage:
Adults: (Oral) 4 mg every 3 to 4 hours. Delayed-release forms: 8 to 12 mg every 12 hours. The 24-hour dosage should not exceed 24 mg.
Children: (Oral) Up to the adult dosage of tablets; 24-hour dosage should not exceed 12 mg.

dimenhydrinate, USP, BP (Dramamine). This agent is used primarily for the relief of motion sickness and is quite successful in this respect if taken a half-hour before air or ground travel. It may be administered parenterally as well, for nonspecific nausea and vomiting.

Dosage:
Adults: (Oral) 50 mg two to four times daily. (IM) 50 mg as necessary.
Children: (Oral) Up to the adult dosage. (IM) 1.25 mg/kg four times daily.

tripelennamine hydrochloride, USP, BP (Pyribenzamine). In addition to its use as an oral antihistamine for mild allergic symptoms, tripelennamine is also available in some topical ointments. Its use as a topical antihistamine is quite disappointing, however, and it is now largely replaced by corticosteroid creams if symptoms warrant local therapy.

Dosage:
Adults: (Oral) 50 mg four times daily.
Children: (Oral) 5 mg/kg/day in four divided doses.

meclizine hydrochloride, USP, BP (Bonine, Antivert). Although long used to control nausea and vomiting of pregnancy, federal regulations now restrict this drug and most other antinausea preparations from use in pregnant women. It is quite effective in the prevention of motion sickness.

Dosage:
Adults: (Oral) 12.5 to 50 mg one to three times daily.
Children: Not recommended.

promethazine hydrochloride, USP, BP (Phenergan). The drowsiness and antisecretory effects caused by promethazine make it particularly useful in preoperative patients. If this drug is administered parenterally with a narcotic agent, the sedative effect is increased. Oral forms and rectal suppositories are available as well.

Dosage:
Adults: (Oral) 25 mg three to four times daily. (IM) 25 to 50 mg as necessary.
Children: (Oral) 6.25 to 12.5 mg three to four times daily. (IM) 0.5 mg/lb as necessary.

brompheniramine maleate, USP, BP (Dimetane, Dimetapp). Very similar in action and uses to chlorpheniramine, this agent is available in tablets as well as delayed-action dosage forms.

Dosage:
Adults: (Oral) One 4-mg tablet every 4 to 6 hours. Delayed-action form: 8 to 12 mg every 8 hours.
Children 6 to 12 years: (Oral) 1 to 2 mg four times daily.

trimethobenzamide hydrochloride, USP, BP (Tigan). This agent is used in the form of capsules, rectal suppositories, and intramuscular injections to control nausea and vomiting in children and adults. It is not recommended for use in pregnant women. Side effects have been infrequent, but occasional hypersensitivity reactions have occurred. Hypotension, coma, disorientation, dizziness, headaches, blurred vision, and opisthotonos have been reported. Because the suppositories contain benzocaine, they should not be administered to individuals known to be sensitive to local anesthetics.

Dosage:
Adults: (Oral) 250 mg three to four times daily. (Rectal suppository) 200 mg three to four times daily. (IM) 200 mg three to four times daily.
Children weighing more than 30 lb: (Oral) 100 mg three to four times daily. (Rectal suppository) 50 to 200 mg three to four times daily. The injectable form is not to be used in children.

cetirizine hydrochloride (Zyrtec). Cetirizine is a long-acting antihistamine used to provide relief of seasonal allergic rhinitis and chronic urticaria.

Dosage:
Adults and children older than 5 years: (Oral) 5 to 10 mg once daily.
Children 2 to 5 years: (Oral) 2.5 mg once daily.

cyproheptadine hydrochloride, USP (Periactin). Generally used for skin reactions such as urticaria or the pruritus of varicella eruptions (chickenpox), this agent is one of the more effective antihistamines for the treatment of dermatologic disorders.

> **Dosage:**
> Adults: (Oral) 4 mg three times daily.
> Children: (Oral) 2 mg three times daily.

NONSEDATING ANTIHISTAMINES

loratadine (Claritin). Loratadine is a long-acting antihistamine that is used for the symptomatic improvement of rhinitis and urticaria in adults and children older than 6 years.

> **Dosage:**
> Adults and children older than 6 years: (Oral) 10 mg once daily.

loratadine plus pseudoephedrine (Claritin D). This combination of 5 mg loratadine and 120 mg pseudoephedrine is formulated in a 12-hour extended-release tablet. It provides decongestant activity as well as the antihistamine effect.

> **Dosage:**
> Adults and children older than 12 years: (Oral) 1 tablet every 12 hours.

desloratadine (Clarinex). This long-acting tricyclic antihistamine is used for once-daily treatment of allergic symptoms in individuals older than 12 years.

> **Dosage:**
> Adults and children older than 12 years: (Oral) 5 mg once daily.

fexofenadine hydrochloride (Allegra). This selective antihistamine exhibits an antihistamine effect within an hour, and is effective in allergic rhinitis.

> **Dosage:**
> Adults and children older than 12 years: (Oral) 60 mg twice daily or 180 mg once daily.

fexofenadine plus pseudoephedrine (Allegra D). This combination contains 60 mg fexofenadine hydrochloride and 120 mg pseudoephedrine and is useful in controlling nasal congestion as well as exerting an antihistamine effect.

> **Dosage:**
> Adults and children older than 12 years: one tablet twice daily.

INTRANASAL ANTIHISTAMINE

azelastine hydrochloride (Astelin). This antihistamine is formulated to be administered intranasally for the treatment of seasonal allergic rhinitis in adults and children older than 5 years. Each spray delivers 137 mcg of azelastine hydrochloride.

> **Dosage:**
> Adults and children older than 12 years: (Intranasal) Two sprays in each nostril twice daily.
> Children 5 to 12 years: (Intranasal) One spray in each nostril twice daily.

ANTIHISTAMINE COMBINATIONS

Antihistamine combinations vary greatly in composition. The proprietary "cold capsules" generally contain a small dose of antihistamine in combination with a decongestant and often aspirin or another salicylate compound. Examples are Allerest, Contac, Coricidin D, Dristan, Novahistine, Sinutab, and Vicks Tri-Span.

Other combinations are available by prescription only and generally have higher doses of the respective drugs.

acrivastine (Semprex-D). This fixed-combination preparation containing acrivastine and pseudoephedrine hydrochloride is used to provide symptomatic relief of seasonal allergic rhinitis.

> **Dosage:**
> Adults and children older than 12 years: (Oral) 8 mg four times daily.

azatadine maleate (Optimine). This preparation, in which azatadine is in a fixed combination with pseudoephedrine hydrochloride, is also used for the symptomatic treatment of seasonal hay fever, rhinitis, and chronic urticaria.

> **Dosage:**
> Adults and children older than 12 years: (Oral) 1 to 2 mg twice daily.

carbinoxamine maleate (Rondec, Andec, Biohist). Also combined with pseudoephedrine hydrochloride, this drug may be used for infants and young children as well as adults for the control of allergic symptoms.

> **Dosage:**
> Adults and children older than 6 years: (Oral) 4 mg four times daily.
> Infants to children up to 6 years: (Oral) 0.5 to 2 mg four times daily.

clemastine fumarate (Tavist). This combination of clemastine with pseudoephedrine can be used in adults and young children with seasonal allergies.

> **Dosage:**
> Adults and children older than 12 years: (Oral) 1.34 mg every 12 hours.
> Children 6 to 12 years: (Oral) 0.67 mg every 12 hours.

THE ROLE OF IMMUNOTHERAPY

Many studies show that **immunotherapy,** or the systematic, repeated exposure to small amounts of an allergen, reduces symptoms of allergic rhinitis in selected patients. It is particularly useful in patients who are unable or unwilling to avoid the allergen, those who experience inadequate relief or intolerable side effects from pharmacologic therapy, or those with comorbid conditions such as asthma. Initially very low concentrations of the allergen are used. The strength of the solution is gradually increased until the symptoms are relieved or a maximum tolerable dose is reached. The possibility of acute allergic reactions to immunotherapy requires careful monitoring. Three to 5 years of continuous treatment is generally required. In some cases the therapy then may be discontinued.

CLINICAL IMPLICATIONS

1. Allergic conditions can best be treated by avoidance of the suspected allergen. Animals should be removed from the home if possible, as should items that collect dust, such as curtains, carpets, and collectibles, particularly in the bedroom.
2. Feather pillows should be avoided and foam pillows used instead. All pillows and mattresses should be covered in vinyl material.
3. Become familiar with the MedicAlert tags and remember to check them for potential drug allergies.
4. The symptoms of a mild allergic reaction include rhinitis, coryza, conjunctival injection, and skin rashes.
5. Anaphylaxis is an acute emergency and has as its onset respiratory distress with wheezing and bronchospasm, leading to edema of the face and extremities, hypotension, and even death.
6. The primary side effect of the antihistamines is drowsiness. The patient should be instructed not to work around machinery or to drive long distances after taking antihistamines.
7. The sleepiness produced by the antihistamines is an individual variation; certain people become rapidly resistant to the drowsiness induced by these agents and can take them routinely without drowsiness.
8. Bed rails and assistance with ambulation may be indicated when an individual, particularly an elderly person, has received an antihistamine.
9. The antihistamines potentiate the central nervous system depression of many other agents, such as alcohol, tranquilizers, sedatives, and hypnotics.
10. Antihistamines are useful in the prevention of motion sickness and should be given 30 minutes before entering the vehicle for optimum effect.
11. Most drugs will have adverse effects as well as the ability to produce allergic reactions.
12. A patient who develops an unusual or unwanted symptom while taking a drug should be questioned about previous drug allergies. The drug should be discontinued until full evaluation of a potential allergic reaction can be made.

Online Resources

For updated drug information and Web activities, go to http://evolve.elsevier.com/Asperheim.

CRITICAL THINKING QUESTIONS

1. The patient has been miserable since his daughter bought a cat. He has coryza, excessive sneezing, and rhinitis. Because his daughter insists on keeping the cat, he wants to control his allergies with antihistamines. What health teaching is indicated here?

2. You have a part-time job in a drugstore as a drug clerk. A pregnant woman comes in and asks your advice as to which over-the-counter antihistamine she can safely take for her spring allergies. How would you respond to this situation?

3. The patient stepped in a nest of fire ants and has a severe local reaction over both lower legs. It is 10 o'clock in the morning, and you detect a strong odor of alcohol on his breath. The physician decides to prescribe Benadryl, 50 mg four times a day, and the man reports that he has to go back to work. What suggestions might be made?

4. The patient has been on Bactrim, a sulfonamide, for 5 days for the treatment of a urinary tract infection. She wants to know which lotion she should buy for this bright red rash on her face and arms.

REVIEW QUESTIONS

1. Symptoms of an allergic reaction may include all except which symptom?
   a. Red, watery eyes
   b. Runny nose
   c. Asthma
   d. Thirst

2. A severe and life-threatening allergic reaction is known as:
   a. epileptic equivalent.
   b. anaphylaxis.
   c. coryza.
   d. urticaria.

3. A drug that may be given orally to treat an allergic reaction is:
   a. loratidine.
   b. epinephrine.
   c. azelastine hydrochloride.
   d. weekly immunotherapy.

4. An example of an intranasal antihistamine is:
   a. Clarinex.
   b. trimethobenzamide.
   c. promethazine.
   d. azelastine hydrochloride.

REVIEW QUESTIONS—cont'd

5. Immunotherapy consists of:
   a. giving increasing doses of antihistamines.
   b. treating asthma aggressively with high doses of drugs.
   c. repeated administration of small amounts of antigen.
   d. introducing allergens in inhalants daily.

6. The primary side effect of diphenhydramine (Benadryl) is:
   a. drowsiness.
   b. jitteriness.
   c. skin rash.
   d. watery eyes.

7. The advantage loratadine has over diphenhydramine is that it:
   a. is less sedating.
   b. is more sedating.
   c. causes fewer skin rashes.
   d. is less expensive.

8. The best approach to the beginning treatment of allergies is to:
   a. begin allergy immunotherapy immediately.
   b. avoid the allergen.
   c. expose the patient to the allergen frequently.
   d. give antihistamines.

9. An agent that may be potentiated or have an increased effect when given with antihistamines is:
   a. penicillin.
   b. rifampin.
   c. alcoholic beverages.
   d. tetracycline.

10. An example of a nonsedating antihistamine is:
    a. trimethobenzamide.
    b. brompheniramine.
    c. cetirizine.
    d. fexofenadine.

Drugs That Affect the Skin and Mucous Membranes

After completing this chapter, you should be able to do the following:

1. Describe the functions of the skin.
2. Describe the effects of emollients, demulcents, and keratolytics on the skin.
3. Understand the uses of the various acne preparations.
4. Describe the action of astringents.
5. Give examples of local anesthetics and the purpose for which each one is used.
6. Identify agents used to treat *Candida* infections.
7. Identify agents used to treat fungal infections.
8. Identify local antiinfectives.
9. Explain how sun-induced skin damage can occur and become familiar with the sunscreens and their action.
10. Recognize the drugs that are photosensitizers.

Key Terms

Acne (ĂC-nē), p. 75
Anesthetics (ăn-ĕs-THĔ-tĭks), p. 72
Astringents (ē-STRĬN-jĕnts), p. 72
Candida albicans (KĂN-dĭ-dē ĂL-bĕ-kănz), p. 73
Candidiasis (KĂN-dĭ-DĪ-ĕ-sĭs), p. 73
Demulcents (dĭ-MŬL-sĕnts), p. 71
Emollients (ĭ-MŌL-yĕnts), p. 71
Moniliasis (MŌ-nĕ-LĬ-ĕ-sĭs), p. 73
Photosensitizer (FŌ-tō-SĔN-sĭ-TĪZ-ĕr), p. 75

The skin is a complex structure that serves many functions. Chief among these are regulation of body temperature, maintenance of electrolyte and water balance, protection, excretion of waste substances, and some metabolic activity, such as formation of vitamin D (the "sunshine vitamin").

Drugs applied to the skin may likewise serve many functions and may be intended for either a local effect or a systemic effect following absorption through the skin. The drugs may be conveniently divided into the following classes.

SOOTHING SUBSTANCES

These agents are applied to irritated and abraded areas to protect them and alleviate itching.

EMOLLIENTS

Emollients are fatty or oily substances applied to soothe the skin or mucous membranes. Irritants, air, and airborne bacteria are excluded by the oily layer, and the skin is rendered softer and more pliable by penetration of the emollient into the surface layers. Emollient substances are used chiefly as vehicles for fat-soluble drugs and as protective agents. Some commonly used emollients are:

Petrolatum
Rosewater ointment (cold cream)
Hydrous wool fat (lanolin)

DEMULCENTS

Demulcents are protective agents employed primarily to alleviate irritation, particularly of mucous membranes and abraded tissue. They are generally applied to the surface in sticky preparations that cover the area rapidly. Demulcents may be incorporated in lozenges to soothe oral and throat mucosa and are swallowed in liquid form as an antidote for corrosive poisons.

A variety of substances possess demulcent properties; some common demulcents are:

Gums and mucilages (e.g., acacia and tragacanth)
Starch
Cream, milk
Egg white

 Considerations for Children

Hexachlorophene

The skin of infants and children is particularly susceptible to absorption of drugs such as hexachlorophene. Therefore, do not use hexachlorophene routinely to bathe infants. Symptoms of neurotoxicity, including seizures, have been observed after systemic absorption of hexachlorophene from the skin. Also, do not apply it to the mucous membranes or abraded skin of patients of any age.

ASTRINGENTS

Astringents precipitate protein but ordinarily do not penetrate beyond cell surfaces; thus the cell remains viable. This action is accompanied by contraction and blanching of skin, and mucus and other secretions may be reduced so that the affected area becomes drier.

These agents are used to arrest minor hemorrhage, check perspiration, reduce inflammation, promote healing, and toughen skin. The principal astringents are:
Salts of aluminum, zinc, and other heavy metals
Tannins (e.g., tannic acid in alcohol, witch hazel)
Alcohols, phenols

IRRITANTS

Irritants produce irritation—the degree of which is determined by the concentration and the duration of action. There are three types of irritants:
Counterirritants—used to irritate unbroken skin to relieve deep pain in muscles, joints, bursae, and other areas
Rubefacients—produce local vasodilation, redness, and a feeling of warmth
Vesicants—cause a strong irritation; blisters may be produced if used in high concentrations or for a prolonged time
The following agents may be either counterirritants, rubefacients, or vesicants, depending upon the concentration used and the length of time of application:
Camphor, menthol, chloroform
Mustard as in a mustard plaster
Oil of wintergreen

KERATOLYTICS

Keratolytics cause sloughing of hardened epithelium. They are used to cauterize ulcers and to destroy excess tissue such as calluses and warts. Common keratolytics are:
Benzoic and salicylic acids
Resorcinol
Lactic acid

LOCAL ANESTHETICS

Anesthetics are substances that cause a loss of sensation. They may have systemic effects, or the effects may be localized. Many ointments contain local anesthetics and are applied topically for minor conditions, such as sunburn and insect bites, as well as for more serious dermatoses, burns, hemorrhoids, and other conditions. These agents may be applied directly to the skin or injected. The following are a few of the local anesthetics.

cocaine, USP, BP. Used especially in ointments and nasal preparations. It is quite habit forming and comes under the restrictions of the Controlled Substances Act.

procaine, USP, BP (Novocain). Used in dentistry and before minor surgery. Because it is not effective topically, it must be injected.

dibucaine, USP, BP (Nupercainal). Applied topically in ointments.

benzocaine, USP, BP. Used in throat lozenges and topical preparations.
Medicone rectal ointment
Unguentine ointment
Surfacaine ointment

ANTIFUNGAL AGENTS

Fungal infections of the skin are a common problem in both warm and temperate climates. They particularly affect areas of the skin that tend to remain warm and moist, such as the feet, the underarms, under the breasts, and the perineal area (*intertrigo*). Topical therapy is often sufficient in uncomplicated infections, but systemic therapy, such as oral griseofulvin, may be necessary to treat long-standing infections.

ketoconazole, USP, BP (Nizoral). This agent is used topically for the treatment of fungal and yeast infections. It is also effective for seborrheic dermatitis. Local application is generally well tolerated, but there may be some local irritation at the site of application.
Dosage:
2% topical cream applied once daily for 2 weeks.

ciclopirox olamine, USP, BP (Loprox). This agent may be applied topically for the treatment of various fungal and yeast infections. It has a low toxicity but some burning may be felt at the site of application.
Dosage:
1% cream or lotion applied topically twice daily for up to 4 weeks.

ciclopirox solution (Penlac Nail Lacquer). This solution may be applied topically directly to the fingernails and toenails in immunocompromised patients for the treatment of fungal infections.
Dosage:
8% topical solution applied to nails daily for 4 weeks.

tolnaftate, USP, BP (Tinactin). When applied twice daily to topical fungal infections, tolnaftate is quite effective against ringworm, athlete's foot, and similar conditions. To prevent recurrences, care must be taken to continue the use of this preparation for 2 weeks after all visible signs of the infection have cleared. Sensitivity reactions are rare.
Dosage:
1% cream, solution, powder, or aerosol twice daily; continue use for 2 weeks after disappearance of visible signs of infection.

zinc undecylenate ointment, USP, BP (Desenex, Undesol, Undex). Zinc undecylenate was one of the first topical antifungal agents and continues to be a popular over-the-counter preparation for the treatment and prevention of athlete's foot. It has been surpassed in effectiveness by tolnaftate and other preparations, however.

Dosage:
20% ointment applied topically twice daily (often in combination with varying amounts of undecylenic acid) for 2-4 weeks.

clotrimazole, USP, BP (Lotrimin). Clotrimazole has a broad spectrum of activity against fungi as well as yeasts. It is available in the form of a solution or cream for topical application. Erythema, blistering, peeling, pruritus, and general skin irritation have been observed in sensitive persons; the application should be discontinued if these symptoms occur.

Dosage:
1% in solution or cream applied topically twice daily for 2-4 weeks.

clioquinol (formerly iodochlorhydroxyquin), USP, BP (Vioform). The antibacterial as well as antifungal properties of this agent make it extremely useful in nonspecific or mixed infections. It is also available in combination with hydrocortisone to suppress local inflammatory reactions. Topical application is helpful in some cases of eczema, athlete's foot, or intertriginous rashes.

Dosage:
3% clioquinol. The combination forms contain 0.5% or 1% hydrocortisone. Applied topically twice daily for 2-4 weeks.

econazole nitrate (Spectazole). A once-daily application of this topical antifungal agent will cure many topical tinea infections. *Candida* (monilial) infections will need twice-daily application.

Dosage:
1% in ointment once or twice daily for 2 weeks. Other antifungal agents are listed in Table 18-1.

ANTIMONILIAL PREPARATIONS

Moniliasis (or **candidiasis**) is an infection caused by *Candida albicans*—a yeast-like organism that infects the skin and mucous membranes. Like fungal infections, topical monilial infections tend to occur in warm, macerated areas. Monilial diaper rash is common in infants, particularly after antibiotic therapy, when the normal intestinal flora is disturbed. Monilial vaginitis and perineal and intertriginous infections tend to occur with increased frequency in diabetic patients and obese individuals.

Mycolog cream and ointment. This commercial preparation consists of a combination of nystatin, neomycin, gramicidin, and triamcinolone acetate. The topical antibiotics and corticosteroid included in this product have been demonstrated to be highly effective in all forms of topical *Candida* infections and aid in clearing secondary infections caused by local irritation and scratching of the areas. When applied two to three times daily, noticeable improvement is seen within 1 week in most cases. Topical sensitivity reactions have been noted but are rare.

Dosage:
100,000 units nystatin, 2.5 mg neomycin, 0.25 mg gramicidin, and 1 mg triamcinolone acetate, per gram of cream or ointment two to three times daily for 1 week or longer.

nystatin vaginal tablets, USP, BP (Mycostatin). Vulvovaginal *Candida* infections may be treated topically with the use of vaginal tablets. Very rarely, irritation or sensitization to this agent may occur.

Dosage:
(Vaginal) 1 tablet containing 100,000 units inserted daily for 2 weeks.

miconazole nitrate vaginal cream (Monistat). This water-miscible cream is indicated for vaginal use in the treatment of vulvovaginal *Candida* infections. Very rarely, vaginal burning, pelvic cramps, hives, skin rash, and headache are observed.

Dosage:
(Vaginal) One applicator of the 2% cream inserted daily for 7 days.

terconazole (Terazol). This agent is used for the treatment of vulvovaginal monilial infections.

Dosage:
(Vaginal) One applicator of the 0.4% cream inserted daily for 7 days, or 1 suppository daily for 3 days.

Table **18-1** | *Other Antifungal Agents*

NAME	USE	HOW SUPPLIED
butenafine hydrochloride (Mentax)	Tinea pedis, corporis	
	Tinea versicolor	1% cream
ketoconazole (Nizoral)	Tinea pedis, corporis, cruris	2% cream or shampoo
miconazole nitrate tincture (Fungoid)	Tinea pedis and corporis	2% solution
oxiconazole nitrate (Oxistat)	Antifungal and antimonilial	1% lotion or cream
terbinafine (Lamisil)	Tinea pedis, corporis	1% cream or lotion

clotrimazole, USP, BP (Lotrimin, Gyne-Lotrimin). This agent is used intravaginally for monilial infections.

> **Dosage:**
>> (Vaginal) One applicator of the 1% cream inserted daily for 7 days, or two 100-mg tablets inserted daily for 3 days.

GENERAL ANTIINFECTIVE AGENTS

ethyl alcohol, USP, BP (alcohol). The alcohol most frequently used as an antiinfective is ethyl alcohol; the optimum antiseptic activity is obtained from a 70% solution. Higher concentrations have a decreased antiseptic action. In addition to its antiseptic activity, alcohol has an astringent effect when applied topically and is frequently used in the treatment of decubitus ulcers; it is commonly utilized to cleanse the skin before giving hypodermic injections and while dressing wounds.

isopropyl alcohol. Isopropyl alcohol is approximately twice as germicidal as ethyl alcohol and is much less corrosive to instruments. Isopropyl alcohol is more toxic, however. It is used in full strength.

benzalkonium chloride, USP, BP (Zephiran Chloride). A rapid-acting, nonirritating antibacterial agent, this compound may be used safely on skin and mucous membranes in concentrations from 1:1000 to 1:10,000. One precaution to be observed with this agent, however, is that all soap or detergent must be completely removed before application of Zephiran, because it is inactivated by anionic agents.

hexachlorophene, USP, BP (incorporated in Gamophen and Dial soaps, Septisol, and pHisoHex). Preparations containing this agent in 3% concentrations are used widely as antiseptic scrubs. When it is used regularly, a residual layer of the antiseptic forms on the skin and reduces the normal bacterial flora. Its activity is lessened by the presence of serum and organic materials. Because hexachlorophene has been found to be systemically absorbed from skin surfaces, it is no longer recommended for the routine bathing of infants. It should be used in its more concentrated forms (e.g., pHisoHex) only on the advice of a physician.

Herb Alert

Aloe

Aloe is commonly rubbed on the skin to soothe minor burns, treat infections, and moisturize dry patches. It has been taken internally as a cathartic but is not generally recommended for this use because, when taken orally, it may produce heart arrhythmias, edema, and nephropathies. It also enhances potassium loss in patients taking diuretics. See Chapter 35 for more information on aloe.

saponated cresol solution, USP, BP (Lysol, Creolin). In strengths of approximately 2%, this solution is used for disinfection of contaminated utensils such as bedpans, basins, and linens. The presence of organic material does not interfere with its action. In very weak dilutions it may be used for vaginal douches.

gentian violet, USP, BP. This antiseptic dye may be applied to surface areas for many infectious conditions. In strengths of 1:1000 to 1:100, it is used to combat impetigo, thrush, fungal infections, cystitis, urethritis, and similar conditions.

iodine tincture, USP, BP. One of the oldest and most effective of the germicides and fungicides, this tincture is used in 2% solution for application to wounds and abrasions. It is not safe for application to large wounds. The agent of choice for application to mucous membranes is a 2% solution of iodine in glycerin.

povidone-iodine solution, USP, BP (Betadine). The iodine content of this preparation furnishes its germicidal activity. The iodine is released more slowly than from the tincture, but the prolongation of action compensates for this in large part. It is used in 1% to 1.5% solutions and has a variety of applications in aerosol, douche, vaginal gel, shampoo, and topical forms.

merbromin solution (Mercurochrome). A mildly active antiseptic, this agent has a variety of uses as a skin antiseptic and as a treatment for urethritis and cystitis. It is used in 2% concentrations. The tincture shows more antiseptic activity than the solution, owing to the added presence of alcohol in the tincture.

hydrogen peroxide solution, USP, BP. The antiseptic activity of this agent results from the liberation of oxygen, which destroys many anaerobic bacteria and produces an effervescent action, which cleans wounds of dead tissue and pus. It deteriorates upon standing, however, and should be stored in a cool, dark place. The 3% solution is most frequently used.

WOUND CARE PRODUCTS

Wounds such as pressure ulcers, venous stasis ulcers, and burns need special care. A variety of products can aid in their treatment. The goal of treatment is to remove any dead tissue (*débridement*), control the level of bacterial growth (cleansing), and provide a moist wound environment while keeping the surrounding intact skin dry.

mupirocin calcium (Bactroban). This topical antibiotic ointment is used for the treatment of local infections, such as impetigo. Few adverse effects occur; burning or local irritation is an indication for discontinuing the drug.

Dosage:

2% ointment applied three times daily for 2-4 weeks.

Over-the-counter antibiotic ointments are readily available and may be used as well.

silver sulfadiazine, USP (Silvadene Cream). This agent has a broad spectrum of antiinfective activity. It is used topically to prevent wound infection in patients with second- and third-degree burns.

Dosage:

1% cream applied topically 1-2 times daily until healing has occured.

mafenide acetate cream, USP (Sulfamylon Cream). This agent is a nonstaining white cream that can be applied topically on second- and third-degree burns.

Dosage:

85 mg mafenide per gram of cream applied topically 1-2 times daily until healing has occured.

SUN DAMAGE TO SKIN

In the past two decades or so, knowledge of sun-induced skin disorders has expanded tremendously. The radiant energy from the sun produces a thermal burn, giving light-skinned persons a coveted tan for short time; over the years, however, sun damage produces premature aging and leathery skin and greatly increased the chances of skin cancer. The potential for sun damage may be increasing with the loss of the ozone layer.

It is now believed that one significant sunburn in early life will measurably increase the risk of skin cancer later. Sun exposure effects are cumulative; thus preventing sun exposure at any age is beneficial.

Many commercial sunscreen products are available. They are labeled with a sun protection factor (SPF) number. The higher the number, the more sun protection there is. To have significant protection, the SPF number should be 15 or higher. Unfortunately, many individuals have become sensitized or allergic to many components of sunscreen. There are *para*-aminobenzoic acid (PABA)–sensitive individuals and those who are allergic to the replacements for PABA, such as the cinnamic acid derivatives.

In addition, the potential for sun damage to the skin may be enhanced by certain drug therapy. Many chemicals and foods act as **photosensitizers**—meaning that they make the skin more susceptible to burning and sun damage. It is not possible to give a complete list, but they include the following:
Cosmetics (lipsticks, many perfumes)
Pigments and dyes in clothes and tattoos
Plants (buttercup, carrots, celery, dill, fennel, figs, limes, mustard, parsley, parsnip)
Some soap deodorants containing hexachlorophene and/or bithionol
Drugs that act as photosensitizers are listed in Box 18-1.

ACNE PREPARATIONS

Acne, an inflammatory eruption of the skin, occurs in most adolescents and many adults and can cause both physical and emotional scars when severe. Many new preparations are available to treat this troublesome disorder.

A variety of factors can aggravate acne. Young women should be counseled to avoid oily cosmetics and creams and choose makeup that is hypoallergenic and water based. The hair should be kept clean and worn in a style off the face. The use of styling gels, creams, or sprays may clog pores.

Dietary theories regarding food's relationship to acne come and go. Seafood contributes iodine, an irritant, to the perspiration and may enhance folliculitis, according to some theories. There may also be an individual intolerance to chocolate or acid fruits when eaten in excessive amounts.

CLEANSING AGENTS

It is recommended that the patient cleanse the face twice daily with a mild, nonirritating soap, such as Dove or Neutrogena, or a product containing triethanolamine. Astringent drying lotions (Stri-Dex Pads, Clearasil Medicated Astringent) help accelerate the resolution of lesions. They may be used for prolonged periods if necessary.

DRUGS USED TO TREAT ACNE

tretinoin (Retinoic Acid, Retin-A). This drug appears to act as a follicular irritant, preventing cells from sticking together. A mild inflammatory reaction is produced, with peeling and extrusion of the comedo. Topical tretinoin has been shown to enhance the repair of skin that has been damaged by ultraviolet radiation. It is used cosmetically for this effect to reduce the wrinkling of aging, sun-damaged skin.

Dosage:

(Topical) Applied once daily at bedtime in the form of a cream, gel, or solution. Strengths of 0.025% to 0.1% are prescribed.

isotretinoin, USP, BP (Accutane). The principal effect of this drug appears to be the regulation of cell proliferation, in addition to exhibiting antiinflammatory and antineoplastic activities. It is used in nodular acne to reduce the size of sebaceous glands and inhibit sebum production. It inhibits the adhesion of epithelial cells and permits them to be sloughed more easily. Its side effects include conjunctivitis, thinning of the hair, photosensitivity, and hyperlipidemia. It is teratogenic to a developing fetus and may not be taken by pregnant women.

Dosage:

Adults and children older than 12: (Oral) 0.5 to 1 mg/kg/day in two divided doses.

benzoyl peroxide, USP, BP (Brevoxyl). Also a peeling agent, benzoyl peroxide is usually applied to the face in the morning after washing. Some irritation or inflammation is

| Box 18-1 | *Drugs Containing Photosensitizers* |

acetazolamide	hydrochlorothiazide
acetohexamide	ibuprofen
amantadine	imipramine
amiloride	indomethacin
amitriptyline	ketoconazole
astemizole	methyldopa
azathioprine	nalidixic acid
barbiturates	naproxen
captopril	nifedipine
carbamazepine	nitrofurantoin
cephalosporin	nonsteroidal antiinflammatory drugs
chlordiazepoxide	nortriptyline
chloroquine	ofloxacin
chlorothiazide	*para*-aminobenzoic acid (PABA)
chlorpromazine	phenothiazine
chlorthalidone	phenylbutazone
contraceptives, oral	promazine
coumarin	promethazine
desipramine	quinidine
diflunisal	retinoic acid
diltiazem	sulfa drugs
diphenhydramine	tetracycline
doxycycline	tolazamide
fluorescein	tolbutamide
fluorouracil	trazodone
furosemide	triamterene
glyburide	trimethoprim
griseofulvin	vinblastine
haloperidol	warfarin

common; if these become severe, the product should be discontinued. It will take 6 to 8 weeks to determine whether treatment is effective.

Dosage:
Applied locally in strengths of 4% or 8% in a variety of vehicles.

erythromycin topical gel (Emgel, Erygel). This antibiotic solution should be applied twice daily for the local treatment of acne. Peeling will occur. Severe dryness and irritation necessitate discontinuing the product.

Dosage:
2% topical gel applied twice daily.

clindamycin phosphate, USP, BP (Cleocin-T, Clindagel). A topical antibiotic applied directly to acneiform lesions, clindamycin has been shown to be effective against *Propionibacterium acnes,* one of the agents contributing to acne. Some systemic absorption does occur, and the side effects of diarrhea and colitis will require the product to be discontinued.

Dosage:
Solution form equivalent to 10 mg of clindamycin per milliliter, to be applied once daily, or as a 1% gel.

benzoyl peroxide plus clindamycin (Benzaclin, Duac). These topical products combine 5% benzoyl peroxide with 1% clindamycin phosphate to be used in the treatment of acne.

Dosage:
Applied twice daily to lesions.

adapalene solution (Differin). This solution is applied topically for the treatment of acne. Some adverse effects such as pruritus, burning, scaling, and erythema may occur in 30% to 60% of patients.

Dosage:
0.1% topical solution applied applied daily for 2-4 weeks.

AGENTS USED IN THE TREATMENT OF ECZEMA/ATOPIC DERMATITIS

Atopic dermatitis is a common skin condition, seen especially in children. Topical steroids may be used for the treatment, but they do have side effects, as discussed in the following section. A few nonsteroidal products are available for this condition.

Table 18-2 *Corticosteroids*

GENERIC NAME	TRADE NAME	HOW SUPPLIED
HIGHEST POTENCY		
betamethasone dipropionate, augmented	Diprolene	0.05% gel, ointment, lotion
clobetasol propionate	Temovate, Temovate-E, Olux	0.5% cream, gel, ointment, foam
diflorasone diacetate	Psorcon	0.05% ointment
halobetasol propionate	Ultravate	0.05% cream, ointment
HIGH POTENCY		
amcinonide	Cyclocort	0.1% cream, ointment, lotion
desoximetasone	Topicort, Topicort LP	0.25%, 0.05% cream, ointment
fluocinonide	Lidex, Lidex-E	0.05% cream, gel, ointment
mometasone furoate	Elocon	0.1% lotion, cream, ointment
INTERMEDIATE POTENCY		
betamethasone valerate	Luxiq	0.12% foam
fluticasone propionate	Cutivate	0.005% ointment, 0.05% cream
hydrocortisone butyrate	Locoid	0.1% cream, ointment
hydrocortisone valerate	Westcort	0.2% cream, ointment
LOW POTENCY		
alclometasone dipropionate	Aclovate	0.05% cream, ointment
desonide	DesOwen	0.05% cream, ointment, lotion
hydrocortisone	Hytone	1% cream, ointment, lotion

tacrolimus (Protopic). This agent is an immuno-suppressant, and is used in other applications to prevent organ rejection. When used for atopic dermatitis, topical tacrolimus has been shown to bind to specific receptors on the T cells, which causes a series of reactions that act to reduce the skin inflammatory response. The most common side effect is a burning of the skin after application.

Dosage:

0.03% or 0.1% ointment applied topically twice daily until symptoms have resolved for 1 week.

pimecrolimus (Elidel). The exact mechanism of action of this agent is not known. It has been shown to be an effective topical treatment for atopic dermatitis in nonimmunocompromised patients.

Dosage:

1% cream applied topically twice daily for as long as symptoms persist.

TOPICAL CORTICOSTEROIDS

The topical corticosteroids have antiinflammatory, antipruritic, and vasoconstrictive properties. They can be absorbed from intact, healthy skin. Occlusion and disease processes enhance the absorption. The potency of the commercially available products varies greatly (Table 18–2).

In general, a lower potency corticosteroid should be used when possible, and discontinued when the desired effect is produced. Predictably the adverse effects—which include skin atrophy, depigmentation of dark skin, and dermatologic absorption of the steroid with possible adrenal suppression—will increase with duration of use and with application of the higher potency steroid preparations.

CLINICAL IMPLICATIONS

1. For the desired effect when topical application of medications is ordered, the skin should be cleansed before application.
2. The site of application should be observed for edema and inflammation. The physician should be informed if the patient complains of discomfort during or after the application of topical medications.
3. Signs of healing in skin lesions are the development of a healthy, pink color and the appearance of granulation tissue.
4. Orders should be followed carefully regarding the application of dressings after administration of topical medications. In some cases, adverse effects can be obtained by bandaging the area after application.
5. To prevent cross-contamination, a different container of a topical medication should be used for each patient.
6. Aerosol containers should be stored in a cool, dry place. The aerosol container should be at least 6 inches from the skin at the time of application. Care should be taken that the aerosol does not spray into the eyes.

CLINICAL IMPLICATIONS—cont'd

7. If improper hygiene contributed to the formation of skin lesions, the patient should be carefully instructed in proper hygiene.

8. Gloves should be worn when applying topical medications to infected areas.

9. The nurse should be aware of the psychological effects of severe and disfiguring skin disorders. Counseling may be advisable in some patients.

10. Many skin disorders are worsened by self-treatment by the patient. If improper application of proprietary medications has occurred, the patient should be counseled against self-treatment.

11. The nurse should become familiar with means to improve acne by proper use of cosmetics and hygienic aids.

12. Topical acne agents have severe side effects in some cases. The nurse should take time to read the product literature on all preparations.

13. Many prescription drugs cause photosensitization. The patient should be advised to avoid prolonged sun exposure and to wear sunscreens.

14. The prolonged use of potent topical corticosteroids should be avoided. The nurse should look for signs of skin atrophy or depigmentation if the product has been used for a long time.

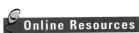

Online Resources

For updated drug information and Web activities, go to http://evolve.elsevier.com/Asperheim.

CRITICAL THINKING QUESTIONS

1. The patient came home from college with a severe case of athlete's foot. What products could be recommended to her? Is there any further advice she could be given?

2. The elderly patient complains of dry, itchy skin. She states that she is a very clean person because she takes a hot bath daily and always uses plenty of soap. What health teaching is indicated?

3. Your roommate returned from the dentist after a tooth extraction. She stated that the dentist gave her a "lot of Novocain." Later in the day her face was markedly swollen. She had difficulty talking and appeared very nervous. On the basis of your knowledge of pharmacology, what do you think might have been the cause of the problem? Is it necessary to call the dentist?

4. The patient comes into the clinic with a fiery red rash over her face and arms. She said the rash developed after she played golf yesterday and she thinks she might be allergic to her medication. Her health is generally good. She has a urinary tract infection and is presently nearly finished with her 14-day supply of trimethoprim-sulfamethoxazole (Bactrim). Do you think it is an allergic reaction? What else could it be?

REVIEW QUESTIONS

1. A use for a counterirritant such as camphor may be to:
   a. relieve allergic symptoms.
   b. treat irritated skin or mucous membranes.
   c. promote healing.
   d. relieve deep muscle pain.

2. Cocaine is an effective local anesthetic for:
   a. nasal mucous membranes.
   b. the gastrointestinal tract.
   c. deep muscle pain.
   d. weeping eczema.

3. Which of the following is not an antifungal agent?
   a. tolnaftate
   b. zinc sulfate
   c. zinc undecylenate
   d. clioquinol

4. Tretinoin (Retin-A) is used in the treatment of:
   a. urticaria.
   b. weeping eczema.
   c. cellulitis.
   d. acne.

5. An agent effective in the topical treatment of monilial infections is:
   a. Chlor-Trimeton.
   b. clotrimazole.
   c. Chloromycetin.
   d. clonidine.

6. A topical agent useful in the treatment of burns is:
   a. miconazole.
   b. Mycolog.
   c. mafenide acetate.
   d. Motrin.

REVIEW QUESTIONS—cont'd

7. The topical corticosteroids have all the following properties except:

    a. enhanced wound healing.
    b. antiinflammatory.
    c. antipruritic.
    d. vasoconstriction.

8. An example of the highest potency topical corticosteroid would be:

    a. hydrocortisone.
    b. desonide.
    c. diflorasone.
    d. alclometasone.

9. An agent used in the treatment of atopic dermatitis is:

    a. Camphor.
    b. lactic acid.
    c. econazole.
    d. pimecrolimus.

10. An indication of the effectiveness of a sunscreen would be the:

    a. PABA content.
    b. emollient ingredients.
    c. SPF number.
    d. photosensitizer ingredients.

19 Drugs That Affect the Respiratory System

After completing this chapter, you should be able to do the following:

1. Understand the function of the respiratory system.
2. Identify important drug groups that produce respiratory depression.
3. Define *expectorant* and give three examples.
4. Become familiar with environmental changes that may reduce the need for asthma medications.
5. Discuss the action of bronchodilators and give three examples.
6. Identify side effects produced by bronchodilators.
7. Recognize which asthma medications are more effective when administered by inhalation.
8. Discuss nursing measures related to assisting patients with respiratory tract disorders.

Key Terms

Asthma (ĂS-mē), p. 81
Bronchoconstriction (brŏng-kō-kŏn-STRĬK-shŭn), p. 82
Bronchodilators (brŏng-kō-DĪ-lā-tĕrs), p. 82
Inflammation (ĬN-flē-MĀshŭn), p. 80
Respiration (RĔS-pē-RĀ-shŭn), p. 80

Respiration is the process of exchanging oxygen and carbon dioxide and is accomplished via the respiratory system. The respiratory system in humans includes the nasal cavity, larynx, pharynx, trachea, bronchi, lungs, muscles of the larynx, intercostal muscles and diaphragm, and the respiratory center in the medulla (Figs. 19–1 through 19–3).

The chief functions of respiration are to supply oxygen to the tissues and remove carbon dioxide as well as to aid in the evaporation of water from the respiratory passages, a function that helps to regulate body temperature. Disruptions to the system can occur when the medulla signals the lungs to breathe too much or too little; when the bronchioles constrict (tighten or narrow), thereby reducing gas exchange; and when inflammation occurs within the lungs. **Inflammation** is a pathologic reaction by the body in response to an injury or abnormal stimulation by a physical, chemical, or biologic agent. When it occurs within the lung

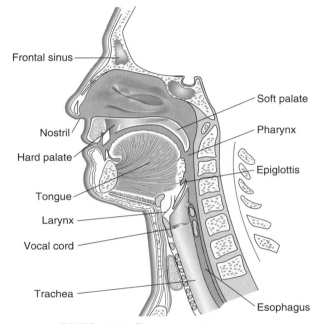

FIGURE 19-1 The upper respiratory organs.

or bronchioles, wheezing, breathlessness, and other symptoms can result.

Drugs that act on the respiratory system may be classified as those that:

1. Act on the respiratory center in the brain
2. Affect the mucous membrane lining of the respiratory tract
3. Affect the size of the bronchioles
4. Act to decrease inflammation in the lungs

DRUGS THAT ACT ON THE RESPIRATORY CENTER IN THE BRAIN

RESPIRATORY STIMULANTS

carbon dioxide, USP, BP. This gas is used as a respiratory stimulant in the treatment of asphyxia of all types. It is the natural respiratory stimulant because it is actually the increase in carbon dioxide in the blood that influences the respiratory center in the brain to cause the individual to take a breath. The lack of oxygen in the tissues does *not* stimulate respiration. During strenuous exercise more carbon

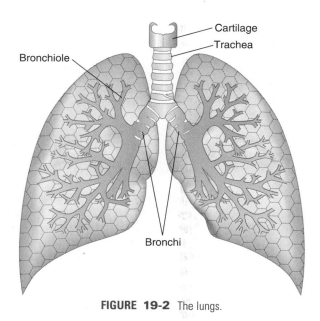

FIGURE 19-2 The lungs.

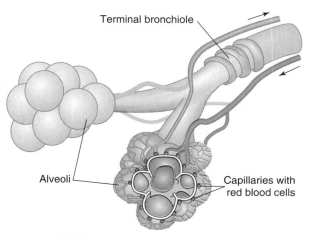

FIGURE 19-3 The terminal respiratory unit.

dioxide is produced, the respiratory center is stimulated, and breathing becomes deeper and more frequent.

doxapram hydrochloride, USP, BP (Dopram). This central nervous system stimulant is used to treat the respiratory depression of chronic obstructive pulmonary disease and, less frequently, neonatal hypoxia. It may also be used to hasten arousal after overdoses of depressant drugs. There is a very narrow margin of safety with this drug, and even small overdoses can lead to convulsions.

Dosage:

Adults and children: (IV) 1 to 2 mg/kg in two initial doses at 5-minute intervals. The dose may be repeated after 1 to 2 hours according to patient response.

RESPIRATORY DEPRESSANTS

The most important of these agents are the central depressants of the opium group (e.g., morphine, codeine) and the barbiturate group (e.g., phenobarbital, secobarbital). Respiratory depression, however, is an undesirable side effect of these drugs. They are not given therapeutically to produce respiratory depression.

DRUGS THAT AFFECT THE MUCOUS MEMBRANE LINING OF THE RESPIRATORY TRACT

Agents in this group are used chiefly to relieve or enable effective coughing. A cough is a reflex action produced by irritation in the upper portion of the respiratory tract. This can be a foreign body (e.g., a particle of food accidentally inhaled), excessive mucus, a malignant growth, and so forth. Treatment of the cough is, of course, only secondary to the treatment of the underlying cause of the cough.

Expectorants are drugs that liquefy the mucus in the bronchi and facilitate the expulsion of sputum. They are used for coughs resulting from the common cold, bronchitis, and pneumonia.

Numerous over-the-counter cough and cold remedies are available, many with the addition of antihistamines or decongestants.

Herb Alert

Red Clover

Red clover is taken internally to treat coughs and respiratory conditions. Externally, it is used for the treatment of chronic skin conditions such as psoriasis and eczema. Red clover exerts a coumarin-like anticoagulant effect; thus it should be used with caution in patients with bleeding disorders or in those taking warfarin, other anticoagulants, or nonsteroidal antiinflammatory drugs. See Chapter 35 for more information on red clover.

Many of the remedies used to treat coughing contain codeine or codeine and morphine derivatives to depress the cough reflex. Suppressing the cough reflex by these agents is desirable in certain circumstances such as a persistent and irritating nonproductive cough.

ASTHMA

Asthma is characterized by variable airflow obstruction and airway hyper-responsiveness. It is a chronic inflammatory disease of the airways in which many inflammatory cell types play a role—in particular, mast cells, eosinophils, and T lymphocytes. In susceptible individuals the inflammation causes recurrent episodes of wheezing, breathlessness, chest tightness, and coughing, particularly at night or in the early morning.

Asthma attacks can be triggered by allergens, physical exertion, and environmental changes, but can also occur with no apparent predisposing event.

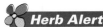

Ephedra (Ma Huang)

The herbal preparation ephedra (not to be confused with the drug ephedrine sulfate) is used to treat colds, asthma, and other respiratory conditions. However, this herb can produce toxic psychosis, life-threatening seizures, tachycardia, hypertension, and heart failure. Life-threatening poisonings occur with very high dosages. It reduces the effects of antihypertensives and the phenothiazines and enhances the effects of theophylline, epinephrine, caffeine, decongestants, and stimulants. Ephedra should be avoided in patients with hypertension, diabetes, psychiatric disorders, and cardiac arrhythmias, and in those taking monoamine oxidase inhibitors. Its use is currently restricted. See Chapter 35 for more information on ephedra.

Pathophysiologic features in the lungs associated with asthma include:
Variable airflow obstruction
Bronchoconstriction
Edema
Airway hyperreactivity
Airway inflammation
Mucus hypersecretion
Impaired mucus clearance
Smooth muscle hypertrophy/hyperplasia
Subendothelial matrix protein deposits
Collagen deposits

ENVIRONMENTAL CONTROL

It is important to educate the patient and his or her family in order to minimize the presence of environmental triggers of asthma.

Allergens bind to mast cells, which in turn release histamine and other allergic and inflammatory mediators. Allergens and noxious agents can cause **bronchoconstriction,** a tightening or narrowing of the lung bronchioles. Control of the environment will assist in lessening these influences.

- Smoke from personal smoking and second-hand smoke should be eliminated, as well as smoke from wood-burning fireplaces.
- Pet dander is a common allergen. Animals should not be present in the home of an asthma patient.
- Dust harbors the dust mite, which is the culprit in triggering asthma.
- Cockroaches should be controlled as much as possible.
- Air filtration and air conditioning should be used to minimize seasonal pollen and mold.
- Seasonal factors should be evaluated, including grass, ragweed, and other plants.
- Occupational concerns must be evaluated. Farmers are around molds and mites in hay and fungal agents in silage. Asbestos, dust, and chemical allergens are implicated. Latex allergies are developing in health care workers and in patients.

- Sports should be chosen that do not involve dusty environments. Swimming is a good sport for asthmatics.

DRUGS THAT AFFECT THE SIZE OF THE BRONCHIOLES

Bronchodilators are agents that dilate, or widen, the bronchioles of the lung by relaxing the smooth muscle of the bronchioles, thus allowing better air exchange.

epinephrine injection, USP, BP (Adrenalin). The rapid action of this drug makes it best for an acute attack. It has a short duration of action, however, so it is not suitable for long-term therapy. It must be given by subcutaneous (subQ) or intravenous (IV) injection. A rapid heart rate and an acute rise in blood pressure may be observed after administration; thus caution must be used when administering this agent.

   Dosage:
      Adults: (subQ, IV) 0.3 mg, often repeated three times at 20-minute intervals.
      Children: (subQ) 0.01 mg/kg as above.

Epinephrine

The elderly often have underlying disorders, such as atherosclerosis and hypertension, that may make them particularly sensitive to the side effects of epinephrine. Tachycardia, premature ventricular contractions, a severe rise in blood pressure, and palpitations may occur after the administration of epinephrine. Cerebrovascular hemorrhage ("stroke" or "brain attack") may occur as a result of a marked increase in blood pressure related to the administration of epinephrine. Administer this drug with extreme caution in older adults.

ephedrine sulfate, USP, BP. Although not as potent as epinephrine, this agent has the added advantages of being active when taken orally and having a longer duration of action. Nervousness and central nervous system stimulation may occur.

   Dosage:
      Adults: (Oral) 25 mg three to four times daily.
      Children: (Oral) 2 to 3 mg/kg/day in four to six divided doses.

terbutaline sulfate, USP, BP (Brethine). Terbutaline has a dilating effect on the smooth muscles of the bronchioles and may be administered for the treatment of acute asthma attacks or chronic obstructive pulmonary disease. Side effects include a rise in blood pressure and heart rate.

   Dosage:
      Adults and children older than 12 years: (Oral) 2.5 mg three to four times daily. (subQ) 0.25 mg with a second dose in 15 to 30 minutes. Other agents should be used if two doses are not effective.

theophylline ethylenediamine (aminophylline), USP, BP. (Theo-24, Theolair, Uniphyl). Various forms of pure theophylline are available commercially. Most of these preparations are designed to prolong theophylline levels in the blood. Although a very effective bronchodilator, this agent has largely been replaced in the treatment of asthma since more effective treatments are available.

The primary side effect is central nervous system stimulation, which may be seen as nervousness, excitation, or tachycardia. Some gastric distress may be produced by oral administration.

Many drugs have interactions with theophylline. It increases the secretion of lithium and may decrease its effectiveness. It may enhance the effects of anticoagulants, cardiac glycosides, ephedrine, and similar sympathomimetic agents.

The dose of theophylline is most accurately controlled by measuring the serum level of the drug. Although texts state that 10 to 20 mcg/mL is generally a safe dose, toxic effects have been noted at levels over 15 mcg/mL.

Dosage:
    Adults: (Oral) 300 to 600 mg two to three times daily. (IV) 500 mg over a 20-minute period. (Rectal) 0.25 to 0.5 gm two to three times daily. Children: (Oral, IV) Initial dose: 5 to 7.5 mg/kg; subsequent administration: 20 to 24 mg/kg/day in divided doses.

albuterol sulfate, USP, BP (Proventil). Albuterol is indicated for the relief of bronchospasm in adults and children older than 2 years with reversible airway obstructive disease. It should be used with caution in patients with coronary disease, because it may have a cardiovascular stimulatory effect.

Dosage:
    Adults: (Oral) 2 to 4 mg four times daily. Children: (Oral) 0.1 mg/kg, increased to 0.2 mg/kg three times daily.

DRUGS THAT DECREASE INFLAMMATION IN THE LUNGS

Asthma is now understood to be an inflammatory condition, rather than a simple constriction of the smooth muscles of the bronchial tree. Current evidence indicates that asthma is a chronic inflammatory disorder of the airways, involving the production of leukotriene and other mediators. Antiinflammatory medications are an essential part of the management of asthma.

montelukast sodium (Singulair). Montelukast is indicated for the prevention of asthma. It is not to be used for the reversal of bronchospasm during attacks. It is to be taken daily even when the patient is asymptomatic. The patient must be advised to have appropriate rescue medications available for an attack.

Dosage:
    Adults: (Oral) 10 mg daily in the evening.
    Children 6 to 12 years: (Oral) 5 mg daily in the evening.
    Children 2 to 5 years: (Oral) 4 mg daily in the evening.

zafirlukast (Accolate). Also used for the prevention of asthma, this agent may be used daily and in some cases may be considered an alternative to daily inhaled corticosteroids or cromolyn. The patient should be advised that zafirlukast will not provide immediate relief from bronchospasm, but it should be continued during an attack along with other rescue medications.

Dosage:
    Adults: (Oral) 20 mg twice daily.
    Children 7 to 12 years: (Oral) 10 mg twice daily.

zileuton (Zyflo). Unlike many other agents used in the treatment of asthma, this agent is an antinflammatory drug. It inhibits the synthesis of leukotriene, an inflammatory mediator. It is used for the prevention and long-term treatment of asthma.

Dosage:
    Adults and children older than 12 years: (Oral) 600 mg 4 times daily.

ADMINISTRATION OF DRUGS BY INHALATION

Various drugs may be administered by inhalation directly to the respiratory tract to exert local bronchodilator or antiiflammatory effects. These agents may be used in the treatment of asthma or chronic obstructive pulmonary diseases such as emphysema.

The availability of metered-dose oral aerosols has simplified the dosing of oral inhalants. The inhaled dose is generally given in terms of the commercially available aerosols. If greater depth within the respiratory tract is desired, the drugs may be administered under pressure by means of an intermittent positive-pressure breathing machine. Respiratory therapists generally monitor the use of these machines. The settings may be varied to obtain the desired pressure (usually 15 to 20 cm of water). The patient should breathe slowly and must be observed for side effects of the drugs, such as nausea, vomiting, dizziness, and tachycardia. Hand-held nebulizers are useful as well.

BRONCHODILATORS

metaproterenol sulfate inhaler, USP, BP (Alupent, Metaprel). When inhaled, this agent produces a direct bronchodilator effect. It is used in the treatment of asthma and emphysema.

Dosage:
    Adults only: (Inhalation) 2 to 3 inhalations (0.65 mg/spray) every 3 to 4 hours. Total daily dosage should not exceed 12 inhalations.

albuterol, USP, BP (Proventil, Ventolin). The onset of action occurs within 15 minutes by aerosol compared with 30 minutes by the oral route. Duration of action is 3 to 4 hours.

> **Dosage:**
> Adults and children older than 12 years: (Inhalation) 2 inhalations (90 mcg/spray) every 4 to 6 hours.

terbutaline sulfate (Brethaire, Bricanyl). The onset of action of this drug is within 5 to 30 minutes and it has a duration of 3 to 6 hours.

> **Dosage:**
> Adults and children older than 12 years: (Inhalation) 2 inhalations (0.2 mg/spray) 60 seconds apart every 4 to 6 hours.

bitolterol mesylate (Tornalate). The onset of action is within 3 to 4 minutes and it will last 5 to 6 hours.

> **Dosage:**
> Adults and children older than 12 years: (Inhalation) 2 inhalations (0.37 mg/spray) 1 to 3 minutes apart every 8 hours.

pirbuterol acetate (Maxair) The onset of improvement is generally within 5 minutes after inhalation.

> **Dosage:**
> Adults and children older than 12 years: (Inhalation) 2 puffs (400 mcg) every 4 to 6 hours.

salmeterol xinafoate (Serevent). Salmeterol is a long-acting bronchodilator used for the prevention of bronchospasm, including exercise-induced bronchospasm. It is administered by oral inhalation; some improvement occurs within 20 minutes, with maximum improvement in 2 hours. It is not intended for use in the treatment of acute asthma attacks, but is used in the long-term maintenance treatment of asthma.

> **Dosage:**
> Adults and children older than 12 years: (Inhalation) 2 inhalations (50 mcg) twice daily.

salmeterol (Serevent Diskus). This form of salmeterol provides the drug in a patented delivery system. The drug is provided in powder form, and each blister on the package contains a dose of the drug.

> **Dosage:**
> Adults and children over 4 years: (Inhalation) 1 dosage unit (50 mcg) twice daily.

formoterol fumarate (Foradil). Formoterol is a long-acting bronchodilator with maximum improvement generally occurring in 1 to 3 hours, with improvement noted for 12 hours. It should not be used to treat acute asthma symptoms, but is used twice daily in the maintenance treatment of asthma and to prevent exercise-induced asthma. The drug is

supplied in the form of a dry powder, intended for use only with its supplied inhaler.

> **Dosage:**
> Adults and children older than 5 years: (Inhalation) 1 dosage unit (the contents of one 12-mcg capsule) every 12 hours.

ANTIINFLAMMATORY AGENTS
Corticosteroids

The corticosteroids are often used for their effect on the respiratory tract, especially in severe asthma attacks. They are used increasingly in the treatment of asthma, particularly by inhalation. When inhaled, they decrease the number and activity of inflammatory cells in the lung tissue, and they act to increase the effects of the bronchodilators, and prevent narrowing of the smooth muscles of the airway. Corticosteroids are discussed further in Chapter 27 (The Endocrine Glands and Hormones).

beclomethasone dipropionate, USP, BP (Beclovent Oral Inhaler). This corticosteroid preparation does not directly relax the bronchioles but acts as an antiinflammatory to aid in the treatment of asthma. It is not used in the primary treatment of asthma because, like all the steroids, it exerts its effect slowly and is generally more useful for its sustained effect.

> **Dosage:**
> Adults: (Inhalation) 2 inhalations (42 mcg/spray) three to four times daily. Maximum daily intake should not exceed 10 inhalations.

Children older than 6 years: (Inhalation) 1 to 2 inhalations three to four times daily.

triamcinolone acetonide (Azmacort). Triamcinolone is indicated for the maintenance treatment of asthma in patients who require systemic corticosteroid medication. Adding this inhaler may reduce the need for systemic corticosteroids.

> **Dosage:**
> Adults: (Inhalation) 2 inhalations (200 mcg) three to four times daily.
> Children: (Inhalation) 1 inhalation three to four times daily.

flunisolide nasal solution, USP, BP (Nasalide, Aerobid). Intended for use as a spray to the nasal mucosa, this antiinflammatory corticosteroid reduces the symptoms of rhinitis and swollen nasal mucous membranes resulting from allergic rhinitis. Although relief is generally apparent after a few days of therapy, it may take as long as 2 weeks before a full therapeutic effect is obtained.

> **Dosage:**
> Adults: (Nasal) 2 sprays (250 mcg/spray) in each nostril two times daily.
> Children older than 6 years: (Nasal) 1 spray in each nostril three times daily.

Combination Bronchodilator/Steroid Inhaler

fluticasone propionate plus salmeterol (Advair Diskus). This agent provides a combination of a corticosteroid (fluticasone propionate) and a long-acting bronchodilator (salmeterol). This combination is now thought to be best for routine prophylactic treatment of severe asthmatics. It is available in three strengths. In each form the salmeterol dosage is maintained at 50 mcg, with a variation in the strength of the fluticasone to deliver 100, 250, or 500 mcg/dose. They are labeled as Advair Diskus 100/50, 250/50, and 500/50, respectively.

Dosage:
> Adults and children older than 12 years: (Inhalation) 1 blister-dose as prescribed every 12 hours.

OTHER AGENTS THAT ACT ON THE RESPIRATORY TRACT

acetylcysteine, USP, BP (Mucomyst). A derivative of the amino acid cysteine, this agent is effective by inhalation when the liquefaction of mucous and purulent material is desired. It loosens pulmonary secretions and aids in their removal by postural drainage.

Dosage:
> Adults and children: (Inhalation) 3 to 5 mL of a 10% to 20% solution three to four times daily.

cromolyn sodium, USP, BP (Aarane, Intal). Although ineffective in the treatment of acute asthma, this drug is useful in the prevention of asthma attacks. It is believed to stabilize the membranes of the mast cells, which are responsible for liberating histamine and initiating the allergic reaction.

Dosage:
> Adults and children: (Inhalation) 20 mg four times daily.

CLINICAL IMPLICATIONS

1. An adequate fluid intake is necessary during the treatment of respiratory infections or wheezing to liquefy mucus and aid in its expulsion.
2. Coughing is beneficial in some cases to clear secretions from the respiratory tract. Antitussives are often prescribed if the coughing is excessive or nonproductive.
3. Because coughing is often increased when the patient is lying flat, greater comfort is attained if the patient is placed in a sitting position.
4. Cough preparations, particularly those with codeine or similar drugs, cause drowsiness. The patient should be cautioned against combining cough preparations with self-prescribed antihistamines, because increased central nervous system sedation may result.
5. In patients with severe, chronic respiratory conditions, such as emphysema or late forms of cystic fibrosis, respiration is stimulated by high blood carbon dioxide levels. High levels of oxygen administered suddenly to these patients may result in respiratory arrest and death.
6. Arterial blood gases are useful in monitoring the severity of an acute asthma attack and are often used as a guideline in adjusting the oxygen and the drug dosage necessary for the treatment of asthma.
7. Cyanosis, particularly on the lips and perioral area, is a sign of decreased blood oxygen level. A decrease in cyanosis and less respiratory distress can be used to quickly assess improvement in the patient's condition.
8. Corticosteroids, when administered for asthma, will have many side effects related to the endocrine system.
9. Prevention of asthma by avoiding or minimizing contact with allergens is always advisable.
10. Nursing measures should be directed toward relief of anxiety in patients with respiratory conditions.
11. The patient should be instructed carefully in the use of her or his asthma medications and should be counseled to be compliant with the dosing schedule.

Online Resources

For updated drug information and Web activities, go to http://evolve.elsevier.com/Asperheim.

CRITICAL THINKING QUESTIONS

1. The patient, 6 years old, is brought to the physician's office after his mother noticed he had some trouble breathing after a strenuous soccer game in the backyard. He has had wheezing a few times after playing outside but has never been brought to his doctor for this. What drugs do you think may be prescribed? What may be his problem?

2. The patient reports she had one of her asthmatic spells last night and spent most of the night in a chair. In the office today she has only scattered and minimal wheezing. Her activities yesterday included vigorous spring housecleaning and grooming her three cats for a show. What medications or other advice may be helpful for this patient?

REVIEW QUESTIONS

1. The chief function of the respiratory system is to:
   a. guard against infections.
   b. supply oxygen to tissues and remove carbon dioxide.
   c. supply carbon dioxide to tissues and remove oxygen.
   d. relax the lung bronchioles.

2. Agents that are known to be respiratory depressants include all of the following except:
   a. phenobarbital.
   b. alcohol.
   c. morphine.
   d. doxapram.

3. Asthma may include all symptoms except:
   a. bronchoconstriction.
   b. bronchodilation.
   c. edema.
   d. airway inflammation.

4. A drug that widens the bronchioles of the lung would be:
   a. carbon dioxide.
   b. oxygen.
   c. montelukast.
   d. epinephrine.

5. A side effect of drugs administered by inhalation may be:
   a. dizziness.
   b. sweating.
   c. bradycardia.
   d. inflammatory response.

6. A long-acting bronchodilator used in the treatment of asthma is:
   a. epinephrine.
   b. zafirlukast.
   c. theophylline.
   d. salmeterol.

7. Advair Diskus contains a combination of:
   a. salmeterol and fluticasone.
   b. salmeterol and epinephrine.
   c. acetylcysteine and fluticasone.
   d. cromolyn and salmeterol.

8. A drug that is used to liquefy thick mucus in the lungs is:
   a. salmeterol.
   b. triamcinolone.
   c. acetylcysteine.
   d. cromolyn.

9. Cyanosis, when observed in an asthma patient, may be a sign of:
   a. increased response to the asthma medication.
   b. increased blood oxygen level.
   c. hypotension.
   d. decreased oxygen level.

10. Respiratory stimulants act on receptors in the:
    a. lining of the lungs.
    b. alveoli.
    c. bronchial tree.
    d. brain.

Objectives

After completing this chapter, you should be able to do the following:

1. Discuss the ways drugs may affect the heart.
2. Identify digitalis preparations.
3. State the action of digitalis.
4. List side effects of digitalis toxicity.
5. Explain the action of antiarrhythmic agents.
6. Explain the action of vasoconstrictors.
7. Explain the action of vasodilators.
8. Identify drugs used to hasten the process of coagulation.
9. Discuss the uses of anticoagulants.
10. Identify the specific antidote for an overdose of sodium heparin.
11. Identify the specific antidote for an overdose of sodium warfarin.
12. Discuss nursing responsibilities related to care of patients taking cardiovascular drugs.
13. Identify the classes of antihypertensive drugs and the general mechanism of action.
14. Become familiar with side effects of antihypertensive drugs.
15. Understand the role of platelets in cardiovascular complications.
16. Identify drugs used in antiplatelet therapy.
17. Identify drugs used as thrombolytic agents.
18. Identify drugs used in antilipidemic therapy.

Key Terms

ACE inhibitors, p. 89
Anticoagulants (ăn-tĭ-kō-ĂG-ū-lănts), p. 95
Antidote (ĂN-tĭ-dōt), p. 88
Antilipidemic (ăn-tĭ-LĬP-ĭ-DĒ-mĭk) **drugs,** p. 98
Antiplatelet (ăn-tĭ-PLĀT-lĭt) **agents,** p. 97
Coagulants (kō-ĂG-ū-lănts), p. 94
Congestive heart failure, p. 89
Diuretics (dī-ū-RĔT-ĭks), p. 90
Inotropic (ĬN-ō-TRŎP-ĭk) **drug,** p. 88
Thrombolytic (THRŎM-bō-LĬT-ĭk) **therapy,** p. 97
Vasoconstrictors (văs-ō-kŏn-STRĬK-tŏrs), p. 92
Vasodilators (văs-ō-DĪ-lă-tŏrs), p. 92

The circulatory system includes the heart and all the blood vessels (Figure 20–1).

The heart is a hollow, muscular organ that is roughly cone shaped; it is situated near the center of the thoracic cavity, in close relation to the lungs. It is divided by partitions (septa) into four chambers: the right and left atria and the right and left ventricles. The left ventricular wall is about twice the thickness of the right ventricular wall because the work the left ventricle must perform is much greater than that performed by the right ventricle.

In normal circulation of blood throughout the body, the oxygenated blood comes into the left atrium from the lungs and passes into the left ventricle upon contraction of the atrium. The ventricle contracts shortly after the atrium, and the blood is forced into the aorta, which branches into other

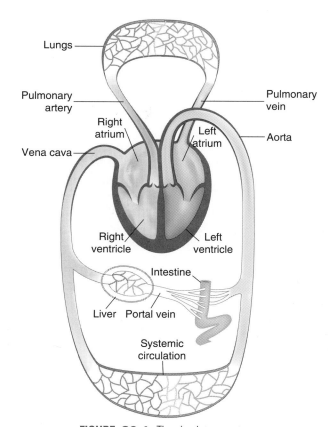

FIGURE 20-1 The circulatory system.

major arteries. The blood is then carried to the gastrointestinal tract, liver, and capillary beds in the systemic circuit. In this capillary region the objectives of circulation are fulfilled: Oxygen and nutritive materials are carried to the tissues, and carbon dioxide and waste products are carried away.

The venous capillaries merge to form larger veins; the blood returns to the heart via the vena cava and enters the right atrium. Contraction of the atrium forces blood into the right ventricle; the ventricle's subsequent contraction forces the blood to the lungs, where it is oxygenated and then returned again to the left atrium to begin the cycle anew.

DRUGS THAT AFFECT THE HEART

Cardiac drugs may affect (1) the heart rate, (2) the rhythm of the heartbeat, (3) the amount of output of blood, or (4) the strength of contraction. In general, there are three main conditions for which the cardiac drugs are used: heart failure, myocardial infarction, and arrhythmias.

HEART FAILURE

Heart failure means that the heart, for one reason or another, is not circulating blood at a satisfactory rate. When a person is in good health, the heart accomplishes the circulation of blood without faltering. Thus it does not allow an abnormal amount of blood to accumulate in the veins of the body, in the chambers of the heart, or in the lungs. The rate of flow is sufficient to provide a normal pressure in the systemic arteries and the veins in the vascular bed of the lungs.

A diseased heart may have such a handicap that it is unable to move the blood satisfactorily. If this defect is moderate, it may occur only during physical exertion (e.g., running or climbing stairs). Under these circumstances, the muscles of the legs need a faster moving bloodstream because of their greater workload. If, by reason of a mechanical handicap (such as leaking or constricted valves), the heart cannot increase its output to meet the demands of the muscles, the body will suffer from the inadequacy. The same is true when the heart is weak because of a diseased condition of its fibers.

The following changes may take place during a period of heart failure:
- The capillaries and all veins contain more than the normal amount of blood.
- The hydrostatic pressure is greater than normal in these areas, forcing fluid into the lungs and body tissues.
- The blood in the periphery retains more carbon dioxide and waste products.
- The blood has less oxygen combined with hemoglobin.
- Respiration in the lungs may be so reduced that the blood pumped into the aorta may contain more carbon dioxide and less oxygen than it should.
- Cyanosis, or bluish discoloration of the skin and mucous membranes, may be present.

- Edema, or swelling caused by abnormal accumulation of fluid in tissues, may occur.

Several classes of drugs are used in the treatment of heart failure. They are often used in combination. An **inotropic drug** (a drug that increases the contractility of the heart), such as digoxin, may be combined with an angiotensin-converting enzyme (ACE) inhibitor, a beta-blocker, and/or a diuretic.

INOTROPIC DRUGS

All inotropic drugs increase the contractility of the myocardium. Digitalis was the first inotropic drug identified and used. The crude digitalis leaf is no longer used because of problems with its standardization. The synthetic form, digoxin, is used exclusively at the present time in oral, intramuscular (IM), and intravenous (IV) formulations.

 Considerations for Older Adults

Digitalis Preparations

Calcium salts, such as calcium carbonate (Os-Cal) and calcium citrate (Citracal), should be used cautiously, if at all, by patients receiving cardiac glycosides (digitalis preparations). The inotropic and toxic effects of cardiac glycosides and calcium are synergistic, and arrhythmias may occur if these drugs are given together. Also, avoid IV administration of calcium in these patients.

digoxin, USP, BP (Lanoxin). The most important action of digoxin on the heart is the strengthening of the heart musculature. The digitalized fibers contract more vigorously and enable the heart to empty more completely. The result is an increase in the amount of blood propelled with any contraction of the ventricles.

The efficiency of the heart is also improved by the slowing of the rate of contraction. This is a desired effect of digoxin, but in overdose the excessive slowing of the heart becomes an untoward effect. The dosage of digoxin should be adjusted so that the pulse remains in the normal range of 60 to 80 beats/minute. Excessive doses of digitalis depress the heart rate still further; therefore, the pulse must always be taken before administering a dose. If the pulse is below 60 beats/minute, the medication should not be given.

Early side effects that warn of overdose of digoxin are nausea, vomiting, and visual disturbances (objects appear brighter than they actually are; green objects may appear almost white). At this point the digoxin dosage is usually decreased or the drug is discontinued for a few days. A lethal dose of digoxin causes death by stopping the heart. The **antidote** (that is, the substance that neutralizes the effects) for digoxin is digoxin immune Fab.

Dosage:
Adults: (Oral, IM, IV) Digitalizing dosage: 8 to 15 mg/kg/day; maintenance, 0.125 to 0.5 mg/day.

Children: (Oral, IM, IV) Digitalizing dosage: 20 to 35 mcg/kg/day; maintenance, 20% to 30% of the digitalizing dosage.

digoxin immune Fab (Digibind). This agent is an antidote for life-threatening digoxin poisoning. It is composed of antigen-binding fragments (Fab) derived from antidigoxin antibodies produced in sheep serum.

Dosage:

(IV) Highly variable, based on the number of tablets ingested and the serum level of digoxin. Tables for dosage calculation are available with the drug literature.

ACE INHIBITORS

Agents that inhibit the angiotensin-converting enzyme have become more important in the treatment of **congestive heart failure,** a condition in which the heart is unable to circulate blood satisfactorily. The benefits that these agents provide for patients with congestive failure have been demonstrated for all levels of left ventricular dysfunction. **ACE inhibitors** are the agents of choice to use for congestive failure, in combination with other agents such as digoxin, thrombolytic agents, aspirin, beta-blockers, and/or nitrites. Their exact mode of action in the treatment of congestive failure is still being debated. They appear to minimize or prevent the left ventricular dilation or dysfunction following a myocardial infarction.

The ACE inhibitors are also used in the treatment of hypertension (blood pressure persistently exceeding 140/90 mm Hg). The ACE enzyme is important in the development of hypertension because it enables angiotensin I (a precursor) to be converted to angiotensin II. Angiotensin II is a vasoconstrictor, meaning that it causes narrowing of the blood vessels, which will increase blood pressure. Inhibiting the production of angiotensin II assists in the treatment of hypertension.

The annoying side effect of a chronic nonproductive cough occurs in a significant percentage of patients. If not severe, it may be simply tolerated for the beneficial effects that the drug has on the heart and blood vessels. When severe, it will be necessary to discontinue the drug. The cough will persist for up to 4 weeks after the drug is discontinued. The other notable side effect, angioedema, is a serious, though infrequent, side effect and is always a reason for discontinuing these agents.

ACE Inhibitors Used in the Treatment of Heart Failure and Hypertension

lisinopril (Prinivil, Zestril)
Dosage for heart failure:
Adults: (Oral) 2.5 mg initially, increased to 10 to 30 mg/day.
Dosage for hypertension:
Adults only: (Oral) 10 to 40 mg daily in one dose.

captopril (Capoten)
Dosage for heart failure:
Adults: (Oral) 6.25 mg three times a day to 25 to 75 mg.

Dosage for hypertension:
Adults only: (Oral) 25 to 50 mg three times daily.

enalapril (Vasotec)
Dosage for heart failure:
Adults: (Oral) 5 mg daily, increased to 10 to 20 mg twice a day.
Dosage for hypertension:
Adults only: (Oral) 5 to 40 mg daily in one or two divided doses.

ACE Inhibitors Used in the Treatment of Hypertension

These agents are used for adults only; no children's dosages have been established.

benazepril (Lotensin)
Dosage:
(Oral) 10 to 40 mg in one or two divided doses daily.

quinapril (Accupril)
Dosage:
(Oral) 10 to 80 mg daily in one or two divided doses.

ramipril (Altace)
Dosage:
(Oral) 2.5 to 20 mg once daily.

fosinopril sodium (Monopril)
Dosage:
(Oral) 10 to 80 mg once daily.

perindopril erbumine (Aceon)
Dosage:
(Oral) 4 to 16 mg once daily.

trandolapril (Mavik)
Dosage:
(Oral) 1 to 4 mg once daily.

moexipril hydrochloride (Univasc)
Dosage:
(Oral) 7.5 to 30 mg once daily.

ANGIOTENSIN II RECEPTOR BLOCKERS

These agents are used for patients who cannot tolerate the ACE inhibitors. They also reduce left ventricular dilation or dysfunction after a myocardial infarction but do so less effectively than the ACE inhibitors. As the name implies, they inhibit the effect of angiotensin II by blocking the receptors for the enzyme. They can be used alone or in combination with a diuretic to treat hypertension; only valsartan is approved for treatment of heart failure, although the others are probably effective.

There is a low incidence of side effects to these agents. The listed side effects include a skin rash, facial edema, insomnia, and myalgia.

losartan (Cozaar)
> **Dosage:**
> Adults: (Oral) 25 to 50 mg daily.

candesartan cilexetil (Atacand)
> **Dosage:**
> Adults: (Oral) 8 to 32 mg daily.

irbesartan (Avapro)
> **Dosage:**
> Adults: (Oral) 150 mg daily.

olmesartan (Benicar)
> **Dosage:**
> Adults: (Oral) 20 to 40 mg daily.

eprosartan mesylate (Teveten)
> **Dosage:**
> Adults: (Oral) 600 to 800 mg in one or two divided doses.

valsartan (Diovan)
> **Dosage for hypertension:**
> Adults: (Oral) 80 to 120 mg once daily.
> **Dosage for heart failure:**
> Adults: (Oral) 40 mg twice daily.

telmisartan (Micardis)
> **Dosage:**
> Adults: (Oral) 40 to 80 mg once daily.

ALDOSTERONE INHIBITORS

Although these agents are helpful in the treatment of congestive heart failure when the preceding two classes of drugs are not tolerated, they cannot be used if the patient has hyperkalemia or reduced renal function. This class can also be used in the treatment of hypertension.

spironolactone (Aldactone)
> **Dosage:**
> Adult (Oral) 25 mg/day.

DIURETICS

Diuretics (drugs that promote the formation and excretion of urine) are used in the treatment of heart failure and in the treatment of hypertension to reduce fluid overload. The symptoms of orthopnea and dyspnea are reduced with treatment. Recording of daily weight changes also is helpful to monitor fluid retention. Diuretics are most helpful in combination with other agents. Furosemide (Lasix) at a dosage of 50 to 200 mg daily, metolazone (Zaroxolyn) at a dosage of 2.5 mg daily,

or hydrochlorothiazide (Hydro-Diuril) at a dosage of 50 mg daily may be used. The dosages are later adjusted as the condition improves.

MYOCARDIAL INFARCTION

Beta-blockers have been recommended for some time for patients who have had myocardial infarctions. The benefit is greatest in those with reduced ejection fractions. Increased survival rates and decreased hospitalizations have long been noted when beta-blockers are added. They are also used alone or in combination with other agents to treat hypertension.

Beta-Blockers Used to Treat Myocardial Infarction and Hypertension

amiodarone hydrochloride (Cordarone, Pacerone)
> **Dosage for infarction:**
> Adults: (Oral) 400 to 800 mg daily. (IV) 50 mg by slow infusion; dosage up to 1000 mg/day.
> **Dosage for hypertension:**
> Children: (Oral, IV) 5 to 15 mg/kg/day.

carvedilol (Coreg)
> **Dosage for infarction:**
> Adults: (Oral) 6.25 mg twice a day.

acebutolol hydrochloride (Sectral)
> **Dosage for infarction:**
> Adults: (Oral) 200 to 400 mg daily.

propranolol hydrochloride (Inderal)
> **Dosage for infarction:**
> Adults: (Oral) 10 to 30 mg three times a day.
> **Dosage for hypertension:**
> Adults: (Oral) Dosages are highly individualized and range from 40 to 160 mg/day. The maximum allowable dosage is 640 mg/day. The long-acting tablets facilitate once-daily dosing.
> Children: (Oral only): 2 to 4 mg/kg/day in two divided doses.

atenolol (Tenormin)
> **Dosage for acute infarction:**
> Adults: (IV) 5 mg over 5 minutes, followed by another 5-mg injection 5 minutes later.
> **Dosage for hypertension:**
> Adults only (Oral) 50 to 200 mg once daily.

Beta-Blockers Used to Treat Hypertension

metoprolol (Toprol, Toprol-XL)
> **Dosage:**
> Adults: (Oral) 100 to 400 mg once daily.

nadolol (Corgard)
> **Dosage:**
> Adults: (Oral) 40 to 240 mg once daily.

timolol maleate (Blocadren)
   Dosage:
      Adults only: (Oral) 10 mg one to two times daily to
      a total daily dose of 40 mg.

betaxolol (Kerlone)
   Dosage:
      Adults: (Oral) 10 to 20 mg once daily.

labetalol (Normodyne, Trandate)
   Dosage:
      Adults: (Oral) 100 to 400 mg in one or two divided
      doses.

CARDIAC ARRHYTHMIAS

The rate of heartbeat and rhythm of the heart are controlled
by the sinoatrial (SA) node, known as the "pacemaker," in
the right atrium. This node generates tiny electrical impulses
to the adjacent muscle of the atria, causing the atria to contract and pump blood into the ventricles.

The impulses sent out by the SA node are received by the
atrioventricular (AV) node, travel down the bundle of His,
and are transported to the ventricular muscles by a network
of nerves. The ventricles contract shortly after the atria. The
SA node as well as the AV node receives autonomic innerva-
tion that controls the rate of the heart to a certain extent.

Any deviation from the normal orderly sequence is a
disturbance of the rhythm and is called an *arrhythmia*.
Sometimes an area of muscle in one of the atria becomes
more excitable than the SA node and fires more rapid
impulses. The rest of the heart then responds to this new
pacemaker, and the resulting arrhythmia is known as atrial
tachycardia.

Such a new focus may discharge impulses at extremely
rapid rates of 180 to 250 impulses per minute. The atria,
instead of beating in unison, are swept by wave upon wave of
contraction and relaxation known as atrial fibrillation.
When fibrillation occurs, the AV node is literally bombarded
with impulses and is unable to let them all through. The
result is that the ventricles, which are the more important
chambers, are irregularly stimulated and, consequently, beat
less efficiently.

Drugs Used to Treat Arrhythmias

quinidine sulfate, USP, BP. This drug is used to decrease the
number of times the atrial muscle can contract in a given
period of time; hence, it is used to treat atrial fibrillation. It
is administered orally or intravenously.
   Dosage:
      Adults: (Oral, IV) 200 to 400 mg three to four times
      daily for 1 to 3 days.
      Children: No standard dosage is established.

procainamide hydrochloride, USP, BP (Pronestyl).
Although also effective in atrial fibrillation, this drug is used
more commonly in ventricular arrhythmias in which premature contractions occur. Generally, it is administered
orally or intravenously.
   Dosage:
      Adults: (Oral) 50 mg/kg/day in divided doses every
      3 hours. (IM) 50 mg/kg/day in divided doses every
      3 to 6 hours. (IV) 50 to 100 mg every 5 minutes, or
      a loading dose of 500 to 600 mg may be given.
      Children: (Oral) 40 to 60 mg/kg/day in divided
      doses. (IV) 2 to 5 mg/kg; repeat in 10 to 30 minutes.

lidocaine hydrochloride, USP, BP (Xylocaine). When
administered intravenously, lidocaine has been shown to be
extremely effective in controlling and preventing ventricular
fibrillation. The drug must be administered by a physician
and must be monitored carefully with electrocardiographic
tracings. It is often used in cardiac intensive care units, particularly in patients who have recently had a severe myocardial infarction, to prevent arrhythmias. Side effects of
lidocaine primarily affect the central nervous system and
include drowsiness, disorientation, confusion, visual disturbances, and, very rarely, convulsions or coma.
   Dosage:
      Adults: (IV) 50 to 100 mg at a rate of 25 to
      50 mg/minute. Maximum dosage per hour is 300
      mg. Prophylactic intravenous infusions are admin-
      istered to deliver a dosage of 1 to 4 mg/minute.
      Children: (IV) Bolus of 0.5 to 1 mg/kg; mainte-
      nance infusions: 10 to 50 mcg/kg/minute.

propranolol hydrochloride, USP, BP (Inderal). Propranolol
is an antiarrhythmic agent that exerts its influence by blocking the effect of circulating norepinephrine on the
myocardium of the heart. It is used for the treatment of life-
threatening arrhythmias, generally in an intensive care unit.
By blocking the receptor sites for norepinephrine, this agent
reduces cardiac irritability. It is used to treat and prevent
atrial flutter and fibrillation and to control extrasystoles.
Side effects include nausea, vomiting, diarrhea, skin rash,
hallucinations, and blood disorders.
   Dosage:
      Adults: (Oral) 10 to 30 mg three times daily. (IV)
      For life-threatening arrhythmias, 1 to 3 mg admin-
      istered slowly at a rate not over 1 mg/minute.
      Children: No children's dosage has been established.

disopyramide phosphate, USP, BP (Norpace). The antiarrhythmic activity of this agent is similar to that of quinidine
and procainamide in the treatment of arrhythmias.
   Dosage:
      Adults only: (Oral) 100 to 150 mg every 6 hours.

nadolol, USP, BP (Corgard). This beta-blocking agent has a
mechanism of action similar to that of propranolol. It is
used to prevent arrhythmias as well as to treat hypertension.
   Dosage:
      Adults only: (Oral) 40 mg once daily, increased as
      necessary to 320 mg daily.

sotalol hydrochloride (Betapace)

Dosage:

Adults: (Oral) 80 to 320 mg daily in two divided doses

amiodarone (Cordarone, Pacerone)

Dosage:

Adults: (Oral, IV) Loading dose of 800 to 1600 mg daily; maintenance dose of 600 to 800 mg once daily.

DRUGS THAT AFFECT THE BLOOD VESSELS

Abnormal conditions affecting the arteries, arterioles, capillaries, and veins are many in number and variety. Drugs may be used to increase or decrease the size of the blood vessels and thus affect the flow of blood through them.

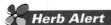 **Herb Alert**

Horse Chestnut

The seeds and leaves of the horse chestnut tree have been used to treat lower extremity edema caused by venous insufficiency. However, this herb enhances the effect of coumarin and must be used cautiously in patients with bleeding disorders, those taking warfarin or other anticoagulants, and those taking nonsteroidal antiinflammatory drugs. Also, long-term use may cause liver and kidney damage. See Chapter 35 for more information on horse chestnut.

VASOCONSTRICTORS

Vasoconstrictors bring about constriction of the muscle fibers in the walls of the blood vessels, either by direct action on the vessels or by stimulation of the vasomotor center in the medulla. They may be used to (1) stop superficial hemorrhage, (2) relieve nasal congestion, (3) raise the blood pressure, or (4) increase the force of heart action.

epinephrine injection, USP, BP; epinephrine solution, USP (Adrenalin). The chief use of epinephrine is to constrict peripheral blood vessels by local application. It is commonly used in the eye for this purpose. Although used to control bleeding from capillaries or small arteries, it does not stop bleeding from a larger vessel.

Given parenterally, epinephrine produces powerful vasoconstriction, which, in turn, causes a marked rise in blood pressure. The heart is stimulated as well, which also contributes to the rise in blood pressure. The peak of this elevation is rarely sustained for more than a few minutes, and the blood pressure returns to normal limits usually within one-half hour after the dose has been given. Because of this transitory action, epinephrine is not the agent of choice when a gradual, sustained elevation of blood pressure is desired. It is quite effective in emergency situations, however. When used

with local anesthetics, the vasoconstricting properties prolong the action of the anesthetic.

Dosage:

Adults: (subQ) 0.3 mg.

Children: (subQ) 0.01 mg/kg.

midodrine hydrochloride (ProAmatine). Midodrine is indicated for the treatment of symptomatic orthostatic hypotension. Because it can cause elevation of supine blood pressure, its use should be restricted to the most severely affected individuals. It is contraindicated in severe organic heart disease, acute renal disease, urinary retention, or thyrotoxicosis.

Dosage:

Adults only: (Oral) 10 mg three times daily.

VASODILATORS

Vasodilators cause the blood vessels to relax or increase in diameter and thereby play a part in the treatment of peripheral vascular diseases, heart conditions, and hypertension. Many vasodilators are used currently.

The Nitrites

These agents cause relaxation of the muscle fibers in the walls of the blood vessels. The relaxation increases the width of the vessels and lowers the pressure of the blood flow through the mucous membranes of the mouth, stomach, or lungs. Many times the tablets are prescribed to be dissolved under the tongue rather than swallowed.

One of the chief uses of the nitrites is in the treatment of angina pectoris (a painful condition caused by spasm of the coronary vessels). The nitrites are also used to relax the smooth muscle spasm in bronchial asthma, to relieve cramps, and to treat hypertension.

glyceryl trinitrate, USP (nitroglycerin). This drug is used in the form of small soluble tablets that are dissolved under the tongue to prevent or relieve attacks.

Dosage:

Adults: (Sublingual) 0.4 mg as necessary.

Children: No standard dosage has been established.

topical nitroglycerin (transdermal systems) (Minitran, Transderm Nitro, Nitro-Dur, Nitrodisc). These transdermal patches should be applied daily to hairless portions of the upper body. The system is designed to last 24 hours.

Dosage:

(Transdermal) Ranges from 0.1 to 0.8 mg/hr.

ANTIHYPERTENSIVE AGENTS

In the United States, about 58 million people suffer from hypertension. Effective treatment of hypertension can reduce the incidence of stroke, myocardial infarction, heart failure, kidney failure, and overall cardiovascular disease, in both morbidity and mortality. Nearly one third of those with hypertension do not take their medication properly, and many stop the medication altogether because of unpleasant side effects. In addition, hypertensive patients, particularly in the early stages of the disease, feel well; thus they have the tendency to take their medication irregularly or not at all. From the patient's point of view, the treatment often seems worse than the illness.

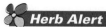

Herb Alert

Garlic

Garlic has been widely promoted for treatment of high cholesterol and high blood pressure. Although it has shown some effectiveness in lowering cholesterol and triglyceride levels and raising high-density lipoprotein (HDL, "good" cholesterol) levels, studies have not shown any impact on lowering blood pressure. Garlic interferes with platelet adhesiveness and thus enhances the antiplatelet effects of nonsteroidal antiinflammatory drugs and warfarin. It also reduces blood sugar levels. See Chapter 35 for more information on garlic.

Lifestyle changes, such as weight reduction, increased exercise, and limiting alcohol and sodium intake, are usually the first treatment options that physicians give their patients. If lifestyle changes do not work, then single-drug therapy is used, beginning with a low dose and gradually titrating upward. Combination drug therapy is used often to reach the target blood pressure, generally in the range of no higher than 120/80 mm Hg.

Although diastolic blood pressure was formerly thought to be the important number to consider when treating the patient, systolic blood pressure is emerging as a more important criterion for diagnosis and decision making, particularly in the middle-aged or older adult who has hypertension. It has been noted that 65% of hypertensive patients older than 60 years have isolated systolic hypertension, defined as a systolic blood pressure over 140 mm Hg with a diastolic pressure under 90 mm Hg. It is now recommended that these patients be treated until the target systolic pressure of 120 is attained. The old-fashioned rule of thumb that an appropriate systolic pressure is "100 plus your age" is incorrect.

The vast majority of patients have "essential" hypertension—that is, no cause is identified. Organic causes of hypertension include renal artery stenosis or other renal abnormalities, pregnancy, use of oral contraceptives, and estrogen replacement therapy.

Several classes of drugs used in the treatment of hypertension are also used to treat cardiovascular disease and were previously discussed. Following are some agents that are used just for hypertension.

Central Alpha Agonists

These agents generally stimulate central alpha-adrenergic receptors, resulting in a decreased sympathetic outflow from the brain to the peripheral circulatory system.

clonidine hydrochloride, USP, BP (Catapres). This agent has a rapid onset of activity, with lowering of blood pressure within 30 to 60 minutes after an oral dose. Dry mouth and drowsiness are the most common side effects.

In addition to its use as an antihypertensive agent, this drug has been found helpful in controlling impulsivity in the hyperactive child or child with attention deficit hyperactivity disorder. It has been used when methylphenidate (Ritalin) has not been helpful with these children. Clonidine, unlike methylphenidate, does not seem to improve school performance and may need to be combined with methylphenidate in some cases. This indication is still under study.

Dosage:
Adults: (Oral) 0.1 to 0.3 mg every 12 hours.
Children: No standard dosage has been established.

clonidine (Catapres TTS). This transdermal delivery system consists of patches of clonidine that may be applied and are effective for 1 week of therapy. The patches are noted as Catapres-TTSB1, B2, or B3 to deliver 0.1, 0.2, or 0.3 mg daily transdermally, respectively.

Alpha-Blockers

The agents in this group are believed to work through blockade of the postsynaptic alpha-adrenergic receptors. This causes a vasodilator effect and a lowering of peripheral resistance. It is usually not accompanied by an increased heart rate. All are given to adults only; no children's dosages have been established.

prazosin hydrochloride (Minipress). Prazosin is generally well tolerated and effective orally, with few systemic side effects after treatment is established. Its most notable problem is the "first-dose effect," a sudden, severe postural hypotension and a sudden syncopal episode or "drop attack." This occurs in a very small percentage of patients and is generally avoided by stressing that the first dose should be taken after the patient has gotten into bed for the night. The drug is generally begun with a lower dose, then titrated upward.

Dosage:
Adults only: (Oral) 1 to 5 mg three times daily to a maximum of 20 mg/day.

terazosin hydrochloride (Hytrin). Action and effects are similar to those of prazosin, including the first-dose effect of postural hypotension. The drug is initiated with a low dose and then slowly titrated upward.

Dosage:
Adults only: (Oral) 1 mg once daily initially; maximum dosage 20 mg daily.

doxazosin mesylate (Cardura). Action and effects are similar to those of prazosin, including the first-dose effect.

Dosage:
Adults only: (Oral) 1 to 16 mg daily in one dose.

The Calcium Channel Blockers

This class of antihypertensive agents acts by blocking the entry of extracellular calcium ions into the myocardial and vascular smooth muscle cells. This leads to reduced cardiac output and reduced total peripheral resistance, with a subsequent reduction in blood pressure. They are also effective for angina pectoris, supraventricular arrhythmias, and cardiomyopathy.

General Considerations

Calcium Channel Blockers

Calcium channel blockers should not be taken with grapefruit juice, which increases the effects of these medications, sometimes resulting in symptoms of overdose. The interaction appears to occur because of an inhibition of the cytochrome P-450 enzyme system by some constituent in the juice. Other juices, such as orange juice, do not have this effect.

nifedipine, USP, BP (Procardia, Adalat). This agent is particularly effective in managing hypertension in patients with coexisting angina or peripheral vascular disease. Hypotension, dizziness, and nausea are included in its side effects.

> **Dosage:**
> Adults: (Oral) 10 mg three times daily. As extended-release capsules, 30 to 60 mg once daily.
> Children: No standard dosage has been established.

verapamil hydrochloride, USP, BP (Calan, Isoptin). This agent is used for hypertension, angina, and tachyarrhythmias. Bradycardia, heart block, and constipation are included in its side effects.

> **Dosage:**
> Adults: (Oral) 120 to 240 mg daily; maximum dosage 480 mg/day. (IV) 0.075 to 0.2 mg/kg, repeated once in 30 minutes.
> Children: (IV) 0.1 to 0.3 mg/kg, repeated in 30 minutes.

diltiazem hydrochloride, USP, BP (Cardizem). This agent is used in hypertension and angina pectoris. Nausea, dizziness, and bradycardia are among its side effects.

> **Dosage:**
> Adults only: (Oral) 60 to 180 mg twice daily.

amlodipine besylate (Norvasc, Lotrel). Amlodipine may be used alone or in combination with other agents for the treatment of hypertension. Its side effects are similar to those of the other agents in this class.

> **Dosage:**
> Adults only: (Oral) 2.5 to 5 mg once daily.

felodipine (Plendil)
> **Dosage:**
> Adults only: (Oral) 5 to 10 mg daily.

isradipine (DynaCirc)
> **Dosage:**
> Adults only: (Oral) 1.25 to 2.5 mg twice a day.

Miscellaneous Agents

methyldopa hydrochloride, USP, BP (Aldomet). This agent's actions are primarily due to its effect on the central nervous system. The hypotensive effect is attributed to a decrease in peripheral vascular resistance with little change in heart rate. Side effects include drowsiness, impotence, and gynecomastia.

> **Dosage:**
> Adults: (Oral) 250 to 500 mg four times daily. (IV) 350 to 500 mg every 6 hours.
> Children: (Oral, IV) 10 to 40 mg/kg/day in divided doses.

DRUGS THAT AFFECT THE BLOOD

COAGULANTS

Coagulants hasten the process of blood coagulation, or clotting.

Calcium Salts

Needed for the reactions in blood coagulation, these salts may be given orally just before surgery to prevent excessive bleeding. Calcium salts may also be given intravenously by slow IV push or diluted in an infusion to treat tetanic convulsions.

calcium gluconate, calcium chloride, calcium lactate
> **Dose:**
> Adults: (Oral, IV) 1 gm as necessary.

Vitamin K

This is a fat-soluble vitamin that is needed for normal blood coagulation. Bile salts must be present in the gastrointestinal tract for absorption of natural vitamin K; hence, in the event of a bile obstruction, an oral preparation of natural vitamin K would be of no use.

phytonadione (vitamin K$_1$ oxide), USP, BP (Mephyton). This emulsion of vitamin K may be given intravenously to control hemorrhage. It is also available in tablet form.

> **Dosage:**
> Adults: (IV) 50 mg two to three times daily by slow IV push or diluted in infusion. (Oral) 5 mg four times daily.

phytonadione injection, USP, BP (AquaMEPHYTON). This colloidal solution of vitamin K has smaller particles that permit this preparation to be given intramuscularly or subcutaneously (subQ) as well as by the intravenous route if other routes are unavailable.

> **Dosage:**
> Adults: (subQ, IM) 10 mg two or three times daily. (IV) (adults only): After being diluted with

5% dextrose in 0.9% saline solution, it should be administered IV at a rate not exceeding 1 mg/minute.

Children: (subQ, IM) 0.5 to 1.0 mg is administered to newborn infants to prevent hemorrhagic disease of the newborn.

ANTICOAGULANTS

Anticoagulants increase the time it takes for blood to coagulate by interfering with thrombin production and subsequent formation of fibrin from fibrinogen. They are used to treat thromboembolic disorders.

Laboratory tests are used to determine the correct dosage of the anticoagulants. The prothrombin time (PT), which is sensitive to plasma concentrations of functional blood coagulation factors, has long been used to evaluate the effectiveness of an anticoagulant, and to guard against overdose. Valid PT determinations can be made if the blood samples are drawn at least 4 to 6 hours after an IV dose or 12 to 24 hours after a subcutaneous dose of heparin. The generally accepted therapeutic value of the PT ratio is 1.5 to 2.5 times the control value in seconds.

A system of standardizing the PT values through determination of an International Normalized Ratio (INR) has been introduced. It is derived from calibrations of commercial thromboplastin reagents against an international reference preparation. An INR of 2.5 to 3.5 corresponds to a PT ratio of 1.4 to 1.6 and is now used as the optimum value for determining the effectiveness of the anticoagulation therapy.

Heparin

sodium heparin injection, USP, BP. Heparin is not active orally and must be given parenterally. The preferred method of administration is by intravenous infusion. In addition, it may be administered by deep subcutaneous (intrafat) injection. It may not be administered IM because of the problems with local reactions and the development of hematomas.

It is used for the prevention and treatment of venous thrombosis and, by extension, prevention and treatment of pulmonary embolism, prevention and treatment of arterial emboli, and treatment of consumption coagulopathies (e.g., disseminated intravascular coagulation). Heparin is the anticoagulant of choice when an immediate effect is desired. An oral anticoagulant (coumarin derivative) is generally started at the same time that heparin is started. After allowing several days for the oral anticoagulant to reach its full effect, heparin can then be discontinued.

The effect of heparin is generally monitored by the PT time, although other clotting factors such as the clotting time and activated partial thromboplastin time (aPTT) are also affected.

Heparin-induced thrombocytopenia (HIT) is a significant side effect to heparin therapy. The heparin induces formation of platelet antibodies. When this occurs, another agent must be used. Platelet counts should be ordered when the patient is receiving heparin, and the drug discontinued if

the platelets drop to 100,000/mm³. The newer low-molecular-weight heparins have less effect on the platelets than does heparin.

Dosage:
Adults: (IV) 5000 units initially, then 20,000 to 40,000 units as a slow infusion over 24 hours.

Low-Molecular-Weight Heparins

Low-molecular-weight forms of heparin are made by peroxide fragmentation of the heparin molecule, with a resulting molecular weight approximately one-half that of heparin. Like the older unfractionated heparin, these agents are used for the prevention and treatment of thromboembolic disorders (disorders in which a blood clot is carried away from its site of origin and blocks a blood vessel). They are administered by deep subcutaneous injection; they are not intended for intramuscular or intravenous injection.

Compared with unfractionated heparins, these agents have a few advantages: they may be given by subcutaneous injection rather than intravenously, they have greater bioavailability after subcutaneous injection, and they have a longer half-life and thus may be administered less frequently. There is a lower incidence of antiplatelet antibody formation and HIT after these heparin forms are administered.

tinzaparin sodium injection (Innohep)
Dosage:
Adults only: (Deep subQ) 175 units/kg once daily.

ardeparin sodium injection (Normiflo)
Dosage:
Adults only: (Deep subQ) 50 units/kg twice daily.

dalteparin sodium injection (Fragmin)
Dosage:
Adults only: (Deep subQ) 2500 units daily.

enoxaparin sodium injection (Lovenox)
Dosage:
Adults only: (Deep subQ) 30 mg twice daily.

Direct Inhibitors of Thrombin

lepirudin (Refludan). Lepirudin, or recombinant DNA (rDNA) for injection, is a highly specific direct inhibitor of thrombin. The natural hirudin was initially extracted from the saliva of the medicinal leech. Although it is structurally and chemically unrelated to heparin, it produces a similar pharmacologic effect through direct interaction with thrombin. It is used for anticoagulation in patients with HIT, to prevent further embolic complications. As with all agents of this class, side effects are primarily associated with hemorrhagic events.

Dosage:
Adults only: (IV) 0.4 mg/kg by infusion over 15 to 20 seconds, followed by 0.15 mg/kg/hr as a slow infusion.

Coumarin Anticoagulants

Like heparin, the coumarin anticoagulants are used in the prevention and treatment of thromboembolic disorders. Their main advantage is that they may be taken orally. Their main disadvantage is that they do not take effect for as long as 2 to 7 days, thus heparin is given initially for treatment while coumarin is being started. Neither administration of large loading doses nor administration by the intramuscular or intravenous route hastens the onset of antithrombotic action. Likewise, the anticoagulant effect lasts for several days after the drug is discontinued.

Coumarin anticoagulants function by altering the synthesis of blood coagulation factors. Coumarin does nothing to hasten the clearance of existing factors from the blood, thus the anticoagulant effect will not occur until depletion of the factors occurs.

The dose of coumarin anticoagulants may be adjusted by using the PT or the INR, a standardized format for reporting thromboplastin values. A therapeutic PT ratio of 1.3 to 2 times the control PT is equivalent to an INR of 2 to 4.

Many drugs have interactions with the coumarins (Box 20–1).

bishydroxycoumarin, USP, BP (Dicumarol). Like heparin, this agent does not affect an already formed clot, but it retards or prevents the extension of one already formed. The main advantage of this drug over heparin is that it may be given orally.

The dosage must be adjusted to the individual patient's needs, and the PT of the blood must be measured at frequent intervals to prevent overdosage. Symptoms of overdosage are nosebleed, small areas of bleeding into the skin, and massive hemorrhage or injury. Overdosage may be treated with vitamin K.

Persons taking warfarin products should not self-treat with herbs or dietary supplements. Many herbs have natural anticoagulants that potentiate the activity of warfarin. Bleeding can occur when warfarin is combined with aspirin or other nonsteroidal antiinflammatory drugs, garlic, dong quai (*Angelica sinensis*), dan shen (*Salvia*), ginseng, vitamin E, and red clover.

Dosage:

Adults: (Oral) 100 mg two to four times daily.

sodium warfarin, USP, BP (Coumadin). Very similar in action to Dicumarol, this agent may be absorbed orally and is used to prevent clot formation and extension. The onset of action is a little faster than that of Dicumarol; Coumadin takes 12 to 18 hours compared with the 24 to 72 hours needed for Dicumarol to take effect. When immediate action is desired, heparin is given intravenously, followed by one of the oral forms for prolonged anticoagulant therapy. Overdosage may be treated with vitamin K. Several herbs and medications can have a cumulative effect with this drug, as mentioned under bishydroxycoumarin.

Box 20-1 | *Drugs That Interact with Coumarin**

DRUGS THAT MAY INCREASE RESPONSE TO COUMARIN	
acetaminophen	streptokinase
allopurinol	sulfonamides
amiodarone	sulindac
azithromycin	tamoxifen
chloramphenicol	tetracyclines
cimetidine	thiazide diuretics
clofibrate	thyroid drugs
diazoxide	tricyclic antidepressants
diflunisal	vitamin E
disulfiram	**DRUGS THAT MAY DECREASE RESPONSE TO COUMARIN**
erythromycin	barbiturates
ethacrynic acid	corticosteroids
fenoprofen calcium	ethchlorvynol
fluoxetine	glutethimide
glucagon	griseofulvin
lovastatin	mercaptopurine
mefenamic acid	nafcillin
metronidazole	oral contraceptives
nalidixic acid	rifampin
nonsteroidal antiinflammatory drugs	spironolactone
propoxyphene	sucralfate
quinolone antibiotics	trazodone
salicylates	vitamin K

*This list is not absolute; be sure to check the most up-to-date drug reference before administering any unfamiliar drug.

Dosage:

Adults: (Oral) 2 to 5 mg daily initially, followed by daily dosage adjustments based on the PT or INR results. Most patients are satisfactorily maintained on 2 to 10 mg once daily.

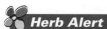 **Herb Alert**

Ginkgo biloba

Ginkgo biloba has been used to relieve the symptoms of intermittent claudication and in the treatment of Alzheimer's disease. Prolonged use has been associated with increased bleeding times and subdural hematomas, and this herb enhances the antiplatelet effects of warfarin and the nonsteroidal antiinflammatory drugs. It should not be used by patients taking tricyclic antidepressants. See Chapter 35 for more information on *Ginkgo biloba.*

THROMBOLYTIC THERAPY FOR MYOCARDIAL INFARCTION

Myocardial infarction, in which a blood clot has formed in a coronary artery, is a life-threatening condition. Advances have been made in aggressively pursuing therapy to dissolve the blood clot before extensive anoxia and tissue damage to the myocardium of the heart occur. **Thrombolytic therapy,** in which blood clots are dissolved, has been shown to rescue myocardium, reduce mortality in patients with acute myocardial infarction, and improve left ventricular function.

streptokinase, USP, BP (Streptase). Streptokinase is a protein produced by group C beta-hemolytic streptococci. It promotes thrombolysis, or dissolution of blood clots. It is used by intravenous infusion to lyse coronary artery thrombi. Benefit has been greatest when therapy has been instituted within 3 to 6 hours of onset of symptoms. Before streptokinase is begun, blood should be drawn for baseline PT, aPTT, thrombin time, and platelet count to determine the baseline status of the patient. The most frequent side effects are hemorrhage, fever, and allergic reactions.

Dosage:

Adults: (IV) 10,000 to 30,000 units given in a bolus with a small volume of diluent, followed by a maintenance infusion of 2000 to 4000 units/minute. The infusion is maintained until lysis occurs or the predetermined maximum dose has been given (around 500,000 units). Note: The dosage may vary individually.

urokinase, USP, BP (Abbokinase). This agent is most effective in lysing recently formed thrombi and should be instituted as soon as possible but no longer than 5 days after clot formation. When used for coronary thrombi, treatment should be given within 6 hours. For pulmonary emboli there is a longer span of effectiveness. Hemorrhage, hypersensitivity, and fever are reported as untoward reactions.

Dosage:

Adults: (IV) For coronary perfusion, 750,000 International Units in 500 mL of diluent. For pulmonary emboli, 4400 International Units/kg over 10 minutes, followed by a continuous infusion of 4400 International Units/kg/hr for 12 hours.

alteplase (Activase, rt-PA, t-PA). This biosynthetic form of the human enzyme tissue-type plasminogen activator (t-PA) is a thrombolytic agent. Unlike streptokinase and urokinase, t-PA is a relatively fibrin-selective plasminogen activator. For maximum effectiveness, it should be administered within 3 to 5 hours after myocardial infarction. The most frequent complication is hemorrhage.

Dosage:

Adults: (IV) 100 mg in a small amount of diluent over a 3-hour period, and a subsequent maintenance infusion of 0.25 mg/kg/hr for the next 2 hours.

ANTIPLATELET THERAPY IN CARDIOVASCULAR DISEASE

Blood platelets are small, granular bodies that number about 250,000 to 350,000 per milliliter of blood. They have three functions:

1. They stick to the inner surfaces of damaged blood vessels, plug up leaks, and cement over injured tissues.
2. When they rupture, they release thromboplastin, a substance that begins a series of reactions that form a blood clot.
3. Once a clot is formed, platelets make it shrink or retract, during which the clot is changed from a soft mass to a firm one. This helps stop bleeding from damaged vessels.

Obviously, platelet activity and blood clot formation are important functions in the body. However, when a patient has atherosclerosis and the linings of many of the blood vessels are ragged with plaques of cholesterol, the formation of clots is unwanted. **Antiplatelet agents** interfere with platelet aggregation on the surface of atherosclerotic plaques, preventing the formation of thrombi and emboli that block blood vessels.

aspirin, USP, BP. By inhibiting enzymes within the platelet, aspirin prevents platelet aggregation. When given daily to patients after a myocardial infarction, there is a reduction in the incidence of recurrent myocardial infarction and cardiovascular death. It may be used daily in low doses to prevent cardiovascular disease. After a transient ischemic attack (TIA), aspirin may be used to prevent further clotting. Aspirin should not be taken when the patient is taking warfarin or other anticoagulants because potentiation of the anticoagulant effect occurs.

Dosage for antiplatelet effect:

(Oral) 65 to 325 mg daily. Higher dosages were not more effective than lower dosages.

dipyridamole, USP, BP (Persantine). Dipyridamole inhibits platelet aggregation caused by platelet-released agents. It is often used in conjunction with aspirin therapy after myocardial infarction.

> Dosage:
>> Adults only: (Oral) 75 to 400 mg daily in divided doses.

ticlopidine hydrochloride (Ticlid). This agent is used to reduce the risk of thrombotic stroke in patients who have previously had a thrombotic stroke or its precursor, a TIA.

> Dosage:
>> Adults only: (Oral) 250 mg twice a day.

tirofiban (Aggrastat). Tirofiban is a selective platelet aggregation inhibitor. It is used to reduce the risk of acute cardiac ischemic events in patients with unstable angina. It may be given concomitantly with heparin, even in the same IV line.

> Dosage:
>> Adults only: (IV) 0.4 mcg/kg/minute for 30 minutes.

clopidogrel bisulfate (Plavix). This inhibitor of platelet aggregation is used for the reduction of atherosclerotic events such as myocardial infarction, stroke, and vascular death in patients with atherosclerosis.

> Dosage:
>> Adults only: (Oral) 75 mg once daily.

cilostazol (Pletal). Cilostazol is used as a platelet aggregation inhibitor, mainly in the treatment of intermittent claudication. It is important to note that grapefruit juice is contraindicated while taking this drug.

> Dosage:
>> Adults only: (Oral) 100 mg twice a day.

ANTILIPIDEMIC DRUGS

The measuring of cholesterol and the definition of "good," or high-density lipoprotein (HDL), and "bad," or low-density lipoprotein (LDL), cholesterol have become a matter of public concern in recent years. As the understanding of the relationship between blood cholesterol levels and atherosclerotic diseases of the blood vessels became known, the "optimum" cholesterol level was moved down to 250, then 225, and then 200 mg/dL. Most recent studies have shown that a level of 160 mg/dL is optimal for vessel health.

The present guidelines recommend obtaining a complete lipoprotein and triglyceride profile every 5 years beginning at 20 years of age.

Individuals are classified as high, medium, or low risk for death by coronary artery disease within 6 years. The classification is made based on cholesterol levels and other factors, such as the presence of coronary artery disease and/or hypertension.

A total cholesterol over 200 mg/dL is an addtional risk factor, as is an HDL level of less than 40 mg/dL or an LDL level of over 100 mg/dL. Individuals in a high-risk category should strive for an LDL level no higher than 70 mg/dL.

A low or normal blood cholesterol level is an unattainable goal for many patients using diet restriction alone, because cholesterol can be manufactured by the body also, and this activity is genetically determined.

After dietary restrictions have been tried, drug therapy is used to attain acceptable cholesterol levels. Many agents, called **antilipidemic drugs,** have been used and continue to be developed.

All drugs in this category are generally contraindicated in pregnant and nursing women. When a woman of childbearing age is a candidate for these agents, a careful history must be taken with regard to childbearing potential.

 Considerations for Pregnant and Nursing Women

Antilipidemic Drugs

All antilipidemic agents are contraindicated for pregnant and nursing women.

cholestyramine for oral suspension, USP, BP (Questran). Cholestyramine is used orally to bind with bile acids in the intestine, forming an insoluble complex that is excreted in the feces. Cholesterol is the precursor of bile acids; thus, when the bile acid loss is accelerated, this stimulates cholesterol to form bile acids, resulting in a net loss of cholesterol from the bloodstream. Cholestyramine is ineffective, and thus contraindicated, in patients with bile duct obstruction. The most common adverse effect is constipation. Abdominal pain and flatulence may also be noted. This may be treated with conventional laxative therapy.

> Dosage:
>> Adults only: (Oral) 15 gm (one packet or one scoopful) two to four times daily.

colestipol granules (Colestid). Like cholestyramine, this agent acts to remove bile acids from the gastrointestinal tract, thus causing more cholesterol to be converted to bile acids and lowering the serum cholesterol level. Constipation is the most common side effect.

> Dosage:
>> Adults only: (Oral) 5 to 30 gm daily in divided doses. It should always be mixed with fluids.

pravastatin sodium (Pravachol). Through a complex mechanism of action involving enzymes and membrane transport complexes, this agent acts to clear the serum of cholesterol and triglycerides. The most significant side effect is alteration of liver function; thus liver enzymes should be tested before therapy and every 6 weeks.

> Dosage:
>> Adults only: (Oral) 10 to 40 mg daily at bedtime for 3 to 6 months.

gemfibrozil (Lopid). This lipid-lowering agent acts to reduce serum levels of triglycerides and very-low-density cholesterol. Renal and liver abnormalities have occurred with prolonged treatment; thus the patient should be followed frequently.

Dosage:

Adults only: (Oral) 1200 mg daily in two divided doses.

lovastatin (Mevacor). This agent was isolated from a strain of *Aspergillus terreus,* a fungus. Through complex enzyme activation, it interferes with the biosynthesis of cholesterol. Liver dysfunction must be guarded against.

Dosage:

Adults only: (Oral) 20 to 80 mg daily in single or divided doses.

simvastatin (Zocor). Also derived from *Aspergillus,* this agent lowers cholesterol by interfering with its biosynthesis. Hepatic, renal, and cardiac complications may occur with prolonged use.

Dosage:

Adults only: (Oral) 5 to 40 mg daily in the evening.

atorvastatin calcium (Lipitor). Atorvastatin is used to lower serum cholesterol, along with dietary control. It may be taken without regard to meals or the time of day.

Dosage:

Adults only: (Oral) 10 to 80 mg once daily.

ezetimibe (Zetia) This agent may be used as monotherapy or in combination with another agent to reduce serum cholesterol.

Dosage:

Adults only: (Oral) 10 mg once daily.

CLINICAL IMPLICATIONS

1. Care should be taken to monitor the pulse of a cardiac patient before each dose of medication. If the pulse is less than 60 beats/minute, digoxin should be withheld and the physician notified.
2. Blood levels of digoxin provide an accurate method of determining the digoxin dose for an individual patient.
3. An increase in urine output is generally seen as an early sign of improvement in a patient being treated for congestive heart failure.
4. A decrease in visible edema from fluid retention is generally noted as a sign of improvement in patients with congestive heart failure.
5. Patients with congestive failure are generally more comfortable in a sitting position and should be placed in this position to minimize dyspnea.
6. Cardiac patients are generally prescribed a low-sodium diet to minimize fluid retention. The patient should be carefully instructed in the importance of the diet.
7. Alterations in the serum calcium and potassium levels will affect the performance of digoxin. Severe changes in the serum concentration of these electrolytes may be responsible for toxic effects from digoxin.
8. The patient should be monitored for any change in the cardiac rhythm during administration of cardiac drugs. An irregular pulse rate should be reported to the physician.
9. The patient should be instructed to take the cardiac medication exactly as prescribed when he or she returns home. He or she should be told to report any weight gain, shortness of breath, or edema to the physician.
10. The prothrombin time (pro time, PT) may be used as a measure of the effectiveness of anticoagulation. The PT is generally believed to be optimum for the anticoagulated patient if it is double the control PT. When the value is more than double the control value, there is a danger of bleeding.
11. Hypertensive agents may have severe side effects. All untoward symptoms should be reported to the physician.
12. Many drugs and herbal remedies have interactions with warfarin. The patient on anticoagulants may not take herbal supplements.
13. The patient on anticoagulants should be instructed to report prolonged bleeding time from cuts and bloody or black bowel movements. Bleeding gums and petechiae may also be signs of elevated anticoagulant activity.

Online Resources

For updated drug information and Web activities, go to http://evolve.elsevier.com/Asperheim.

CRITICAL THINKING QUESTIONS

1. The patient is admitted to the hospital emergency room with shortness of breath; cold, clammy skin; a heart rate of 100 beats/minute; and a cough producing pink, frothy sputum. A probable diagnosis of heart failure and pulmonary edema has been established. What nursing procedures might be taken immediately to make her more comfortable? What drugs are likely to be needed?

2. The patient comes into the emergency room in a state of extreme anxiety, expressing a fear that he is dying. His pulse is thready, rapid, and irregular with a rate of 150 beats/minute. A probable diagnosis of atrial fibrillation is established. What drugs are likely to be needed? What other techniques are known to be useful in stopping an attack such as this?

3. The patient appears chronically ill. He has recurrent chest pain and reports shortness of breath. The probable diagnosis is angina. What drugs are likely to be useful in managing his condition?

4. After a heart attack, the patient was placed on warfarin (Coumadin), 10 mg a day. He has returned to work and feels well. However, he is annoyed that he has to have periodic blood tests and checkups. Could you help him understand the need for these tests?

5. The patient comes to the office to have his rash checked. He fears he may be allergic to his warfarin (Coumadin). You see that he has large, deep-red spots on his forearms, some measuring 10 cm in diameter. What is the cause of the rash? What should be done?

REVIEW QUESTIONS

1. Heart failure means that the heart:
   a. has stopped beating.
   b. has stopped circulating blood.
   c. has stopped circulating blood efficiently.
   d. has lower hydrostatic pressure than normal.

2. A drug commonly used to increase the contractility of the heart is:
   a. digoxin.
   b. disopyramide.
   c. lidocaine.
   d. nitroglycerin.

3. Which of the following is used in the treatment of angina pectoris?
   a. midodrine
   b. digitalis
   c. glyceryl trinitrate
   d. felodipine

4. An agent that may be given intravenously to control hemorrhage is:
   a. phytonadione.
   b. felodipine.
   c. glyceryl trinitrate.
   d. perindopril.

5. An example of an ACE inhibitor is:
   a. amiodarone.
   b. olmesartan.
   c. isradipine.
   d. enalapril.

6. An antiplatelet drug may be used in the treatment/prevention of:
   a. hemophilia.
   b. hypertension.
   c. hemorrhage.
   d. transient ischemic attacks.

7. An advantage of low-molecular-weight heparins over the traditional heparin is:
   a. shorter half-life.
   b. less bioavailability.
   c. subcutaneous injection rather than intravenous injection.
   d. intravenous injection only.

8. Bishydroxycoumarin is used for:
   a. coagulation.
   b. anticoagulation.
   c. hypertension.
   d. antidote for heparin overdose.

9. Gemfibrozil may be used to treat:
   a. hypertension.
   b. hypotension.
   c. constipation.
   d. hyperlipidemia.

10. A common problem when treating hypertensive patients is:
   a. increase in the cholesterol level in the blood.
   b. compliance with taking the medications.
   c. rapid lowering of the blood pressure.
   d. congestive heart failure.

Drugs That Affect the Central Nervous System

Objectives

After completing this chapter, you should be able to do the following:

1. Classify and give examples of drugs that affect the central nervous system.
2. Differentiate between the narcotic and nonnarcotic analgesics.
3. Identify the three narcotic analgesics.
4. State the precautions to be observed when narcotic analgesics are administered.
5. List the symptoms of drug dependence.
6. Explain the action of general anesthetic agents.
7. Identify drugs used to prevent and treat migraine headaches.
8. Become familiar with the different types of epilepsy and the drugs used to treat each type.
9. Identify drugs used to treat attention deficit hyperactivity disorder.
10. Identify drugs used to treat Parkinson's disease.

Key Terms

Addiction, p. 104
Analgesia (ăn-ăl-JĒ-zē-ă), p. 105
Anesthesia (ăn-ĕs-THĒ-zē-ă), p. 102
Anticonvulsants (ăn-tī-kŏn-VŬL-sănts), p. 109
Barbiturates (băr-BĬCH-ū-rătes), p. 103
Narcotic (năr-KŎT-ĭk), p. 105
Opiates, p. 105
Opioids (Ō-pē-oids), p. 105
Tolerance, p. 124

The nervous system, including the peripheral nerves, constitutes the body's equipment for rapid coordination of many of its activities. These activities must often be set into motion and coordinated to the body's needs in a fraction of a second. An example is the very rapid closing of the eyelids when the eyes are unexpectedly touched (e.g., by a grain of sand). We move ourselves at will by sending electrical signals from the central nervous system through the peripheral nervous system to our skeletal muscles.

The central nervous system (CNS) is composed of the brain and spinal cord; together they coordinate many functions such as blood pressure, heart rate, the flow of saliva and gastric juices, skin temperature, and sensations such as pain.

In addition, the brain serves to store knowledge and to cause conscious and unconscious reactions to stimuli and conditions on the basis of past experience. Our awareness of our environment, our satisfaction or dissatisfaction with it, happiness, love, and all emotions or moods are seated in the brain.

It has long been known that the brain can be both depressed and stimulated. The use of alcoholic beverages and plants with depressant effects has its origin in antiquity. The discovery of anesthesia may be cited as one of the greatest boons to humankind, for it made possible lifesaving surgical procedures that were hitherto unthinkable.

A noteworthy advance of the 20th century has come in its last decade—the discovery of drugs that give truly effective treatment to the mentally ill. After centuries of study, the first big steps have been taken in unraveling the mysteries of mental illness. Although Chapter 23 is devoted exclusively to drugs used in the management and treatment of mental illness, many of the agents discussed in this chapter have also been used therapeutically in this area.

CENTRAL NERVOUS SYSTEM STIMULANTS

Central stimulants are drugs that increase the activity of the brain and spinal cord. A common use of the central stimulants is to treat attention deficit hyperactivity disorder (ADHD). It is recognized more frequently in children, and it is known to last into adulthood in many individuals. Nonmedicated children with ADHD often suffer from the cumulative effects of a lifetime of ADHD-associated behaviors. Distractibility, talkativeness, and inappropriate impulsive behavior make life difficult for the child and his or her associates.

Herb Alert

Ginseng

Ginseng has been used as a stimulant, as a tonic, and to treat menopausal hot flashes. It is claimed to enhance cognitive function, but this has not been substantiated. Ginseng should not be used with warfarin or nonsteroidal antiinflammatory drugs because it enhances the anticoagulant effect of these agents. Ginseng enhances the effects of phenelzine and should not be used by patients with diabetes or those taking monoamine oxidase inhibitors. See Chapter 35 for more information on ginseng.

The diagnosis of ADHD is made by a clinical exam. In addition to medical treatment for ADHD, there may be some associated learning disabilities that require educational adjustments.

amphetamine salts (Adderall) This mixture of the salts of amphetamine is used to treat ADHD and narcolepsy. Peripheral effects of this agent include raising of the blood pressure and a weak bronchodilator action. Heart palpitations, restlessness, dizziness, insomnia, anorexia, and weight loss may occur as adverse side effects.

> **Dosage:**
> Adults and children older than 12 years: (Oral) 5 to 60 mg daily.
> Children 6 to 12 years: (Oral) 5 mg daily, dosage adjusted as necessary.

dextroamphetamine sulfate (Dexedrine) Dextroamphetamine may be used instead of amphetamine because its increased potency permits the use of a lower dosage. The side effects are similar to those of amphetamine.

> **Dosage:**
> Adults: (Oral) 5 mg two to four times daily.

doxapram hydrochloride, USP, BP (Dopram). This central stimulant acts on all levels of the CNS but is used primarily as a respiratory stimulant to hasten arousal in individuals who have taken depressants, or after anesthesia. There is a narrow margin of safety with this agent, and hypertension, tachycardia, and seizures have occurred with its use.

> **Dosage:**
> Adults and children: (IV) 1 to 2 mg/kg for the first two doses at 5-minute intervals and then repeated as necessary at 1- to 2-hour intervals, diluted with intravenous (IV) fluids.

methylphenidate hydrochloride, USP, BP (Ritalin). The primary use of methylphenidate is in the treatment of ADHD, attention deficit disorder (ADD), or other syndromes. Although the drug is a central stimulant, it causes a kinetic slowing of the hyperactive individual and increases the ability to concentrate. It is occasionally used in the treatment of narcolepsy and mild depressive states. The drug is short acting, generally taking effect within one-half hour, and the dose will last 4 hours. A midday dose is necessary to sustain the effect during the school day. The side effects, when they occur, are generally mild and include nervousness, headache, and insomnia. They can generally be controlled by alteration of the dosage.

> **Dosage:**
> Adults and children: (Oral) 5 to 20 mg two to three times daily.

methylphenidate hydrochloride, extended-release tablets (Concerta). This extended-release form of methylphenidate eliminates the need for a midday dose for the school-age child, and thus avoids the perceived stigma of taking

 Considerations for Children

methylphenidate (Ritalin)

Methylphenidate (Ritalin) should be used with caution in children with a history of seizures or an abnormal electroencephalogram (EEG). There is some evidence that the seizure threshold is lowered in patients receiving methylphenidate.

the drug at school. The tablet must be taken whole, not crushed.

> **Dosage:**
> Adults: (Oral) 36 mg once daily in the morning, up to maximum of 54 mg daily.
> Children: (Oral) 18 mg once daily in the morning. Dosage may be individually adjusted.

pemoline (Cylert). Like methylphenidate, this agent is used in the treatment of ADD and ADHD. It has a gradual onset of action, however, and therapeutic effects may not be evident for 2 to 3 weeks. It has the advantage of being taken once daily instead of in divided doses.

> **Dosage:**
> Adults and children: (Oral) 37.5 mg daily in the morning. The dosage may be increased at weekly intervals to a maximum of 112.5 mg daily.

atomoxetine hydrochloride (Strattera) This agent is used for the treatment of ADD and ADHD, as are the drugs listed above, but is different in that it is NOT strictly a central stimulant and is NOT a controlled substance. Growth should be monitored in a child taking this agent because it has been shown to decrease the appetite. In addition, increases in blood pressure and heart rate, and abdominal pain have been reported with use.

> **Dosage:**
> Adults: (Oral) 40 to 100 mg once daily.
> Children: (Oral) 0.5 mg/kg initially, then increased to 1.2 mg/kg/day.

CENTRAL NERVOUS SYSTEM DEPRESSANTS

The action of central nervous system depressants may be general, depressing the CNS more or less as a whole, or they may act in a more specific way on one or more centers of the brain. **Anesthesia,** a pharmacologic CNS depressant, produces a loss of sensation, which also might be general, or systemic, or localized.

GENERAL ANESTHETICS

The general anesthetics produce a loss of sensation throughout the body by cutting off all sensory impulses to the brain, thus causing unconsciousness. General anesthetics are most commonly administered by inhalation, although a few, such as sodium pentothal, are administered intravenously (Tables 21–1 and 21–2).

Stages of Anesthesia

The stages of anesthesia provide guidelines regarding the level or depth of anesthesia. The anesthetist controls the depth of anesthesia for various procedures by observing the stages. All stages of anesthesia are passed through during induction; the order is then reversed during the recovery period.

I—**Analgesia.** This stage begins when the anesthetic is administered and lasts until loss of consciousness. It is characterized by analgesia, euphoria, perceptual distortions, and amnesia.

II—**Delirium.** This stage begins with loss of consciousness and extends to the beginning of surgical anesthesia. There may be excitement and involuntary muscular activity. Skeletal muscle tone increases, breathing is irregular, and hypertension and tachycardia may occur.

III—**Surgical Anesthesia.** This stage lasts until spontaneous respiration ceases. It is further divided into four planes based on respiration, the size of the pupils, reflex characteristics, and eyeball movements.

IV—**Medullary Depression.** This stage begins with cessation of respiration and ends with circulatory collapse. The pupils are fixed and dilated, and there are no lid or corneal reflexes.

LOCAL ANESTHETICS

The local anesthetics are presented in this section for completeness and clarity, but they are not central depressants. Rather, local anesthetics interfere with nerve conduction from an area of the body to the CNS. In this way they interfere with pain perception by the CNS. Table 21–3 presents a summary of the local anesthetics.

HYPNOTICS AND SEDATIVES

Hypnotic and sedative agents generally may be used in smaller doses for daytime sedation and in larger doses for the induction of sleep at bedtime.

Patients who are taking these agents must be cautioned not to take other central depressants, such as alcohol. The antihistamines, with their side effect of drowsiness, can also produce adverse effects when administered concurrently with these agents. In some cases when these agents are used for their hypnotic effect, a morning "hangover" or sedative effect may be experienced. In many cases this can be minimized by using one of the shorter acting hypnotics or reducing the dose.

Barbiturates

These agents are prescribed more frequently than any other class to produce sedation of the CNS. **Barbiturates** are derivatives of barbituric acid and act by depressing the respiratory rate, blood pressure, and temperature as well as the

Table 21-1 | *Volatile Anesthetics*

GENERIC NAME	TRADE NAME	USES	CONCENTRATION
enflurane, USP, BP	Ethrane	General use	1.5–4 vol %
ether, USP, BP	—	Major surgical procedures	10–15 vol %
halothane, USP, BP	Fluothane	Major procedures, particularly when vasoconstriction is desired	1–3 vol %
methoxyflurane, USP, BP	Penthrane	Obstetrics, short procedures	2–3 vol %
nitrous oxide, USP, BP	—	Short procedures	80 vol %
vinyl ether, USP, BP	Vinethene	Major procedures	2–4 vol %

Table 21-2 | *General Anesthetics Administered Intravenously*

GENERIC NAME	TRADE NAME	USES	DOSAGE OR CONCENTRATION
diazepam, USP, BP	Valium	Anticonvulsant, induction aid, preoperative medication	Adult: 2–10 mg slow IV push Child: 1–10 mg slow IV push
ketamine hydrochloride, USP, BP	Ketalar	Obstetrics, short procedures	2%–3% solution
midazolam hydrochloride	Versed	Sedation anesthetic for short procedures	Adult: 10–50 mcg/kg IV initially, then 20–100 mcg/kg/hr Child: 100–150 mcg/kg IV initially, then as necessary
thiopental sodium, USP, BP	Pentothal	Short procedures or to facilitate induction with volatile anesthetics	2.5% solution

Table 21-3 | *Local Anesthetics*

GENERIC NAME	TRADE NAME	USES	CONCENTRATION
bupivacaine hydrochloride, USP, BP	Marcaine	Epidural or caudal block, local nerve block	0.25%–0.5% solution subQ
chloroprocaine hydrochloride, USP, BP	Nesacaine	Epidural, caudal, or local nerve block	1%–2% solution subQ
cocaine hydrochloride, USP, BP	—	Mucous membranes of the nose and throat	1%–20% topically
etidocaine hydrochloride	Duranest	Epidural or peripheral nerve block	1% solution subQ
lidocaine hydrochloride, USP, BP	Xylocaine	Local nerve block	1%–2% solution subQ
mepivacaine hydrochloride, USP, BP	Carbocaine	Dental and local block	1% solution subQ
prilocaine hydrochloride	Citanest	Peripheral nerve block	4% solution subQ
procaine hydrochloride, USP, BP	Novocain	Local nerve block	0.25%–2% solution subQ
tetracaine hydrochloride, USP, BP	Pontocaine	Spinal anesthesia	1% solution subarachnoid

subQ, Subcutaneously.

Considerations for Older Adults

Hypnotics and Sedatives

The dose of sedatives and hypnotics may need to be reduced for older adults. The metabolism of these drugs is often impaired in older adults, and their excretion also may be slower in older adults than it is for younger people. Symptoms of overdose may occur at or below standard doses.

Herb Alert

Valerian

Valerian is used as a sedative to treat insomnia. It enhances the effects of sedatives, hypnotics, antihistamines, and benzodiazepines. Its use should be avoided during pregnancy and lactation. See Chapter 35 for more information on valerian.

CNS. The response to the barbiturates may be mild sedation, hypnosis, or general anesthesia, depending on the dose and the method of administration. The barbiturates are not analgesics, however, and cannot be depended on to produce sleep when insomnia is caused by pain.

These drugs are definitely habit forming and will produce **tolerance,** that is, the power of resisting the action of a drug, or the ability to take large doses without adverse effects. They may lead to **addiction** (habitual dependence on a substance that is beyond voluntary control) if large doses are taken over a long period of time. The symptoms of barbiturate poisoning are similar to those of chronic alcoholism. There is impairment of mental efficiency, confusion, belligerence,

blurred speech, and tremors. The skin is clammy and cyanotic, the temperature drops, and respiratory depression continues, causing death.

Severe poisoning results at 5 to 10 times the hypnotic dose, and death results at 15 to 20 times the hypnotic dose. The treatment of barbiturate poisoning is accomplished by using dialysis. The patient's blood is passed through an artificial kidney in which the barbiturate is diffused out of the blood.

There are many commonly used barbiturates. They differ in onset of action, duration of action, and method of administration, but for all practical purposes the pharmacologic effects on the body are the same.

phenobarbital, USP, BP (Luminal)
   Dosage:
      Adults: (Oral, IM, IV) 30 mg four times daily.

pentobarbital, USP, BP (Nembutal)
   Dosage:
      Adults: (Oral) 100 to 200 mg at bedtime.

secobarbital, USP, BP (Seconal)
   Dosage:
      Adults: (Oral) 100 to 200 mg at bedtime.

butabarbital, USP, BP (Butisol)
   Dosage:
      Adults: (Oral) 30 mg four times daily.

Nonbarbiturate Sedative-Hypnotic Agents

chloral hydrate, USP, BP. Sleep is produced in a relatively short time after administration of this drug and lasts from 5 to 8 hours. The sleep greatly resembles natural sleep, and the patient can be awakened without difficulty. There is no analgesic effect from this drug, so it is not used when the restlessness or insomnia is due to pain.

> **Dosage:**
> Adults: (Oral) 500 mg at bedtime.
> Children: (Oral) 50 mg/kg at bedtime.

flurazepam hydrochloride, USP, BP (Dalmane). This agent is used to treat all types of insomnia and is a hypnotic of moderate activity.

> **Dosage:**
> Adults only: (Oral) 15 to 30 mg at bedtime.

OPIATES AND OPIOID ANALGESICS

In ancient times, **analgesia** (the relief of pain) was attributed to the opium poppy. Opium is described in Chinese literature written long before the time of Christ. It is obtained from the hardened, dried juice of the unripened seeds of the species of poppy grown in Asia Minor. Three alkaloids derived from opium are in use today: morphine, codeine, and papaverine. Any drug derived from opium, or its synthetic analogs, is termed a **narcotic.** Drugs derived from opium are known as **opiates,** whereas drugs with actions similar to those of opium, but not derived from opium, are called **opioids.**

Although undoubtedly the most powerful and effective pain relievers known to humans, these agents are also the most addicting. After repeated doses, the dose must be continually increased to obtain relief of pain. In the case of the narcotic addict, the desired euphoria is also subject to dose tolerance, and the dosage levels must be continually increased to obtain the desired effect.

Addiction to opiates or opioids is characterized by tolerance, physical dependence, and habituation. Repeated doses of these drugs lead not only to marked tolerance but also to a very strong desire for the drug that the victim seems powerless to resist. The results vary in individuals, but long use leads to depression and weakness not only of the body but also of the mind and morals. The patient suffers a loss of appetite and various other digestive disturbances and, before long, becomes thin and anemic. The addict seems particularly incapable of telling the truth and will resort to almost any method to obtain the drug. Ill health, crime, and low standards of living are the result not of the effects of morphine itself but of the sacrifices of money, social position, food, and self-respect made to obtain the daily dose of the drug.

Opiates

All agents in this class are narcotics and are controlled by narcotics prescribing regulations.

morphine sulfate, USP, BP (Oramorph, MS Contin, MSIR, Roxanol). Morphine depresses the cerebral cortex; sensation and perception are dulled. Anxiety and apprehension disappear, and euphoria may occur. When administered for painful situations, such as postsurgery, the drug is most effective if administered before the pain becomes severe. As long as time intervals are strictly observed and the drug dose is reduced as the pain becomes less severe, addiction is not seen as a frequent problem in short-term indications for this agent. Some of the other effects of morphine include the following:

- The respiratory center is depressed, which is seen as the most dangerous effect of drug overdose.
- The pupils contract and become "pinpoint" in size.
- The emptying time of the stomach is delayed.
- Peristalsis is decreased (this and the previous effect explain why the patient may often experience abdominal pain, distention, and constipation when given morphine for pain).
- The cough center is depressed, and coughing is lessened.
- The patient may experience interference with motor coordination. He or she may have difficulty handling a glass of water, may misjudge distances when attempting to pick up articles, and may stagger when walking.

Some of the uses of opium and its derivatives are as follows:

- The chief use, as before stated, is as a potent pain reliever.
- As a preliminary medication before general anesthesia, morphine is usually given with atropine. Atropine is used mainly to prevent excessive salivation and respiratory tract secretion, but it also antagonizes the depressant action of morphine upon the respiratory center and tends to speed the heart. This combination promotes a relaxed state, which favors a more satisfactory induction of anesthesia and decreases the amount of general anesthetic needed for the induction.
- Opium derivatives are frequently used in cough preparations. These syrups or expectorants usually contain codeine, dihydrocodeinone, or dihydromorphinone, but paregoric has been found useful as well.
- To treat diarrhea, paregoric (camphorated opium tincture) may be used alone or in combination with an absorbent. Laudanum (opium tincture) has also been used, as well as synthetic derivatives of opium (Lomotil).
- Because of the relaxant effect of morphine on the smooth muscles, opium derivatives may be used as antispasmodics.

Poisoning caused by opium or morphine results from overdoses that have been taken with a therapeutic or suicidal intent. Death usually results from asphyxia brought on by respiratory failure. The pupils are constricted at first and later become dilated as asphyxia deepens. As a rule, the patient perspires freely and increasingly as poisoning advances. The body temperature falls, and the skin feels cold and clammy and appears cyanotic or gray. Attention must be focused especially on respiration in the treatment of poisoning. Naloxone is the treatment of choice for overdoses.

The toxic dose of morphine is 60 mg in a normal individual, and the fatal dose is about 240 mg. Addicts become tolerant of the drug, however, and can take much higher doses without severe toxic effects.

> **Dosage:**
> Adults: (SC, IM, IV) 10 mg, repeated up to six times daily.
> Children: (SC, IM, IV) 0.1 mg/kg, up to six times daily.

Note that doses necessary may be much higher if tolerance develops.

naloxone (Narcan). This agent is a competitive narcotic antagonist used in the management and reversal of overdoses of morphine and synthetic opioids. It antagonizes all the effects of morphine.

Dosage:
Adults: (IV) 0.4 to 2 mg. May repeat every 2 to 3 minutes up to 10 mg if needed.
Children: (IV) 1 to 2 mcg/kg every 2 to 3 minutes, up to 0.2 mg.

codeine phosphate, USP, BP; codeine sulfate, USP, BP. Codeine, like morphine, is a narcotic regulated under the Controlled Substances Act. It is a mild analgesic, but the respiratory depression in overdose and the potential for drug abuse require that the usual precautions for narcotic analgesic therapy be taken. It is often prescribed in a combination form with aspirin, acetaminophen, or other analgesic agents. Its antitussive activity is well known; thus it is included in many cough preparations.

Dosage:
Adults: (Oral, subQ) 30 mg/kg four to six times daily.
Children: (Oral, subQ) 0.5 mg/kg four to six times daily.

Opioids

meperidine hydrochloride, USP, BP (Demerol). This is one of the synthetic substitutes for morphine. It does cause addiction, but tolerance develops at a slower rate and the withdrawal symptoms are not as severe as those of morphine. Unlike morphine, it does not produce sleep but is an effective analgesic agent. Because the respiratory depression produced is less than that caused by morphine, it is preferred to morphine in obstetrics. Meperidine is a narcotic and is subject to regulation under the Controlled Substances Act.

Dosage:
Adults: (Oral, subQ, IM) 50 to 100 mg every 3 to 4 hours. (IV) 15 to 35 mg/hr.
Children: (Oral, subQ, IM) 1 mg/kg four to six times daily.

fentanyl transdermal system (Duragesic). This transdermal delivery system consists of patches that are applied to the skin and provide a continuous systemic delivery of fentanyl, a potent opioid narcotic. All the different sizes of patches have the same concentration of drug per area of patch. Increased doses are obtained by using the larger patches for greater surface area of delivery. They may be used for acute and chronic pain conditions, such as cancer and Paget's disease of bone. After removal of the patch, serum concentrations of fentanyl decline gradually and reach an approximate 50% reduction 17 hours after removal. The patch should be applied to a nonirritated area of skin on a flat surface or the upper torso. Each patch is to be worn for 72 hours. Side effects are similar to those associated with opioids, along with the potential for addiction.

Dosage:
(Topical) Patches deliver 25, 50, 75, or 100 mcg/hr. A patch is applied every 72 hours.

oxycodone (Roxicodone, OxyIR, OxyFAST, OxyContin). This opioid is used orally to relieve mild to moderate pain. It is available in many combinations with acetaminophen or aspirin and in extended-release forms that facilitate pain control.

Dosage:
Adults: (Oral) 5 mg every 6 hours.
Children 6 to 12 years: (Oral) 0.61 mg every 6 hours.
Children 12 years and older: (Oral) 1.22 mg every 6 hours.

oxymorphone hydrochloride (Numorphan). Also an opioid, this agent may be given rectally, subcutaneously, intramuscularly (IM), or IV. The onset of action is within 5 to 10 minutes after IV administration.

Dosage:
Adults or children older than 12 years: (IM, subQ) 1 to 1.5 mg every 4 to 6 hours. (IV) 0.5 mg every 4 to 6 hours. (Rectal) 5 mg every 4 to 6 hours.

sufentanil citrate (Sufenta). Sufentanil is primarily administered IV but may be given IM as well. It is used alone for general anesthesia in some cases, but generally is administered along with another anesthetic.

Dosage:
Adults: (IV) 10 to 50 mcg/kg.
Children: (IV) 10 to 25 mcg/kg.

tramadol hydrochloride (Ultram). This agent is used as an analgesic for moderate to mild pain.

Dosage:
Adults and children older than 16 years: (Oral) 50 to 100 mg every 4 to 6 hours.

butorphanol tartrate (Stadol). A synthetic agent, butorphanol is structurally related to morphine. It is used for moderate to severe pain such as that associated with cancer, burns, renal colic, and migraine headaches.

Dosage:
Adults: (IM, IV) 1 to 2 mg every 3 to 4 hours. (Nasally) Metered pump, 1 mg per spray.

NONNARCOTIC ANALGESICS

Although some remain habit forming, the drugs of this category generally do not have the addicting properties of the narcotic analgesics. They also are not as effective as the narcotic agents in their analgesic activity.

acetaminophen, USP, BP (Tylenol, Tempra). Acetaminophen has been shown to be an effective and safe analgesic and antipyretic. Unlike aspirin, however, it has no antirheumatic or antiinflammatory activity; thus it is of limited benefit in the treatment of pain arising from joint disorders. It is not as irritating to the gastric mucosa as aspirin, so it is useful in patients who do not tolerate aspirin well.

Acetaminophen has been found to be of great benefit in the treatment of fevers in infants and young children. It is not associated with Reye's syndrome, which has been noted in young children who have received aspirin products.

Sensitivity reactions are rare, and acetaminophen is usually well tolerated by patients sensitive to aspirin. The dosage limits should be carefully observed with acetaminophen. Overdoses lead to serious hepatic toxicity.

Dosage:
Adults: (Oral) 325 mg every 4 hours as necessary.
Children: (Oral) 60 to 120 mg four times daily.

propoxyphene hydrochloride, USP, BP (Darvon). Propoxyphene is a synthetic analgesic that is chemically related to the narcotics. It has an analgesic activity similar to that of codeine and is administered orally for the relief of mild to moderate pain. It has been shown to have some addicting properties, although not to the extent of the opioids.

It is often combined with aspirin (Darvon with ASA) or with aspirin, phenacetin, and caffeine (Darvon Compound) for enhancement of its analgesic effect. In combination with acetaminophen, the trade name is Wygesic. Propoxyphene napsylate, when combined with acetaminophen, has the trade name Darvocet-N.

Side effects are mild and are usually limited to mild allergic symptoms. Patients sensitive to aspirin should not be given the combination products containing aspirin. It is not recommended for children.

Dosage:
Adults: (Oral) 65 mg four times daily.

pentazocine hydrochloride, USP, BP (Talwin). Pentazocine is a very effective nonnarcotic analgesic that may be used for moderate to severe pain. It is effective orally and parenterally. It should not be stopped suddenly after prolonged use, because some withdrawal effects may occur. The oral preparations of this drug are combinations:
pentazocine with aspirin (Talwin Compound)
pentazocine with naloxone hydrochloride (Talwin NX)
pentazocine with acetaminophen (Talacen)

Dosage:
Adults: (Oral, subQ, IM, IV) 30 mg every 3 to 4 hours.

nalbuphine hydrochloride (Nubain). Although it is believed to be equivalent to morphine on a milligram-to-milligram basis for analgesia, this agent does not produce euphoria.

Dosage:
Adults only: (subQ, IM, IV) 10 mg every 3 to 6 hours.

sumatriptan succinate (Imitrex). Sumatriptan succinate acts by binding to a specific type of receptor, 5-hydroxytryptamine (5-HT, serotonin), which is found on blood vessels and on sensory nerves. It appears to constrict blood vessels in the carotid vascular bed and also blocks nerve fibers that conduct pain. The agent is administered by self-injection or taken orally for the treatment of vascular or migraine headaches.

At first hailed as "the most" effective drug in migraine therapy, it has proved disappointing in many cases, probably because many so-called migraines are not vascular headaches at all, but are tension, cluster, or muscular contraction types instead. Thus the drug may work beautifully for some headaches, but not all headaches that the patient may have. A positive response, defined as being pain free 2 hours after the drug is administered, has ranged from 50% to 60%.

It effectively causes vasospasm, thus relieving the vascular headache, but its side effects also relate to vasospasm: angina pectoris, hypertension, and Raynaud's phenomenon have been reported. It should be avoided in pregnancy.

When sumatriptan fails to give the desired relief from migraine headaches, one of the second-generation triptans, such as rizatriptan and zolmitriptan, may give a beneficial effect.

Dosage:
Adults only: (Oral) 25 mg initially. If necessary, after 2 hours a second dose of up to 100 mg may be given. Maximum daily oral dosage is 300 mg. (subQ) 6 mg self-administered. A second dose may be given in 1 hour, but no more than 12 mg in 24 hours.

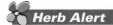 **Herb Alert**

Feverfew

Feverfew is used in the prevention of migraine headaches, and some new studies appear to confirm its effectiveness. Its effectiveness as a digestive aid and as a local anesthetic, and for the treatment of intestinal parasites, arthritis, and menstrual cramps, has not been confirmed. Feverfew enhances the antiplatelet action of nonsteroidal antiinflammatory drugs and warfarin. Its use should be avoided during pregnancy and lactation. See Chapter 35 for more information on feverfew.

rizatriptan benzoate (Maxalt). This second-generation triptan also binds to the 5-HT receptors. This agent crosses the blood-brain barrier, however, and has enhanced activity at the 5-HT receptors within the CNS. It has better bioavailability and is successful with more patients than is sumatriptan. Notably, it may be effective in patients who have had a previous drug failure with sumatriptan. Nausea, dizziness, and insomnia are the usual side effects. It may raise the blood pressure, and thus should be avoided in hypertensive patients. It should not be given to patients with a history of heart trouble because of its vasoconstrictive effects.

Dosage:

Adults only: (Oral) 5 to 10 mg at the onset of a migraine headache. A repeat dose may be taken in 2 hours. No more than 30 mg should be taken in 24 hours.

zolmitriptan (Zomig). Also a second-generation triptan, this drug has enhanced bioavailability and does cross the blood-brain barrier to act on the 5-HT receptors in the brain. It is used to treat migraine headaches and may be effective when the other triptans have not treated the migraine headaches satisfactorily. Its side effects are similar to those of rizatriptan.

Dosage:

Adults only: (Oral) 2.5 to 5 mg at the onset of a migraine headache. Dose may be repeated after 2 hours, not to exceed 10 mg in 24 hours.

ALCOHOL

Alcoholic beverages have been prepared and used by humans as both beverages and medicinal agents since ancient times. At one time alcohol was thought to be a remedy for practically all diseases. During the past century, therapeutic usefulness has diminished greatly because of the availability of more effective and efficient agents, but its abuse as a beverage has become both a medical and a sociologic problem.

Ethyl alcohol (grain alcohol) is obtained by fermentation. It is formed by the growth of yeast in fruit and vegetable juices containing sugar or starch. Undistilled beverages such as wines and beers contain less than 14% alcohol; distilled liquors such as whiskey, brandy, rum, and gin contain about 50% alcohol.

When consumed, alcohol depresses the cells of the cerebral cortex. In large quantities, its depressant action extends to the cerebellum, the spinal cord, and the respiratory center of the medulla. Alcohol kills by paralyzing the respiratory center, which controls breathing.

One effect of alcohol on the cerebral cortex is depression of inhibitory behavior. Small amounts often produce a feeling of well-being, talkativeness, greater vivacity, and increased confidence in one's abilities. Large quantities may cause excitement and impulsive speech and behavior. The special senses become dulled, and the person cannot hear normally and thus talks louder. This sense of freedom from inhibitions has given alcohol a false reputation as a stimulant. For this reason a sedative should not be given to an individual under the influence of alcohol, because it would add to the depression of the CNS.

Therapeutic uses of alcohol include the following:
- Dilation of peripheral blood vessels in vascular disease
- Improvement of appetite and digestion
- Hypnotic effect in some individuals
- Local antiseptic and astringent
- Analgesic when injected in or around the sensory nerve trunks for pain relief

The condition known as epilepsy is as old as the written pages of the history of humankind. It was the "royal illness" of Egyptian pharaohs. Descriptions of the convulsive seizure, the sinister cry, and the loss of consciousness can be traced back to the earliest medical records. Paracelsus described epilepsy as the "disease of lightning," for the individual was struck down as if by a bolt from the sky. Actually, the disease is characterized by an increase in electrical discharges from the brain, producing an irregular pattern. It is a chronic disorder caused by a brain dysfunction, associated with some alteration of consciousness and variable movement. The brain wave patterns obtained by taking an electroencephalogram permit diagnosis of the disease.

TYPES OF EPILEPSY

Major Motor Epilepsy (Grand Mal Seizures)

The seizures are often preceded by an aura and are characterized by a cry, loss of consciousness, and tonic-clonic movements. There is often loss of bladder and bowel control. The attack lasts 2 to 5 minutes and may be followed by deep sleep.

Absence Attacks (Petit Mal Seizures)

A quick loss of consciousness for only 1 to 30 seconds may not be noticeable by others. The patient may not even realize the extent or number of seizures he or she has during the day.

Complex Partial Seizures

This seizure is characterized by a brief loss of contact with the environment or by repetitive motions. The patient is generally confused for a minute or two after the attack.

Epileptic Equivalents

Episodes that resemble seizures may be caused by hypoglycemia, tetanus, poisoning, fluid overload, anaphylaxis, tremors, or drug withdrawal.

ANTICONVULSANTS AND OTHER DRUGS USED TO TREAT EPILEPSY

The first step taken to control epilepsy was in 1857, when Sir Charles Locock gave large doses of bromides to 14 epileptic patients. In nearly all of his cases the frequency and severity of the seizures was diminished. Bromides produced many toxic effects when given over an extended period of time, however, which caused their use to be restricted to some extent.

In 1912, phenobarbital was found to be even more effective than bromides in producing depression of the motor cortex and reducing the number of seizures. Phenobarbital has the disadvantage of depressing the sensory areas of the brain along with the motor areas.

The next advance was made in 1921, when one compound related to the barbiturates was found to depress the motor cortex only and not the sensory areas of the brain. This compound was diphenylhydantoin (now called phenytoin). Since that time, other analogs of this drug have been made and have brought epilepsy under excellent control. As yet there is no cure for epilepsy, but the disease may be controlled through the use of **anticonvulsants.**

phenytoin, USP, BP (Dilantin). This drug causes depression of the motor cortex without depression of the sensory areas of the brain. It is used to a great extent for major motor epilepsy and often is combined with phenobarbital for more effective therapy.

The principal adverse reactions to phenytoin are dizziness, muscular incoordination, gastric distress, weight loss, and skin rashes. None of these symptoms is severe, however, and they may be overcome by temporarily decreasing the dosage or perhaps stopping the drug for a short period of time.

Plasma concentrations of phenytoin are used to regulate the dosage of this drug most effectively. Therapeutic concentrations are 7.5 to 20 mcg/mL. The steady-state serum level may not be achieved until about 1 week of therapy.

There are two types of phenytoin capsules:
- Phenytoin prompt: rapidly absorbed and gives a peak activity in 1 to 3 hours.
- Phenytoin extended: formulated to be more slowly absorbed and produce peak concentrations in 4 to 12 hours. Only this type of phenytoin may be used for once-daily dosage plans.
  Dosage:
  Adults: (Oral) 100 mg three to four times daily (prompt) or 300 mg once daily (extended). (IV) Rate of administration should not exceed 50 mg/minute.
  Children: (Oral) 5 mg/kg/day in three divided doses.

fosphenytoin sodium (Cerebyx). This synthetic agent is intended for parenteral administration. Its active metabolite is phenytoin, hence the therapeutic effect is that of phenytoin. Like phenytoin, it is used for the treatment of major motor epilepsy.

Each vial contains 75 mg of fosphenytoin, which is equivalent to 50 mg of phenytoin. The dose of this drug is expressed as phenytoin equivalents (PE) to avoid the need to calculate the equivalent dose of phenytoin each time this drug is used.

It is used for short-term parenteral administration when other means of phenytoin administration are unacceptable. It is used for the control of status epilepticus and for the prevention and treatment of seizures during neurosurgery.
  Dosage:
  Adults: (IM, IV) 10 to 20 mg PE/kg.

carbamazepine, USP, BP (Tegretol). This agent is used in the management of major motor seizures and complex partial seizures. It is ineffective in petit mal seizures. In addition, it may be useful in controlling the pain of trigeminal neuralgia and other forms of neuritis. The side effects of this agent may be dangerous and include aplastic anemia, liver toxicity, congestive heart failure, acute urinary retention, nausea, vomiting, and gastric distress. It should not be used for the control of seizures that respond to other, less toxic, agents.
  Dosage:
  Adults: (Oral) 200 to 400 mg four times daily.
  Children: (Oral) 10 to 20 mg/kg/day in divided doses.

clonazepam, USP, BP (Klonopin). Clonazepam is used in the management of absence attacks and complex partial seizures. The most frequent side effects are drowsiness, ataxia, and behavioral disturbances. Tolerance to this drug may occur.
  Dosage:
  Adults: (Oral) 1.5 to 20 mg daily in three divided doses.
  Children: (Oral) 0.01 to 0.03 mg/kg/day.

ethosuximide, USP, BP (Zarontin). This agent is used in the management of absence attacks. The most common side effects are nausea, vomiting, gastric distress, anorexia, drowsiness, ataxia, and irritability. Very rarely, blood disturbances, including aplastic anemia, have occurred.
  Dosage:
  Adults: (Oral) 20 mg/kg/day in a single dose. Dose should not exceed 1.5 gm daily.

ethotoin (Peganone). Ethotoin is used to manage major motor and complex partial seizures. It is both less effective and less toxic than phenytoin. It is often combined with other agents for more effective seizure control. Reported side effects include blood dyscrasias, vomiting, diarrhea, chest pain, and nystagmus.
  Dosage:
  Adults: (Oral) 1 to 3 gm daily.
  Children: (Oral) 500 mg to 1 gm daily.

methsuximide, USP, BP (Celontin). Used in the control of absence attacks, this agent is often combined with other antiepileptic agents, such as phenytoin or phenobarbital, for the management of combined types of epilepsy. It has very rarely been associated with blood dyscrasias. Minor personality changes and fluid retention have been reported.
  Dosage:
  Adults and children: (Oral) Initially 300 mg/day, then increased at weekly intervals until seizure control is obtained to a maximum dose of 1.2 gm daily in divided doses.

paramethadione, USP, BP (Paradione). This agent is used in the management of absence attacks that have been found to be refractory to other agents. It is not helpful in the control of other forms of epilepsy, except as an adjunct to other drugs in the treatment of combined types. Severe blood dyscrasias have been reported. Skin rashes, drowsiness, visual disturbances, and alopecia have occurred.

Dosage:

Adults: (Oral) 900 mg to 2.4 gm/day in divided doses.

Children: (Oral) 300 to 900 mg/day in divided doses.

phenacemide, USP, BP (Phenurone). Phenacemide is used in the control of severe seizure disorders that have not responded to other agents. It may be used with other agents to treat combined forms of epilepsy. This drug is highly toxic, and its use must be monitored carefully. Aplastic anemia, fatal liver necrosis, and acute psychotic states have been reported. Anorexia and weight loss, drowsiness, paresthesias, skin rashes, and headaches are commonly observed.

Dosage:

Adults: (Oral) 1.5 to 5 gm/day in divided doses.

Children older than 5 years: (Oral) 250 mg three times daily.

phensuximide, USP, BP (Milontin). Phensuximide is used in the management of absence attacks, although its effects often decrease during long-term therapy. Skin rashes, alopecia, and muscle weakness have occurred. No severe blood dyscrasias have been reported with this agent.

Dosage:

Adults and children: (Oral) 500 mg to 1 gm two to three times daily.

primidone, USP, BP (Mysoline). This agent is used primarily in the treatment of complex partial seizures, but it has been used in major motor seizures as well. Mild toxic effects such as drowsiness, nausea, vomiting, ataxia, and dizziness are reported. Serious toxic effects are rare.

Dosage:

Adults: (Oral) 250 mg to 2 gm/day in two to four divided doses.

Children: (Oral) 125 to 750 mg/day in divided doses.

trimethadione, USP, BP (Tridione). Trimethadione is used in the management of absence attacks refractory to ethosuximide and may be combined with other agents for the treatment of combined forms of epilepsy. It has been associated with severe blood disorders, but these are rare. Skin rashes, drowsiness, visual disturbances, and alopecia have been reported.

Dosage:

Adults: (Oral) 300 mg three times daily. It may be increased to 2.4 gm daily in divided doses.

Children: (Oral) 100 to 300 mg three times daily.

valproic acid, USP, BP (Depakene). This agent has been shown to be extremely useful in the management of epilepsy. It may be used alone or with other agents in the management of absence attacks, and it may be used with other agents for the control of multiple seizure types. The most frequent side effects are nausea, vomiting, and increased appetite with weight gain. Drowsiness, skin rashes, and decreased platelet counts have been observed.

Dosage:

Adults: (Oral) 15 mg/kg/day to a maximum dosage of 30 mg/kg/day. It may be given once daily or in divided doses.

felbamate (Felbatol). This agent is believed to raise the seizure threshold and reduce seizure spread. It is used primarily in complex partial seizures.

Dosage:

Adults and children older than 14 years: (Oral) Up to 2.4 gm/day in divided doses.

Children younger than 14 years: (Oral) 15 mg/kg/day in divided doses.

gabapentin (Neurontin). Gabapentin is generally used in combination with other agents for the control of complex partial seizures. It is also used the treatment of many peripheral neuropathies and for postherpetic neuralgia.

Dosage:

Adults and children older than 12 years: (Oral) 900 mg to 1.8 gm daily in three divided doses.

lamotrigine (Lamictal). This agent is structurally different from most anticonvulsants. It is believed to act by stabilizing neuronal membranes. It is used primarily for the management of complex partial seizures.

Dosage:

Adults and children older than 12 years: (Oral) 25 mg daily. May be increased to 400 mg daily.

Children younger than 12 years: (Oral) 0.15 mg/kg/day.

tiagabine hydrochloride (Gabitril). This anticonvulsant is used primarily in combination with other agents for the control of complex partial seizures.

Dosage:

Adults and children older than 12 years: 4 to 8 mg/day in divided doses.

topiramate (Topamax). Topiramate is generally used in combination with other agents in the management of complex partial seizures in children and adults.

Dosage:

Adults: (Oral) 200 to 400 mg/day.

Children: (Oral) 1 to 3 mg/kg/day.

phenobarbital, USP, BP. Its long duration of effect after oral administration makes phenobarbital useful in a once-daily dose for the management of all forms of epilepsy except absence attacks. It may be given to prevent febrile seizures and to treat acute seizure states. However, it has a relatively slow onset of action even when administered intravenously. It is often combined with other agents for control of seizures. The primary side effect is drowsiness. However, this is often minimized by a once-daily dose administered at bedtime. There is some rather alarming evidence that the sedation or lowering of intelligence may be cumulative and progressive when this agent is used for a long period of time. It seems to be reversible if phenobarbital is discontinued, however.

Dosage:

Adults: (Oral) 100 mg once daily. (IV) For status epilepticus, 200 to 300 mg slowly.

Children: (Oral) 3 to 5 mg/kg/day once daily. (IV) 15 to 20 mg/kg over 10 to 15 minutes.

diazepam, USP, BP (Valium). The injectable form of diazepam has been used intravenously with remarkable success for the control of seizures from various causes. It may be administered to halt status epilepticus, seizures secondary to brain damage, or tetany. Valium is of little value in the long-term control of epilepsy, however. Respiratory arrest may occur with intravenous infusion; thus resuscitation equipment should be available. Its oral use as a tranquilizer is discussed in Chapter 23.

Dosage:

Adults: (IV) 2 to 10 mg slowly.

ANTIPARKINSONIAN AGENTS

Parkinson's disease is a clinical syndrome characterized by lesions of the basal ganglia in the brain. The lesions cause abnormalities in motor activities. About 1% of the population over 65 or about 1 million people in the United States, are believed to have Parkinson's disease.

Parkinson's disease has no known cause, but it seems to be related to depletion of dopamine in the brain. The disease causes alterations in muscle tone, disturbances in postural stability, and abnormal involuntary movements. A resting tremor, described as a pill-rolling motion of the fingers, is characteristic of the condition.

Secondary parkinsonism may be caused by drugs such as the phenothiazines and lithium, by toxins such as methanol or carbon monoxide poisoning, and by degenerative diseases such as Alzheimer's disease. Secondary parkinsonism is treated with the same agents.

Treatment is generally individualized and may be delayed in the early stages of the disease, when physical therapy may provide enough assistance.

DOPAMINERGIC AGENTS

The following agents are used only in adults.

levodopa (Dopar, Larodopa). This agent is an isomer of dihydroxyphenylalanine and is the metabolic precursor of dopamine. It is converted to dopamine in the basal ganglia. It is used to treat Parkinson's disease and to control the symptoms of parkinsonism. It should be used with caution in patients who have a history of myocardial infarction or ventricular arrhythmias. In addition, gastrointestinal hemorrhage, psychiatric disorders, and bronchospasm have been reported as adverse effects of this drug.

Dosage:

Adults: (Oral) 500 mg to 1 gm/day in divided doses.

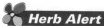 **Herb Alert**

Kava Kava

Kava kava is used to relieve anxiety and stress and promote sleep. It reduces the effects of levodopa and other antiparkinsonian drugs. It enhances the effects of sedatives, hypnotics, antihistamines, alcohol, and alprazolam. Its use should be avoided in patients with depressive disorders and during pregnancy and lactation. See Chapter 35 for more information on kava kava.

carbidopa (Lodosyn). Although available alone, this agent is generally used in combination with levodopa because it inhibits the metabolic breakdown of levodopa and makes more of the drug available to the brain.

Dosage:

Adults: (Oral) 25 mg three times daily.

levodopa plus carbidopa (Sinemet, Atamet). These combinations generally have either a 1:4 or a 1:10 ratio of carbidopa to levodopa. The combinations work well in many cases to reduce the number of medications that have to be taken each day.

Dosage:

25 mg carbidopa/100 mg levodopa three times a day.

OTHER AGENTS USED TO TREAT PARKINSON'S DISEASE

Other drugs used in the treatment of Parkinson's disease are listed in Table 21–4.

Table 21-4 | *Other Agents for Treatment of Parkinson's Disease*

GENERIC NAME	TRADE NAME	ADULT DOSAGE, ORAL
benztropine mesylate	Cogentin	1–4 mg/day, divided
bromocriptine mesylate	Parlodel	1.25–15 mg/day, divided
pergolide mesylate	Permax	0.05–3 mg/day, divided
pramipexole dihydrochloride	Mirapex	0.125–1.5 mg 3 times daily
procyclidine hydrochloride	Kemadrin	2.5–5 mg 3 times daily
ropinirole hydrochloride	Requip	0.25–6 mg 3 times daily
tolcapone	Tasmar	100–200 mg 3 times daily
trihexyphenidyl hydrochloride	Artane	1–6 mg 3 times daily

CLINICAL IMPLICATIONS

1. Central nervous system stimulants are generally given early in the day because they may interfere with the patient's sleep pattern.
2. Central nervous system stimulants may aggravate other medical conditions such as hypertension, cardiovascular disease, and hyperthyroidism.
3. The opioid analgesics are the most effective for pain relief.
4. All patients should have a full realization of the addicting potential of the opioid analgesics and should be cautioned not to overuse the drugs.
5. Central stimulants such as methylphenidate (Ritalin) have a calming effect on persons with attention deficit hyperactivity disorder.
6. Preanesthetic agents to promote sedation aid in the successful induction of general anesthetics. Efforts should be made to maintain the patient in a calm mental condition before surgery.
7. The nurse should be available to explain the actions of the preanesthetic medication and to answer any questions the patient may have about anesthetic induction.
8. Local anesthetics may have as a side effect central nervous system stimulation and irritability. In some cases stimulation may be severe enough to produce seizures.
9. Hypnotics are given to produce restful sleep in unfamiliar surroundings such as hospitals. Nursing measures such as a back rub and the maintenance of a quiet environment may be used to promote restful surroundings as well.
10. Hangovers or continued sedation the day after a hypnotic medication should be noted. Elderly persons are particularly susceptible to sedation from these agents and may need shorter acting hypnotics.
11. Guardrails are often used to prevent accidental injuries when a patient has been prescribed a sedative or hypnotic. The patient should be instructed not to get out of bed without assistance after administration of these agents.
12. When analgesics are prescribed, the nurse should give the medication within the prescribed time frame but ideally before the patient experiences severe recurrence of pain. Small, frequent doses are sometimes more effective than longer spacing of larger doses.
13. Addiction is generally not a problem when narcotics are prescribed for relief of a temporary painful situation, such as postoperatively.
14. The epileptic patient should be cautioned against driving until seizures are controlled for 1 year and should be cautioned against working around machinery. He or she should not swim unattended.
15. Parkinson's disease is a degenerative disease of the central nervous system. A similar condition, parkinsonism, may be due to the side effects of certain drugs.

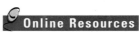

Online Resources

For updated drug information and Web activities, go to http://evolve.elsevier.com/Asperheim.

CRITICAL THINKING QUESTIONS

1. The patient in his second postoperative day was observed to have slow, shallow respirations and "pinpoint" pupils. His hand shook when he reached for a magazine on his overbed table, and he seemed to be less alert than before surgery. What medications do you think he had received for pain? What steps should be taken to handle this situation? Should the physician be called?

2. The patient is brought to his pediatrician's office with a temperature of 104° F and a draining left ear. The mother states that she did not have any acetaminophen (Tylenol) to give the child to control the fever. The child had a generalized seizure during the examination. What do you think caused the temperature elevation? What caused the seizure? Are there any other measures that the mother could have taken to reduce the fever? Does the child need medication for seizures?

3. A patient was brought to the emergency room after taking an overdose of phenobarbital. She is unconscious. What is the most important consideration in meeting this emergency situation?

4. It has been reported that a patient in your unit has not been swallowing her sleeping pills; instead, she is hoarding them in her drawer. She has been very depressed lately. What is the nurse's responsibility when administering any medication? Does the nurse have other responsibilities for this patient? What would you do in this situation?

REVIEW QUESTIONS

1. A major difference between the opioid and nonopioid analgesics is their:
   a. potential for addiction.
   b. there is no difference.
   c. effect on the blood pressure.
   d. effect on the heart.

2. A symptom of chronic opioid use/abuse is:
   a. dilated pupils.
   b. agitation.
   c. diarrhea.
   d. constricted pupils.

3. Codeine is the opioid most often used in:
   a. intravenous pain relief.
   b. preoperative medication.
   c. postoperative medication.
   d. cough preparations.

4. A medication that is effective when administered in a transdermal patch is:
   a. codeine.
   b. morphine.
   c. fentanyl.
   d. meperidine.

5. An example of a nonnarcotic analgesic is:
   a. tramadol.
   b. oxycodone.
   c. butorphanol.
   d. propoxyphene.

6. An agent often used in the treatment of major motor epilepsy is:
   a. phenytoin.
   b. methylphenidate.
   c. levodopa.
   d. cocaine.

7. An absence attack is another name for:
   a. an episode in which the person has amnesia for a whole day.
   b. a convulsive seizure.
   c. absent blood pressure.
   d. loss of consciousness for less than a minute.

8. An agent that is used in the treatment of Parkinson's disease is:
   a. phenobarbital.
   b. phenytoin.
   c. diazepam.
   d. levodopa.

9. Which agent may be used to treat an overdose of morphine?
   a. naloxone
   b. nadolol
   c. codeine
   d. meperidine

10. Which of the following is not used to treat attention deficit hyperactivity disorder?
    a. methylphenidate
    b. dextroamphetamine
    c. ethotoin
    d. pemoline

22 Pain Medications

Objectives

After completing this chapter, you should be able to do the following:

1. Take a careful history of the patient's pain.
2. Understand the sources of chronic pain and the different types of treatment available.
3. Realize that it is the patient's assessment of pain that is most important.
4. Recognize that negative responses on the part of health care workers are inappropriate when assisting patients with chronic pain.
5. Understand that approaches to pain management may use drugs of varying potency.
6. Understand that tolerance to opioids may occur if the patient is treated over a long period of time, and that this is accepted.
7. Become aware of the methods used to prevent illegal use of the narcotic medications.

Key Terms

Coanalgesic (KŌ-ăn-ăl-JĒ-sĭk), p. 118
Physical dependence, p. 118
Pseudoaddiction (SŪ-dō-ăd-DĬK-shŭn), p. 118
Withdrawal, p. 118

The relief of pain and suffering has always been an important goal in patient care. Pain is a problem for many people with many medical conditions, and it is the most feared symptom of any medical problem. Pain hurts; it makes you lose your appetite and become irritable, and it interferes with the quality of life.

Our medical care system is designed to focus on acute care, but it is now necessary to manage many patients with incurable and disabling illnesses that progressively worsen over time. Chronic pain is one of the most common complaints in the primary care facility, and many patients complain that their pain has persisted for over 5 years, either as a constant discomfort or as frequent flare-ups. Frequently depression accompanies painful syndromes and may require separate medication and attention for the pain management to be effective.

In spite of new and effective medications and new treatment procedures, pain is often undertreated. There are many reasons for this:

- The opioids have a well-known potential for abuse and addiction.
- Drug seekers make up all sorts of excuses to obtain narcotic medications that they do not need for any medical conditions.
- Some drug seekers are not truthful.
- Some abusers obtain medications from multiple physicians and clinics.
- Some pain medications are diverted to other persons.
- Some practitioners refuse to write prescription refills for all of these reasons. Meanwhile truly painful conditions are undertreated.

In the terminal patient who is expected to have only a short time to live, tolerance and addiction to the pain medication must be of no concern, and the medications should be dispensed according to increasing need, to provide as much comfort as possible.

For the nonterminal patient with a painful condition, however, the goals must be somewhat different. Some issues to be considered in pain management for these patients may include the following:

1. A realistic goal for therapy. Total freedom from pain is rarely possible as a goal. Instead the patient should be questioned as to his or her needs and expectations. For example, one patient may wish to do simple housework and care for her children without excessive pain. Another patient may accept some pain, but want to remain alert enough to drive his car. A condition that has progressed to a more severe level may require more pain relief at night so that the patient can get a good night's sleep in order to be more alert during the day. It is important to discuss and think through the goals of therapy, and then use them to assess progress.

2. A means of evaluating and describing pain. Because pain is totally subjective (determined by the patient's perception), a method of measuring and communicating issues related to pain must be found that is meaningful to both the patient and the health care worker. Often a pain intensity scale ranging from zero to 10 is used. With this scale, 10 represents the most pain that could be experienced while conscious, and zero represents no pain, is used.

3. The progression of analgesia. Analgesic therapy should start with the agents that have lower potency and

addiction potential, then progress to the more potent agents.

4. Agreements with regard to the patient's responsibility for the pain medication and the physician's responsibility to prescribe the medication. This is often in the form of a written contract, to be discussed in more detail later in this chapter.

ETIOLOGY OF PAIN

Visceral pain from internal organs is generally poorly localized and is more often due to an underlying condition such as cancer. Chronic pain that is not caused by cancer is generally one of two types: *somatic pain,* which arises by activation of the pain receptors in the skin and musculoskeletal tissue, and *neuropathic pain,* which is caused by a disease or injury to the peripheral nerves or their ganglia (groupings of nerve junctions) in the central nervous system.

Somatic pain is often due to back problems and degenerative joint disease. Osteoporosis in the elderly is often associated with collapsed vertebrae and stress fractures, which are acutely painful. Degenerative joint disease is readily apparent in most instances with signs of local inflammation. More troublesome is the diagnosis of fibromyalgia, a musculoskeletal disorder that has no clear diagnostic markers.

Neuropathic pain would include pain resulting from a herpes eruption or diabetic complications, as well as many other conditions that cause inflammation or degeneration of nerves.

INVESTIGATION OF THE CAUSES OF PAIN

A careful history of pain is most important. This should include the history of the condition that is causing the pain, a record of all previous diagnostic procedures, the names of all previous treating practitioners, a determination of the level of the pain, and an understanding of how the pain interferes with the patient's quality of life. It is important to remember that pain is subjective. The physical examination is extremely important in making the diagnosis, but it cannot be relied upon to determine the amount of pain that the patient is experiencing.

Chronic pain causes limitations, both physical and psychological, in the patient's ability to manage his or her daily activities. A careful psychological history should be taken, investigating for signs of depression; if these are found, the depression should also be treated.

Although it is important to diagnose and treat the underlying cause of the pain, in many cases it is equally important to treat the pain itself, even when the diagnosis remains in doubt. Early and aggressive treatment of pain reduces the patient's risk of developing a chronic pain syndrome.

ASSESSMENT OF THE PAIN

Pain needs to be assessed before a plan can be made for management. Considerable effort must be made to gather information on the type, location, and severity of the pain, as well as its impact on the patient's ability to function and on the quality of life. Psychological, spiritual, social, and family histories are important in the assessment.

Because pain is subjective, the patient's assessment of the severity and quality of pain should be accepted. Family members tend to overestimate the pain of their loved ones, and health care workers tend to underestimate it. Nevertheless, insight is gained by including all parties in the evaluation. The observation of grimacing, wincing, limping, profuse sweating, hypertension, pallor, or tachycardia is useful but not diagnostic. In the end, the clinician must accept the patient's report of pain—pain is what the patient says it is.

Pain should be assessed for severity, for factors that ease the pain or make it worse, and for the timing and characteristics of the pain. The history should include any previous painful situations or diagnoses of painful conditions, recent attempts at cure, issues and concerns of substance abuse, and previous response to various methods of pain control. The patient's beliefs about the origin of pain should be assessed and included in the history.

Other issues involve how the pain affects the patient, and how the patient responds to pain. What makes the pain worse, and what improves it? Does it interfere with sleep? It is extremely important to assess the way in which the pain interferes with the activities of daily living, work, hobbies, and social roles. The relationship between high levels of pain and distress and psychological illness should not be ignored in the assessment of the pain. Depression and anxiety can magnify the expression of pain.

Quality-of-life assessment tools are useful in addressing physical well-being as well as underlying problems. For example, fatigue is almost universal as a symptom in pain patients.

It should be remembered that particular care should be taken when assessing patients unable to communicate well. This includes young infants and children, as well as elderly or mentally incompetent patients, the emotionally disturbed, and those who speak only a foreign language. Children may be reluctant to report pain for fear of undergoing further painful diagnostic procedures. Often agitation, fear, and other unusual symptoms are the only way these patients can express their pain. In some cases they are given sedatives when their pain should be addressed instead.

Patients may fear becoming addicted to controlled substances, and many health care workers reinforce that fear. Patients may fear being labeled a "problem patient," and so they may not complain to their physicians about pain and/or inadequate pain relief. Negative responses by health care workers may make patients describe their pain as less severe than what they actually feel.

Effective communication with the patient is extremely important. *The most common reason for unrelieved pain in the American health care system is the failure of staff to routinely and accurately assess pain and pain relief.* Many patients silently tolerate unrelieved pain, especially if they are not specifically asked about it. Thus the key to delivering high-quality pain management is effective communication. All team members must consistently communicate changes in patient status and become aware of treatment plans. Patients and their families value effective communication and an individualized approach to pain management and palliative care. Even patients with severe pain report greater satisfaction with their pain management if they have had good communication with their physician and can experience reduction if not total relief of pain.

PROGRESSIVE LEVELS OF PAIN RELIEF

The approach to the treatment of pain may be considered in three steps: the treatments for mild, moderate and severe pain. A general rule is that, when pain increases, a sustained-release form of a narcotic may be administered by mouth, and a shorter acting "rescue drug" may be given for breakthrough pain between doses. Frequent use of the rescue drug should be noted; if it is necessary for the patient to take the rescue drug more than three or four times a day, a larger dose of the baseline sustained-action drug should be given. The usual dose of the short-acting drug should be equivalent to 5% to 15% of the 24-hour dose of the long-acting drug.

Patients should be told the name of the medication, and they should clearly understand how it is to be taken. If there are restrictions with regard to food or water or combining the pain reliever with other medications, those should be clearly explained. The side effects should be mentioned and any concerns of the patient should be addressed. The patient should be encouraged to ask questions and to participate in her or his care.

Adult dosages are provided for all drugs listed below. Pediatric dosages may be obtained in the respective chapters where the drugs are covered in more detail. All are oral doses unless otherwise specified.

MILD PAIN

This pain can generally be treated with a nonsteroidal anti-inflammatory drug (NSAID) or a nonopioid analgesic. Unless contraindicated, any regimen should include one of these mild analgesics, even when pain is severe enough to require the addition of an opioid. Parenteral and rectal forms of some of these agents are available if the patient is unable to take oral medications.

The potential for gastric ulcer formation needs to be considered with the NSAIDs. The addition of misoprostol or a proton pump inhibitor may be considered. Aspirin may cause bleeding tendencies.

Drugs for Mild Pain

acetaminophen (Tylenol)
Dosage:
Up to 3 to 4 gm/day; also rectal.

aspirin
Dosage:
Up to 3 or 4 gm/day; also rectal.

celecoxib (Celebrex)
Dosage:
Up to 400 mg/day.

diflunisal (Dolobid)
Dosage:
Up to 1500 mg/day.

etodolac (Lodine)
Dosage:
Up to 1000 mg/day.

ibuprofen (Motrin)
Dosage:
Up to 2400 mg/day.

indomethacin (Indocin)
Dosage:
Up to 200 mg/day.

ketorolac tromethamine (Toradol)
Dosage:
Up to 120 mg/day; also IM, IV. Limit treatment to 5 days.

naproxen sodium (Naprosyn, Anaprox)
Dosage:
Up to 1650 mg/day.

sulindac (Clinoril)
Dosage:
Up to 400 mg/day.

valdecoxib (Bextra)
Dosage:
Up to 40 mg/day.

MODERATE PAIN

These short-acting agents for relief of moderate pain may be administered alone or in combination with a nonopioid analgesic as pain increases. Agents in this class are also used when breakthrough pain occurs, or the patient may need step-up therapy using all stronger analgesics. Starting dosages are given in most instances, which may be increased.

Drugs for Moderate Pain

codeine sulfate, combined
Dosage:
30 to 200 mg every 3 to 4 hours.

hydrocodone bitartrate (Dilaudid)
Dosage:
   30 mg every 3 to 4 hours.

oxycodone hydrochloride, combined (Percodan, Percocet)
Dosage:
   30 mg every 3 to 4 hours.

pentazocine (Talwin)
Dosage:
   50 mg every 4 hours; also IM.

propoxyphene (Darvon) combined
Dosage:
   65 to 130 mg every 4 hours.

tramadol hydrochloride (Ultram)
Dosage:
   50 to 100 mg every 4 to 6 hours (to 400 mg/day).

SEVERE PAIN

Some agents for severe pain may need to be administered parenterally. Dosages are given for the beginning range used when these medications become necessary. Tolerance may bring the dosages well above the levels listed below if the medications are used over a period of time. The milder analgesics are often continued with these drugs, and the use of the shorter acting moderate drugs for breakthrough pain is often necessary as well.

Drugs for Severe Pain

butorphanol (Stadol)
Dosage:
   (Parenteral) 2 mg every 4 hours.

morphine sulfate
Dosage:
   (Oral or Parenteral) 30 to 60 mg every 3 to 4 hours.

morphine sulfate controlled release (Oramorph SR, MS Contin)
Dosage:
   (Oral) 90 to 120 mg every 12 hours.

fentanyl citrate (Duragesic, Actiq)
Dosage:
   (Topical patch) 25 to 100 mcg/hr. (Parenteral) 0.1 mg/hr. (Oral) as lozenge, 0.2 to 1.6 mg.

hydromorphone hydrochloride (Dilaudid)
Dosage:
   (Oral) 7.5 mg every 3 to 4 hours. (Parenteral) 1.5 mg every 3 hours.

levorphanol tartrate (Levo-Dromoran)
Dosage:
   (Oral) 3 mg four times daily. (Parenteral) 2 mg every 6 hours.

meperidine hydrochloride (Demerol)
Dosage:
   (Oral or Parenteral) 100 to 500 mg every 3 to 4 hours; limit use to 1 to 2 days.

methadone hydrochloride (Dolophine)
Dosage:
   (Oral or parenteral) 10 to 20 mg every 6 hours.

nalbuphine (Nubain)
Dosage:
   (Parenteral) 10 mg every 4 hours.

oxycodone (OxyContin, OxyIR, OxyFAST)
Dosage:
   (Oral) 30 to 160 mg every 12 hours.

oxymorphone hydrochloride (Numorphan)
Dosage:
   (Parenteral) l mg every 3 to 4 hours.

OPIATES AND OPIOIDS

As discussed in Chapter 21, an opioid is a synthetic drug made to imitate opium derivatives; examples include meperidine, hydromorphone, and oxycodone. Morphine, codeine, and papaverine are opium derivatives, and thus correctly termed *opiates*. However, most narcotics currently in use are synthetic in part or whole, so for ease of use we will use the term *opioids* to discuss the narcotic drugs. Unless stated otherwise, it should be assumed that the opiate characteristics are identical to those discussed for opioids.

EQUIVALENT DOSES OF OPIOIDS

For comparison purposes, the oral doses of the opioids that are equivalent to a dose of 10 mg of morphine administered intramuscularly are shown in Table 22–1.

LONG-TERM EFFECTS OF THE OPIOIDS

Early in the process of analgesia, severe pain appears to counteract the sedative effects of the opioids. Certainly tolerance develops to the sedating effects of opioids, but the mechanism for developing dose-related tolerance when these agents are used for analgesia is more poorly understood. The need for dosage increases certainly develops more slowly when the drugs are given for true pain relief than when they are taken by addicts for the euphoria effect. There is no true ceiling or maximum dose for the opioids. Extremely large doses may be necessary to relieve severe pain.

   Physical dependence is a condition in which the patient requires continued use of a drug for proper functioning, and would experience withdrawal symptoms if it were discontinued. It is a physiologic phenomenon that occurs following regular use of opioids for more than 2 weeks and thus should be expected. Physical dependence also

Table 22-1 *Doses of Various Opioids That Are Equivalent to Morphine 10 mg Intramuscularly*

DRUG	EQUIVALENT DOSE
ORAL ANALGESICS	
morphine	60 mg
codeine	200 mg
hydrocodone	40 mg
hydromorphone	7.5 mg
levorphanol	4 mg
meperidine	300 mg
methadone	20 mg
oxycodone	30 mg
TRANSDERMAL EQUIVALENT	
fentanyl	25-mcg patch equivalent to 45 to 135 mg/day of oral morphine

occurs following administration of steroids, beta-blockers, and other antihypertensive drugs for an extended period of time. This is not to be considered the same as drug addiction, which is generally driven by a desire for the euphoria associated with the drug and may involve criminal behavior.

The fear of opioid addiction should not be a primary concern when implementing appropriate therapy for acute pain and cancer pain. However, there are still patients who attempt to obtain opioids for illegal use by trying to pass themselves off as patients with legitimate need. The use of drug screens, looking for appropriate levels of the prescribed drug as well as for other illegal agents, may assist in identifying these individuals.

Pseudoaddiction is a term that has been used to describe the drug-seeking behaviors that may occur when a patient's pain is undertreated. Patients may "clock watch," may become focused on obtaining medication, and may otherwise seem to be inappropriately "drug seeking." This behavior resolves when the pain is adequately treated.

Many patients with acute pain are anxious, but are calmed when the pain is relieved with analgesics. Antianxiety agents may be necessary as adjunctive medication.

Withdrawal (a syndrome that occurs when a drug-dependent person discontinues the drug suddenly) must be prevented, and can be avoided if the drugs are tapered gradually. The time course of the withdrawal symptoms is a function of the half-life of the opioid. With short half-life drugs such as morphine and hydromorphone, the symptoms may appear in 6 to 12 hours and peak at 24 to 72 hours. With longer half-life drugs such as methadone and levorphanol, symptoms may be delayed for several days and are generally less severe.

SIDE EFFECTS OF THE OPIOIDS

Respiratory depression is an effect of the opioids, particularly with higher doses. There are always precautions against combining the opioids with other sedating drugs. Alcohol is additive and thus should be avoided also.

Opioids may cause constipation, sleepiness, dry mouth, nausea, and vomiting. To manage the constipation, the patient should be instructed to drink several 8-ounce glasses of fluid per day and eat foods high in fiber, such as beans, lentils, and dried or fresh fruits. A stool softener should be given routinely when the patient requires daily opioids. Senna tablets or other laxatives may become necessary and should be taken as needed.

Antihistamines such as over-the-counter cold preparations are additive for the sleepiness and dry mouth side effects, and thus should be avoided if possible. Alternatively, the side effects should be anticipated and managed.

Except in unusual cases, the nausea and vomiting associated with opioid therapy generally go away within a short time.

COANALGESICS

A **coanalgesic** is any of a group of drugs that may be used to enhance pain relief. A number of other classes of drugs may be used to increase the effects of opioids or NSAIDs, and some may have independent analgesic properties as well.

TRICYCLIC ANTIDEPRESSANTS

Examples: amitriptyline, desipramine, imipramine, nortriptyline

These agents are used for the treatment of neuropathic pain and for their antidepressant activity. Use of these agents alone is generally not effective; they should be combined with other analgesics. Anticholinergic effects such as dry mouth, urinary retention, constipation, sedation, and orthostatic hypotension must be considered as potential side effects. Administration of these agents at bedtime may promote a better night's sleep and may minimize the daytime side effects. They are discussed more completely in Chapter 23 (Tranquilizers and Antidepressants).

BENZODIAZEPINES

Examples: diazepam, lorazepam, clonazepam

These tranquilizers may be useful for treating anxiety. They are discussed more completely in Chapter 23 (Tranquilizers and Antidepressants).

ANTICONVULSANT DRUGS

Examples: gabapentin, carbamazepine, oxcarbazepine, topiramate, sodium valproate, tiagabine, phenytoin, lamotrigine

These agents reduce the spontaneous "firing" of central motor neurons that causes seizures. The success of this pharmacologic action led researchers to see if they also decreased spontaneous firing of sensory neurons associated with neuropathic pain. They are useful in the treatment of trigeminal neuralgia, posttraumatic neuralgia, and postherpetic neuralgia. In some cases they are also being used to treat painful conditions "off label" (without full approval by the Food and Drug Administration because of inadequate research data). They are discussed more completely in Chapter 21 (Drugs That Affect the Central Nervous System).

LOCAL ANESTHETICS

Examples: lidocaine, capsaicin

Topical lidocaine patches and nerve blocks have been used extensively in acute pain management. Epidural and intravenous infusions of local anesthetics may be useful acutely, but not for ongoing therapy. They are discussed in Chapter 21 (Drugs That Affect the Central Nervous System). Capsaicin is an enzyme found in hot peppers. When applied topically in an ointment formulation, it relieves neuropathic pain and arthritic pain. These nonprescription formulations may be useful as adjunctive therapy.

GLUCOCORTICOIDS

Examples: prednisone, dexamethasone

These agents have many concurrent uses in pain management. They may directly break up certain tumors and may relieve nerve or spinal cord compression by reducing edema in tumor and nerve tissue. They may increase euphoria and increase appetite in severely ill patients. Chronic use produces weight gain, cushingoid appearance, osteoporosis, myopathy, and psychosis, but these are largely disregarded in the chronically ill patient. The glucocorticoids should be gradually withdrawn rather than abruptly stopped when therapy is discontinued. These agents are discussed more completely in Chapter 27 (The Endocrine Glands and Hormones).

SKELETAL MUSCLE RELAXANTS

Examples: carisoprodol, cyclobenzaprine, orphenadrine

These agents may be useful in preventing the pain from muscle spasms. They are sedating and may have anticholinergic side effects as well.

AGENTS USED FOR METASTATIC BONE PAIN

Examples: bisphosphonates, radiotherapy

Pamidronate disodium (Aredia) inhibits reduction of bone mass and has been shown to reduce skeletal complications such as pathologic fractures in metastatic bone lesions. It may be administered in an intravenous infusion. Widespread bony metastases may be irradiated for pain relief or targeted with localized radiation therapy using a radioactive isotope such as strontium, which may be taken up by the bony metastasis.

THE PATIENT'S MEDICATION USE AGREEMENT

A written agreement made between the prescriber and the patient has become a useful tool in pain management. It has been found that a written agreement reinforces the serious nature of the patient's condition and points out the conse-

quences if the patient does not comply with the agreed-upon goals and conditions for long-term pain management. These agreements are generally written by the prescriber according to the needs of his or her practice, and may include the statements shown in Figure 22–1.

Informed consent is an essential part of the documentation. These agreements are particularly recommended for patients with a history of substance abuse, or those taking higher doses of opioids.

Random drug testing may not be necessary for every patient, but it may be extremely helpful for patients at risk for drug diversion activities or whose behavior seems unusual. Drug testing confirms that the patient is indeed taking the medications prescribed to him or her, and is not taking other controlled or illegal substances as well. Before discussing unusual drug test results with the patient, it may be helpful to speak to the laboratory technician to confirm the proper interpretation of the results. Drug testing techniques must follow acceptable standards to avoid mismanagement of samples.

CLINICAL IMPLICATIONS

1. All members of the health care team are important when assessing the patient's pain and her or his response to medication.
2. Negative personal opinions concerning patients taking chronic pain medications must be avoided.
3. Concurrent conditions such as depression or anxiety may need to be treated separately.
4. Apparent drug-seeking behavior may occur as a result of inadequate pain control rather than addictive behavior.
5. The use of analgesic medications should be progressive in nature, beginning with the milder analgesics and moving to stronger agents as the severity of pain increases.
6. The patient should be encouraged to talk about his or her pain, including whether or not it is satisfactorily relieved, and should be taught to evaluate pain on a scale of zero to 10.
7. A realistic goal for therapy is essential for the chronic pain patient.
8. Patients should become familiar with actions of their medications, the names of the medications, and the potential for side effects.
9. The patient may require a frank discussion of the differences between addictive behavior, generated by a search for euphoria, and the use of these agents for pain relief.
10. Physical dependence on an opioid may occur if it is used for over 2 weeks. This is an expected effect and is not a matter of concern when treating chronic pain.
11. When an agent is discontinued, gradually decreasing the drug minimizes the withdrawal symptoms.
12. Methods of guarding against abuse of the opioids may include a medication use agreement as well as periodic drug testing.

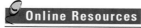

Online Resources

For updated drug information and Web activities, go to http://evolve.elsevier.com/Asperheim.

```
******************************
```
Medication Agreement

1. I, _____ understand that I have pain that has not been adequately controlled, and I understand that the purpose of pain management will be to relieve the pain. I understand that it may not be possible for the complete elimination of the painful condition.

2. I understand that the pain medication will only be prescribed by _____ on the agreed upon schedule. I will not seek pain medication from any other practitioner, and will not take other medications without the knowledge and permission of _____ .

3. Medication refills will be provided as written prescriptions only. No refills will be given prior to the next scheduled appointment date. No-show appointments may be cause for terminating the agreement. Forged or altered prescriptions, or diversion of the medications to any other person will be cause for terminating the agreement.

4. Lost or stolen medications will not be replaced under any circumstances. It is my responsibility to secure my medication.

5. If recommended to see another specialist or take some other form of therapy I understand it is my obligation to cooperate with these endeavors.

6. I agree to undergo random drug testing whenever it is requested.

7. I agree to fill my prescriptions only at the following pharmacy: _____ , address _____ . If I change pharmacies for any reason I will call the health care provider's office and inform him or her. I understand I cannot use more than one pharmacy at any one time. A copy of this agreement will be given to the pharmacist.

8. I understand that this agreement may be terminated if I am no longer receiving a reasonable therapeutic benefit from the medication, or if it is determined that I am no longer a good candidate to receive the medication.

9. I understand that by signing this agreement I must abide by the rules stated above and that failure to abide by these agreements will result in the possible termination of services from my health care provider.

(Patient)_____

Date_____

(Health Care Provider)_____

```
******************************
```

FIGURE 22-1 Sample medication use agreement.

CRITICAL THINKING QUESTIONS

1. The patient appears chronically ill and requests pain medication. He is pale and diaphoretic and was observed to be favoring his left leg when walking in. What questions would be important in the initial evaluation of his painful condition?

2. The patient is nervous and distracted, and cannot answer most of the questions about his medical history. What additional considerations may be made with regard to his treatment?

3. The patient comes in with a grocery bag of medications. You notice there are many herbal remedies, cold products, antihistamines, and medications from several doctors. How would you approach this medical history?

4. The patient strongly resists a standard drug test as part of his medication agreement. He feels this means he is not trustworthy. How would you counsel him?

REVIEW QUESTIONS

1. A patient who watches the clock for each dose of pain medication may be:
   a. a definite drug addict.
   b. overtreated with pain medication.
   c. undertreated with pain medication.
   d. ignored.

2. With regard to an objective assessment of the patient's pain, the health care worker often:
   a. overestimates the pain.
   b. underestimates the pain.
   c. needs the scale of zero to 10 to assess the pain.
   d. is totally accurate in her or his assessment.

3. An agent that may be given for an initial trial of pain control is:
   a. morphine.
   b. codeine.
   c. ibuprofen.
   d. fentanyl.

4. A narcotic that can be given by the transdermal route is:
   a. pentazocine.
   b. ketoralac.
   c. codeine.
   d. fentanyl.

5. A dose of oral oxycodone that is equivalent to 10 mg of morphine intramuscularly is:
   a. 10 mg.
   b. 20 mg.
   c. 30 mg.
   d. 60 mg.

6. A coanalgesic is an agent that:
   a. can be used instead of narcotics for relief of severe pain.
   b. is responsible for codependency.
   c. can be used to make the patient cooperate with pain relief.
   d. can be used to potentiate pain relief.

7. A mechanism that avoids inappropriate use of or dependence on narcotics is:
   a. the use of a medication agreement between the patient and physician.
   b. periodic drug testing.
   c. the use of only one pharmacy for the prescriptions.
   d. all of the above.

8. The person best qualified to assess the patient's pain is the:
   a. patient.
   b. health care worker.
   c. family.
   d. doctor.

9. An agent that may be used for short-term breakthrough pain when a patient is already on a long-acting narcotic is:
   a. Tylenol.
   b. hydrocodone.
   c. OxyContin.
   d. rofecoxib.

10. An agent that is often necessary when a patient is on daily opioids is:
    a. a laxative.
    b. an antidiarrheal agent.
    c. an antihistamine.
    d. an anticholinergic agent.

23 Tranquilizers and Antidepressants

After completing this chapter, you should be able to do the following:

1. Become familiar with the conditions for which the tranquilizers and antidepressants are used.
2. Become familiar with the various types of drugs used to treat psychiatric disorders.
3. Distinguish between a monoamine oxidase inhibitor and a tricyclic antidepressant and give two examples of each type.
4. Discuss adverse effects of the phenothiazine type of antipsychotic drugs.
5. Discuss important uses for the phenothiazine type of antipsychotic agents.
6. List indications for the temporary use of the tranquilizers.
7. List the symptoms of a major depressive disorder.
8. Summarize important responsibilities of the nurse related to administration of monoamine oxidase inhibitors.
9. Summarize important responsibilities of the nurse related to administration of antidepressants.

Key Terms

Antidepressant (ăn-tī-dē-PRĔS-ănt), p. 125
Anxiolytic (ĂNGK-sē-ō-LĬT-ĭk) **agents,** p. 128
Depression, p. 125
Monoamine oxidase inhibitors (MAOIs), p. 126
Sedatives, p. 122
Selective serotonin reuptake inhibitors (SSRIs) (SĔR-ĕ-TŌ-nĭn rē-ŬP-tāk), p. 125
Tranquilizers (TRĂNG-kwĕ-LĪZ-ĕrs), p. 122

Many agents have become available for the temporary and long-term treatment of psychosomatic illnesses. The most satisfactory management of this problem would be aimed, of course, at the prevention of emotional and mental disorders, but achieving this goal will take an unknown length of time, for many and varied reasons. Until we provide a happy, peaceful environment for ourselves and our offspring, devoid of practices that lead to emotional trauma and instability, we will have man-made illnesses. The religious, sociologic, educational, and political factors involved in rectifying the basic problems are so numerous and complicated that progress in the prevention campaign will undoubtedly be very slow. A much more practical solution would be to learn to adjust to our problems and difficulties rather than constantly seeking to be rid of them.

As research continues in the field of mental illness, more information is obtained about the direct effect of hormone levels on the brain and the mood of the individual. Current research is developing many new drugs that are known to function by altering brain chemistry.

Psychotherapy and psychoanalysis, with or without concomitant drug therapy, have been used to help patients uncover the underlying causes of their illnesses. Other treatments include electroconvulsive shock therapy for patients who do not respond to the pharmacologic agents.

Among the first drugs used for these illnesses were the simple **sedatives,** which served to calm or quiet nervous excitement and sometimes induced sleep. The treatment was merely a symptomatic approach, however, for it did nothing to remove the conditions causing the illness in the first place, nor did it help the patient to adjust to the circumstances.

TRANQUILIZERS

As a group, the **tranquilizers** were developed to calm or tranquilize individuals without making them too sedated to perform their activities of daily living.

chlorpromazine hydrochloride, USP, BP (Thorazine). The quieting, relaxing effect of this drug was quickly appreciated, and it has been used extensively. It shows great tranquilizing effects in emotional upsets, such as anxiety and tension; in conditions characterized by hyperactivity, agitation, and similar manifestations of emotion; and in certain types of schizophrenia. The important feature of this and similar agents is that they make the patient more amenable to psychotherapy. Treatment may have been all but impossible because of the inability even to communicate with the patient, much less reason with him or her, but upon administration of the drug the patient is able to discuss problems and fears in a calm and sensible manner. However, overuse of these agents can lead to dependence when the patient has reached a stage in which he or she should be able to adjust to problems without reliance upon drugs.

Chlorpromazine is useful in alleviating nausea and vomiting caused by certain conditions such as carcinoma, acute infections, radiation sickness, ingestion of certain drugs (e.g., nitrogen mustard), and postoperative effects.

Some of the side effects that may occur are tachycardia, hypothermia, dryness of the mouth, parkinsonism, jaundice, liver damage, blood dyscrasias, and rashes.

Dosage:
Adults: (Oral, IM, Rectal) 10 to 50 mg three or four times daily.
Children: (Oral, IM, Rectal) 0.55 mg/kg four times daily.

prochlorperazine maleate, USP, BP (Compazine). Although effective as a tranquilizing agent, prochlorperazine is rarely used for long-term therapy because of its high incidence of extrapyramidal symptoms, such as gait disturbances, restlessness, and aberrations in muscle contraction. Occasionally, opisthotonos occurs even on the first dose of this drug, with arching of the back, inability to speak, and loss of muscle control. This reaction has been confused with a certain type of epileptic seizure but is seen to differ from it upon close observation. This drug is used primarily for its antinauseant effects, particularly postoperatively. It may be given orally or intramuscularly (IM).

Dosage:
Adults: (Oral, IM) 5 to 10 mg three to four times daily.
Children: (Oral, IM) 0.1 mg/kg four times daily.

trifluoperazine hydrochloride, USP, BP (Stelazine). This drug is also chemically quite similar to chlorpromazine but is more potent; thus it can be given in lower doses. Lower doses are given to outpatients; higher doses are usually reserved for hospitalized patients.

Dosage:
Adults: (Oral, IM) 1 to 10 mg two times daily.
Children over 6 years: (Oral) 1 mg one to two times daily.

triflupromazine hydrochloride (Vesprin). This agent is used for the symptomatic management of psychotic disorders.

Dosage:
Adults: (IM or IV) 60 mg daily in divided doses.
Children: (IM or IV) not to exceed 10 mg daily in divided doses.

thioridazine hydrochloride, USP, BP (Mellaril). The wide range of doses and the relatively low incidence of side effects experienced with this compound make it very useful as a tranquilizer. It is used for the same purposes as chlorpromazine is used.

Dosage:
Adults: (Oral) 20 to 800 mg/day in divided doses.
(IM) 1 to 2 mg every 4 to 6 hours.

Children: (Oral) 0.25 mg/kg four times daily. (IM) 1 mg one to two times daily.

meprobamate, USP, BP (Equanil). This drug has a depressant effect on the transmission of nerve impulses inside the spinal cord and possibly in certain areas of the brain. It has a relaxant action on the skeletal muscles because of this depressant action. It is effective as a tranquilizer in moderately tense and anxious patients. Side effects are rare and of the minor type. They include skin eruptions, fever, chills, weakness of skeletal muscles, and, occasionally, a drop in blood pressure. There is a mild addiction with prolonged use of this drug, but withdrawal effects are minimal if the drug is tapered off rather than discontinued suddenly.

Dosage:
Adults: (Oral) 400 mg three to four times daily.
Children older than 6 years: (Oral) 100 to 200 mg two to three times daily.

chlordiazepoxide hydrochloride, USP, BP (Librium). Completely unrelated to other tranquilizers chemically and pharmacologically, this agent is indicated whenever fear, anxiety, and other emotional upsets complicate the medical picture. In low oral doses, it is effective in mild to moderate anxiety and tension. It is used for premenstrual tension, chronic alcoholism, and behavior disorders and in gastrointestinal, cardiovascular, gynecologic, or dermatologic disorders. It is regulated by the Controlled Substances Act. Drowsiness, confusion, and ataxia (impaired coordination) have been reported in some patients after administration of this drug, but such effects can be avoided in almost all instances by proper dosage control.

Dosage:
Adults: (Oral) 5 to 25 mg three to four times daily.
(IM, IV) 50 to 100 mg every 2 to 4 hours.
Children older than 6 years: (Oral) 5 to 10 mg two to four times daily.

hydroxyzine hydrochloride, USP, BP (Atarax, Vistaril). This drug is used for mildly anxious and tense patients and in the treatment of dermatologic conditions thought to be induced by a psychogenic component. It is quite effective in the relief of itching.

Dosage:
Adults: (Oral, IM) 25 to 100 mg three to four times daily.
Children: (Oral) 50 mg daily in divided doses. (IM) 0.5 mg/kg every 6 hours.

diazepam, USP, BP (Valium). Diazepam is useful in the treatment of anxiety reactions stemming from stressful circumstances or whenever illness is complicated by emotional factors. It may be given to patients in psychoneurotic states manifested by anxiety, tension, fear, and fatigue as well as in acute agitation resulting from alcohol withdrawal. It appears to be of some use in the alleviation of muscle spasms associated with cerebral palsy and athetosis. It is of little use in psychotic patients. It has a tendency to be habit forming. Side effects include drowsiness, nausea, dizziness, blurred vision, headache, incontinence, slurred speech, and skin rash. It is contraindicated for infants, patients with a history of convulsive disorders, and patients with glaucoma.

Dosage:
Adults: (Oral, IM, IV) 2 to 10 mg two to three times daily.
Children: (Oral, IM, IV) 1.0 to 2.5 mg three to four times daily.

clorazepate dipotassium (Tranxene). Chlorazepate is used in the treatment of mild anxiety and tension states. It is not recommended for severely depressed or psychotic individuals. Side effects include dizziness, nervousness, headache, ataxia, dry mouth, skin rashes, and decreases in blood pressure. The possibility of dependence must be considered when this agent is prescribed for a long period of time.

Dosage:
Adults: (Oral) 7.5 mg four times daily.
Children: No standard dose is established.

fluphenazine hydrochloride, USP, BP (Permitil, Prolixin). This agent, a structural derivative of the phenothiazine agents, may be administered orally or intramuscularly to relieve the agitation associated with schizophrenia. This agent has a slight increase in extrapyramidal side effects compared with the earlier phenothiazines. Sedation, nausea, polyuria (excreting large amounts of urine), headache, glaucoma, and urinary and fecal retention occur with use.

Dosage:
Adults and children older than 12 years: (Oral) 0.5 to 10 mg daily in divided doses. (IM) 12.5 to 25 mg. For prolonged therapy, the dose may be given every 2 to 4 weeks.

haloperidol, USP, BP (Haldol). This phenothiazine derivative is primarily used as a treatment for schizophrenia. Side effects resemble those of fluphenazine.

Dosage:
Adults: (Oral) 0.5 to 1.5 mg two to three times daily. (IM) 3.0 to 5.0 mg. Additional doses may be administered every 30 to 60 minutes until control is obtained.
Children: No standard dose is established.

haloperidol decanoate (Haldol). This injectable form of haloperidol is used for long-term parenteral treatment of schizophrenia and psychotic states. After IM injection there is a slow and sustained release of the medication, with plasma concentration reaching a peak after 6 days from the time of the injection. The half-life is about 3 weeks.

Dosage:
Adult: (IM) 50 to 100 mg IM every 4 weeks.

aripiprazole (Abilify). This agent is used in the treatment of schizophrenia. It should be used with caution in combination with other centrally acting drugs. It is not a controlled substance.

Dosage:
Adults: (Oral) 15 mg once daily.

lithium carbonate, USP, BP (Eskalith, Lithane, Lithonate). Lithium carbonate has been found highly effective in the control of bipolar disorder. Although the exact mechanism of action is not known, it is believed to alter the metabolism of norepinephrine in the brain. The full effect of this drug is not seen until after 6 to 10 days of treatment; thus other pharmacologic agents with a more rapid onset of action are often prescribed with this drug in the early phase of treatment. Serum lithium levels should be measured frequently to avoid toxic levels of this drug. Fine hand tremor, polyuria, thirst, nausea, and diarrhea are seen at therapeutic levels of this agent. At toxic levels, serious neurologic and cardiovascular effects are seen. A list of drugs that interact with lithium is presented in Table 23–1.

Dosage:
Adults and children older than 12 years: (Oral) Initially 600 mg three times daily, then reduced to 300 mg three times daily.
Children: Not recommended for those younger than 12 years.

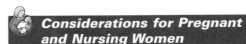

Considerations for Pregnant and Nursing Women

Lithium
Lithium can cause fetal toxicity when administered to pregnant women. Administration of the drug to pregnant and nursing women is appropriate only in life-threatening situations or with severe disease for which safer drugs are ineffective. When possible, lithium should be withdrawn for at least the first trimester. Monitor serum lithium concentrations carefully during pregnancy.

OTHER TRANQUILIZERS

loxapine (Loxitane)
Dosage:
Adults: (Oral) 10 mg twice daily.

Table 23-1 *Drug Interactions with Lithium*

DRUG	EFFECT ON LITHIUM LEVEL	MANAGEMENT
Thiazide diuretics	Increased	Monitor, adjust dosage
NSAIDs	Increased	Monitor, adjust dosage
ACE inhibitors	Increased	Monitor, adjust dosage
Calcium channel blockers	Increased or decreased	Monitor, adjust dosage

ACE, Angiotensin-converting enzyme; NSAIDs, nonsteroidal antiinflammatory drugs.

mesoridazine besylate, BP (Serentil)
Dosage:
    Adults: (Oral) 10 mg three times daily. (IM) 25 mg; may be repeated in 30 to 60 minutes.

molindone hydrochloride (Moban)
Dosage:
    Adults: (Oral) 5 to 15 mg three to four times daily.

olanzapine (Zyprexa)
Dosage:
    Adults: (Oral) 5 to 10 mg daily. (IM) 5 to 10 mg one or two times daily. (IV) Diluted 1-mg doses every 1 to 2 minutes for a maximum of 5 mg. Parenteral therapy is used for only 24 to 48 hours, and then the patient is changed to oral therapy.

pimozide (Orap)
Dosage:
    Adults: (Oral) 1 to 2 mg/day.
    Children: (Oral) 0.05 mg/kg/day.

quetiapine fumarate (Seroquel)
Dosage:
    Adults: (Oral) 25 mg twice daily to a maximum of 400 mg daily.

risperidone (Risperdal)
Dosage:
    Adults (Oral) 1 mg twice daily to a maximum of 8 mg daily.

thiothixene, USP, BP (Navane)
Dosage:
    Adults: (Oral) 2 mg three times daily to a total of 15 mg/day. (IM) 4 mg two to four times daily.

ANTIDEPRESSANTS

Depression is a mental state characterized by feelings of sadness, often accompanied by psychomotor retardation. Clinical depression must be separated from despondency or sadness that is the direct result of life events. The latter is generally founded in difficult situations; it is temporary, and it is naturally reversed in time.

Endogenous depression, or depression without obvious external causes, is greatly underdiagnosed in the population. Fearing the social stigma of mental illness, people would much rather blame their malaise on physical symptoms such as back pain, allergies, abdominal distress, headaches, fatigue, ulcers, and other disorders. The treatment of the secondary disorder is rarely completely successful if an underlying depression is not first discovered and treated.

The tendency to see a patient's disease as a puzzle to be solved, and not to see the concerns of the patient, is unfortunately common in all aspects of health care. Diseases are not independent and separate from the patient as a person. Depression particularly can alter the success of many treatments.

One in six people in the United States will have a major episode of depression at some point in their lives. Except for coronary artery disease, no chronic physical illness results in more disability than depression.

Diagnostic criteria for major depression are as follows:
1. Depressed mood
2. Anhedonia (loss of interest or pleasure)
3. Recurrent thoughts of death or suicide
4. Indecisiveness or decreased concentration
5. Fatigue
6. Feelings of worthlessness or guilt
7. Overall slowness or agitation
8. Insomnia or hypersomnia
9. Significant weight loss or gain

A patient must have five of these nine symptoms to be diagnosed as having depression.

An **antidepressant** is any agent used to counteract depression. Running can be used as a simple antidepressant. The production of natural endorphins after vigorous exercise has been shown to give an antidepressant or even euphoric effect. This is known as the "runner's high." Some institutions are now experimenting with vigorous physical exercise as an adjunct to the treatment of mental illness.

 Herb Alert

St. John's Wort

St. John's wort has been used to treat mild to moderate depression. It is now a component of various herbal remedies for the treatment of anxiety and depression. St. John's wort reduces the effects of theophylline, coumarin, digoxin, indinavir, cyclosporine, and oral contraceptives. It appears to enhance the effects of SSRIs and tricyclic antidepressants. It should be avoided in patients taking MAOIs. See Chapter 35 for more information on St. John's wort.

The antidepressant drugs, because they work indirectly by raising or lowering the levels of certain naturally occurring brain hormones, may take 2 to 3 weeks to exert their effect. These agents should be used with caution when other therapeutic agents are administered, because there are many drug interactions and untoward side effects in such combinations.

SELECTIVE SEROTONIN REUPTAKE INHIBITORS

The main effect of all **selective serotonin reuptake inhibitors (SSRIs)** is the specific and potent inhibition of serotonin reuptake on the presynaptic neuron, which increases serotonin availability at the synapse. This causes increased concentration of serotonin in the central nervous system, and this is believed to be responsible for the antidepressant effect. The antidepressant effect, then, is due to an increased supply of an intrinsic, or naturally occurring, brain hormone.

The SSRIs are generally tolerated well. They are simple in their dosage requirements—starting slowly and gradually increasing the dose to the desired effect—and they are generally trouble free. There is generally no advantage to starting immediately at a high dose, because the adverse effects may become evident before enough time has elapsed to see whether the agent is effective against the depression. If no response occurs to an agent by about 8 weeks, then it is best to switch to another drug in the same class. Long-term treatment appears to produce the most stable remission rates.

Side effects long recognized include gastrointestinal disturbances, particularly at the beginning of treatment, as well as headache, sexual dysfunction, and anorexia. Recently some symptoms have been recognized when the drug is abruptly stopped after the patient takes it for several months. These include vertigo, gastrointestinal symptoms, anxiety, crying spells, flulike symptoms, and insomnia. These are generally mild and usually resolve in 2 weeks. The dose should be tapered over at least 5 to 7 days when an SSRI is withdrawn to avoid or minimize these symptoms.

In addition to depression, other indications for the SSRIs include obsessive-compulsive disorder, panic disorder, post-traumatic stress disorder (PTSD), and premenstrual syndrome (PMS). Drugs in this class are summarized in Table 23–2. Table 23–3 lists drugs that interact with SSRIs.

Considerations for Older Adults

Paroxetine (Paxil)

There is evidence that older patients taking paroxetine may develop hyponatremia and a transient syndrome of inappropriate secretion of antidiuretic hormone (SIADH). Monitor serum sodium concentrations in older adults taking paroxetine, particularly in the first few months of therapy.

MONOAMINE OXIDASE INHIBITORS

Monoamine oxidase inhibitors (**MAOIs**) inhibit monoamine oxidase, a naturally occurring hormone that is involved in the breakdown of several neurotransmitters in the brain, including epinephrine, dopamine, and serotonin. They are effective antidepressants but have many untoward reactions with food substances. MAOIs may not be taken with foods that are high in amines, such as Chianti wine, cheeses such as Swiss and cheddar, chicken liver, avocados,

Table 23-3 | *Drug Interactions with the SSRIs*

DRUG	INTERACTION	MANAGEMENT
alprazolam (Xanax)	Increased alprazolam level	Monitor, reduce dosage
warfarin (Coumadin)	Increased warfarin level	Monitor, adjust dosage
phenytoin (Dilantin)	Possible phenytoin toxicity	Monitor phenytoin level
carbamazepine (Tegretol)	Increased carbamazepine level	Monitor and adjust dosage
cimetidine (Tagamet)	Increased SSRI level	Monitor clinically and adjust
Beta-blockers	Increased beta-blocker effects	Adjust dosage

pickled herring, figs, and alcoholic beverages. If these are combined with a MAOI, a severe increase in blood pressure occurs.

phenelzine sulfate, USP, BP (Nardil). The best results obtained with this drug are seen when it is used for the true depressive states: patients who are sad, worried, and sleepless and who have gloomy thoughts and feel useless. This agent takes 1 to 2 weeks to attain the full therapeutic effect. Optic damage, constipation, urinary retention, hypotension, liver damage, and skin rashes have been observed with the use of this agent.

> **Dosage:**
> Adults only: (Oral) 15 mg three times daily.

tranylcypromine sulfate, USP, BP (Parnate). This antidepressant, like phenelzine, is a MAOI, and its actions, effects, and side effects are similar. The food and wine restrictions mentioned above apply to the use of this drug also.

> **Dosage:**
> Adults only: (Oral) 20 to 30 mg/day in divided doses.

TRICYCLIC ANTIDEPRESSANTS

The term *tricyclic* merely describes the chemical structure of these compounds. They are composed of two aromatic hydrocarbon rings connected by a seven-member ring.

imipramine hydrochloride, USP, BP (Tofranil). Although similar in effect to phenelzine, this agent has the singular property of not stimulating the central nervous system unless the individual is actually depressed. It has very little or no effect on the normal individual. Because of this property, it has been used frequently for routine treatment of the elderly. On days when an elderly individual is depressed, this agent has a mood-brightening effect; when the individual is not depressed, it does not produce overstimulation. It has been used with variable success in the treatment of enuresis (uncontrolled passing of urine).

Table 23-2 | *Selective Serotonin Reuptake Inhibitors*

GENERIC NAME	TRADE NAME	DOSAGE
citalopram	Celexa	10–60 mg/day
escitalopram	Lexapro	10–20 mg/day
fluoxetine	Prozac, Sarafem	20–80 mg/day
fluvoxamine	Luvox	25–300 mg/day
paroxetine	Paxil	10–60 mg/day
sertraline	Zoloft	50–200 mg/day

Transient atropine-like effects, especially dryness of the mouth, are rather common during the initial phase of therapy, but they disappear with continued administration. Tachycardia, constipation, dizziness, and parkinsonism occasionally occur.

Improvement is often seen within 3 to 4 days, and the maximum effect is seen within 2 weeks.

Dosage:
> Adults: (Oral) 75 to 300 mg daily in divided doses. (IM) 100 mg/day in divided doses.
> Children older than 6 years, for enuresis: (Oral) 25 to 50 mg once daily 1 hour before bedtime.

amitriptyline hydrochloride, USP, BP (Elavil). In addition to serving as a mood elevator, this agent has a tranquilizing component that helps alleviate the anxiety that often accompanies depression. Many physicians customarily treat anxious or agitated and depressed patients with a combination of an antidepressant and a tranquilizer. This is seldom necessary when this agent is used. Side effects, when they occur, are usually mild. Dizziness, nausea, excitement, hypotension, tremors, headache, heartburn, dryness of the mouth, and blurring of vision have been reported.

Dosage:
> Adults and children older than 12 years: (Oral) 25 to 150 mg/day once daily or in divided doses. (IM) 20 to 30 mg four times daily.
> Children younger than 12 years: Not recommended.

doxepin hydrochloride, USP, BP (Sinequan, Adapin). Doxepin has been shown to be of benefit as an antidepressant and antianxiety agent and is recommended in the treatment of alcoholism, depression neuroses, anxiety associated with various organic diseases, and some forms of insomnia. The maximum effect may not occur for 2 weeks after therapy is begun. Side effects are drowsiness, tachycardia, hypotension, extrapyramidal symptoms, nausea, vomiting, and paresthesias. It is administered orally.

Dosage:
> Adults: (Oral) 25 to 50 mg three times daily, or the entire daily dose may be administered at bedtime.
> Children: No standard dose is established.

desipramine hydrochloride, USP, BP (Pertofrane). This antidepressant is useful in the treatment of mild to moderate depressive states. Side effects include blurred vision, urinary retention, weakness, lethargy, nightmares, and euphoria.

Dosage:
> Adults and children older than 12 years: (Oral) 75 to 300 mg/day in divided doses.

nortriptyline hydrochloride, USP, BP (Aventyl, Pamelor). Like desipramine, this agent is used in the treatment of mild to moderate depressive states. Side effects resemble those of desipramine.

Dosage:
> Adults and children older than 12 years: (Oral) 75 to 300 mg/day in divided doses.

protriptyline hydrochloride, USP, BP (Vivactil). The action and effects of this agent resemble those of desipramine.

Dosage:
> Adults and children older than 12 years: (Oral) 15 to 30 mg/day in divided doses.

trimipramine maleate (Surmontil). This agent is indicated for the treatment of depression. Side effects include hypotension, tachycardia, and paresthesias of the extremities.

Dosage:
> Adults: (Oral) 75 mg daily initially in divided doses, increased as necessary to 200 mg daily.

OTHER ANTIDEPRESSANTS

venlafaxine hydrochloride (Effexor). The advantage of this drug is its relatively short onset of action, showing some antidepressant activity in about 4 days rather than the 14 to 21 days that are common with other agents. It is well tolerated by most patients, including the elderly; occasional headaches and dry mouth have been reported.

Dosage:
> Adults: 75 to 350 mg orally daily in three divided doses.

bupropion hydrochloride (Wellbutrin, Zyban). This agent, chemically unrelated to the other antidepressants, is used as a long-term antidepressant. It has been shown effective as an adjunct to smoking cessation as well. When it is discontinued, it does not need to be tapered.

Dosage:
> Adults: (Oral) 150 to 300 mg daily.

mirtazapine (Remeron). Mirtazapine is used in the treatment of major depressive disorders. Its activity is similar in potency to that of the tricyclic antidepressants, although it is not related chemically.

Dosage:
> Adults: (Oral) 15 mg, up to a maximum of 45 mg, once daily at bedtime.

nefazodone (Serzone). This agent is indicated for use in the treatment of depression. Side effects reported include priapism, hepatotoxicity, postural hypotension, and mania.

Dosage:
> Adults: (Oral) 100 to 300 mg daily.

NONPSYCHIATRIC USES OF ANTIDEPRESSANTS

In recent years it has become evident that the concomitant use of antidepressants may help many patients cope with pain. The mechanism of antidepressant drug action in chronic pain syndromes is unclear. The increased serotonin level that these drugs produce is somehow associated with increased analgesia, and decreased serotonin with hyperalgesia. Antidepressants can be only one component of a comprehensive therapeutic program, and it is essential that the chronic pain patient have other goals as well (i.e., returning to work, hobbies, or other daily activities).

Currently, there are insufficient data to support the choice of one antidepressant over another for certain types of pain. Amitriptyline and doxepin have been studied most thoroughly.

The antidepressants have also been used prophylactically to prevent migraine headaches and PMS. In addition, they are used along with other agents in the treatment of other painful conditions such as shingles (varicella zoster), cancer, fibrositis, postherpetic neuralgia, and diabetic neuropathy.

ANXIOLYTIC AGENTS

The **anxiolytic agents** relieve anxiety and are used primarily for disorders caused by anxiety. These agents are generally less sedating than the tranquilizer class of agents and lend themselves to more long-term treatment with fewer side effects.

buspirone hydrochloride (BuSpar). The principal pharmacologic effect of this drug is relief of anxiety. It has no anticonvulsant or muscle-relaxing properties, does not significantly depress psychomotor function, and has little sedative effect. For these reasons it is generally the drug of choice for the elderly patient.

It is used for the management of anxiety disorders and has been shown to be useful for long-term therapy without losing its effectiveness. Dizziness, headache, nausea, and tachycardia have been reported in some patients. It has a slow onset of action, requiring 3 to 4 weeks before optimum clinical results are noted.

Dosage:

Adults only: (Oral) 10 to 30 mg daily in divided doses.

 Considerations for Older Adults

Buspirone

Buspirone is the agent of choice as a tranquilizer for the elderly because it is nonsedating and is not associated with memory impairment.

THE USE OF ANTICONVULSANTS IN ANXIETY DISORDERS

Despite progress in the understanding of the pharmacotherapy of anxiety disorders, the response rate to drug therapy remains suboptimal in many cases. The anticonvulsants, which are used to treat epilepsy, are a class of agents with an

emerging role in the treatment of anxiety disorders. The anatomic center for anxiety appears to be in the hippocampus and amygdala. The sensory input that is sent via the thalamus to the amygdala is known to be critical for the evaluation of stress and fear, and appears to be involved in some of the anxiety disorders. The anticonvulsants are being used in the treatment of anxiety disorders as well as PTSD.

carbamazepine (Tegretol)
   Dosage:
      Adults: (Oral) 800 to 1200 mg/day.

divalproex (Depakote)
   Dosage:
      Adults: (Oral) 1000 mg/day (serum level 70 mcg/mL).

gabapentin (Neurontin)
   Dosage:
      Adults: (Oral) 1190 mg/day.

topiramate (Topamax)
   Dosage:
      Adults: (Oral) 400 mg/day.

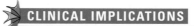 **CLINICAL IMPLICATIONS**

1. Psychotherapeutic agents are among the most over-prescribed medications.
2. Natural, temporary situations promoting sadness, anxiety, or restlessness need not always be treated by a psychotherapeutic agent.
3. Endogenous depression, or a generalized sadness and listlessness without apparent cause, may be alleviated by antidepressants.
4. A proper diet, vigorous physical exercise, and a pleasant environment are not to be ignored in the treatment of emotional disorders.
5. Anxiety that interferes with normal functioning may be effectively treated with a tranquilizer.
6. The nurse should be available to discuss the patient's anxiety about his or her condition or reason for hospitalization. Many times the patient's fears can be calmly discussed and alleviated. Patients may fear that the physician is not telling them everything and that the condition is worse than they are being told.
7. Elderly persons generally require lower doses of psychotherapeutic agents and may experience excessive sedation when these drugs are administered.
8. Guardrails and assistance in ambulation should be added to a patient's care when tranquilizers are first administered.
9. Self-administered medication such as antihistamines and cough preparations may cause excessive sedation when combined with tranquilizers.
10. Alcohol or sedatives should not be combined with tranquilizers.
11. Antidepressants require 2 to 3 weeks to exert their therapeutic effect in most instances. The patient

should be advised of this delay when these agents are administered.

12. The potential for abuse and addiction is high when tranquilizers are administered for an extended period of time.

13. The patient should not take more than the prescribed dose when these agents are administered. He or she should be counseled to this effect, particularly when ready for discharge from the hospital.

14. Monoamine oxidase inhibitors may cause life-threatening reactions if combined with wine, cheese, or other substances containing amines.

15. Combining two or more psychotherapeutic agents may cause many untoward effects.

16. Current information on drug interactions may be obtained from the pharmacist. Information on untoward effects is computerized, constantly updated, and available to pharmacists online. They should be consulted when the patient is taking many different medications.

Online Resources

For updated drug information and Web activities, go to http://evolve.elsevier.com/Asperheim.

CRITICAL THINKING QUESTIONS

1. The patient has been hospitalized in the state mental hospital for 6 months and is considerably improved after therapy and treatment with Thorazine. He has begun to walk with an increased shuffle lately, and at rest his fingers have a pill-rolling movement. Is this serious? Does the medication need to be discontinued? What could help him?

2. The elderly patient has been crying and upset since the sudden death of her husband. She states that her fatigue is increasing daily, and many days she does not even get out of bed and dress. She doesn't feel like cooking for herself and usually just has tea and toast during the day. What medication could be of benefit? Any other suggestions?

3. The patient recently lost his executive position as a result of company downsizing. His wife brought him in to the office today. In contrast to his previous appearance, he is now unshaven, his clothes are in some disarray, and he sits sullenly on the examining table, answering very few questions and then only in monosyllables. What medicine could be beneficial?

4. The patient began sobbing hysterically. She states that she and her husband are having marital troubles, her teenage son has been experimenting with drugs and is now at the Drug Abuse Center, and, in addition, her in-laws are coming to stay for 2 weeks. She feels that if she could just get by the next few weeks, things may straighten themselves out. What medication might be of benefit here?

5. The patient describes herself as having too many "highs" and "lows." Last night she did not sleep at all, and instead reorganized all her closets and cleaned the house from top to bottom. At other times she says she can hardly get out of bed for most of the day. What condition does she describe? What drug may help?

REVIEW QUESTIONS

1. What property does buspirone have that makes it useful in the elderly?
   a. More sedating
   b. Less sedating
   c. Antiparkinsonian effect
   d. Antipsychotic

2. Which drug would not be expected to interact with lithium?
   a. hydrochlorothiazide
   b. ibuprofen
   c. propoxyphene
   d. enalapril

3. Serotonin levels may be increased by which drug?
   a. nortriptyline
   b. amitriptyline
   c. phenobarbital
   d. citalopram

4. An antidepressant that is used in smoking cessation therapy is:
   a. buspirone.
   b. bupropion.
   c. nortriptyline.
   d. sertraline.

5. An anticonvulsant that is used in the treatment of anxiety disorders is:
   a. gabapentin.
   b. buspirone.
   c. fluoxetine.
   d. doxepin.

6. When treating an elderly person with a sedative, the dose may need to be:
   a. higher.
   b. lower.
   c. unchanged.
   d. combined with another drug.

7. Lithium is prescribed for the treatment of:
   a. schizophrenia.
   b. chronic depressive disorders.
   c. hyperactivity in children.
   d. bipolar disorder.

8. Parkinsonism has been observed as a side effect of:
   a. diazepam.
   b. buspirone.
   c. bupropion.
   d. chlorpromazine.

9. Which tranquilizer is also effective as a muscle relaxant?
   a. chlorpromazine
   b. diazepam
   c. nefazodone
   d. trifluoperazine

10. A side effect of chlorazepate may be:
    a. hypertension.
    b. hypotension.
    c. hypersalivation.
    d. diarrhea.

Prostaglandins and Prostaglandin Inhibitors

After completing this chapter, you should be able to do the following:

1. Recognize the drugs that are known as prostaglandins and understand their effects in the body.
2. Recognize the effect that a prostaglandin inhibitor will have on a given body tissue.
3. Understand bodily functions that are carried out by prostaglandins.
4. Recognize inflammation as a function of prostaglandins.
5. Become familiar with the antiinflammatory effects of prostaglandin inhibitors.
6. Become familiar with the COX-2 inhibitors as antiinflammatory agents and recognize their advantages.

Key Terms

COX-2 inhibitors, p. 134
Cyclooxygenase-2, p. 134
Nonsteroidal antiinflammatory drugs (NSAIDs), p. 132
Prostaglandin (PRŌS-tă-GLĂN-dĭn) **inhibitor,** p. 132
Prostaglandins (PRŌS-tă-GLĂN-dĭns), p. 131

Prostaglandins are potent unsaturated fatty acids that act in exceedingly low concentrations on local target organs. They are physiologically active substances and are found in many tissues. The drugs in this class of pharmacologic agents were at first believed to exert their effects through the central nervous system because many of these agents exhibit analgesic and antiinflammatory effects. Early drugs, such as aspirin, were long believed to be central nervous system analgesics, but are now known to exert their effects through the prostaglandin system.

The first report of the prostaglandins was made in the 1930s when New York gynecologists Kurzrok and Lieb noted that human semen had an ability to produce strong contraction or relaxation of the uterus. It was soon found that this unknown substance, named prostaglandin because it was believed to be produced by the prostate gland, could affect other types of smooth muscle as well.

It was later found that the term *prostaglandin* was a misnomer because these substances were widely distributed in many tissues and body fluids. They are produced close to

their sites of action and are rapidly metabolized when circulating through the body.

For simplicity, these agents are named alphabetically—prostaglandin A, B, C, and so forth—and abbreviated as PGA (prostaglandin A), PGB, and so on.

ACTIONS OF THE PROSTAGLANDINS

In this section, the known prostaglandins are discussed according to the body system that they affect.

REPRODUCTIVE TRACT

In men, prostaglandins are believed to assist in the emptying of the seminal vesicles, thus aiding in ejaculation.

In women, prostaglandin release is believed to aid in uterine contraction during menstruation. The commercial prostaglandins are used to induce uterine contractions in elective abortions.

dinoprostone (Prostin E$_2$ Suppositories). This prostaglandin is generally administered in a vaginal suppository. It is given to terminate a pregnancy from the 12th to the 20th week of gestation. It may also be used to evacuate a uterus when a missed abortion or fetal death has occurred. Adverse effects include dizziness, vomiting, diarrhea, urine retention, headache, and cardiac arrhythmia.
   Dosage:
      (Vaginal) 20 mg by suppository every 3 to 5 hours.

dinoprostone (Prepidil Cervical Gel). When administered inside the cervix, this agent stimulates the pregnant uterus to contract. It is indicated for "ripening" the cervix at or near term when there is an obstetric need for induction of labor. It causes the cervix to soften, shorten, and dilate in preparation for birth. Maternal gastrointestinal upset and headaches are common side effects.
   Dosage:
      One 3-gm syringe applied to the cervix.

CIRCULATORY SYSTEM

Cardiac output is generally increased by prostaglandins E, F, and A, but the therapeutic use of these agents has not been perfected as yet.

The primary purpose of prostaglandin E has been to keep the ductus arteriosus open (patent) in newborn infants. Infants with certain congenital heart deformities rely on the patent ductus arteriosus to supply oxygenated blood until they are old enough or stable enough to undergo corrective heart surgery. (Conversely, prostaglandin inhibitors such as indomethacin, discussed later in the chapter, are used to close the patent ductus arteriosus when natural processes fail to do so in an otherwise healthy infant. This has greatly reduced the necessity for surgery in many infants.)

alprostadil sterile solution (Prostaglandin E, Prostin VR Pediatric). This agent is administered by intravenous infusion to keep the ductus arteriosus open. Infants with certain congenital heart deformities rely on the patent ductus arteriosus to supply oxygenated blood until they are old enough or stable enough to undergo corrective heart surgery. This agent should not be used in infants with respiratory distress syndrome. It has been noted to cause cortical proliferation of the long bones with long-term use.

Dosage:
   (IV) As a continuous infusion providing 0.1 mcg/kg/minute.

GASTROINTESTINAL TRACT

misoprostol (Cytotec). This synthetic analog of prostaglandin E (alprostadil) is a gastric antisecretory agent with protective effects on the gastric mucosa. It is used for the prevention of NSAID-induced gastric ulcers. It should be administered for the duration of the NSAID therapy. It is an abortifacient (causes abortion), thus it is contraindicated in pregnancy.

Dosage:
   200 mcg four times daily with food.

URINARY TRACT

alprostadil (MUSE). Alprostadil is a naturally occurring form of prostaglandin E. It is a vasodilating agent and a platelet aggregation inhibitor. It is used in a transurethral delivery system and is administered as needed to obtain an erection. The onset of action is within 5 to 10 minutes; the duration of action is 30 to 60 minutes. Local discomfort is reported to be mild and transient. Urethral burning, bleeding, and testicular pain are reported as side effects.

Dosage:
   Adults only: (Transurethral) 125 to 1000 mcg inserted into the urethra.

ALLERGY AND IMMUNOLOGY

It has been shown that prostaglandins prevent the release of histamine from sensitized cells. Very low doses of prostaglandins, however, provoke the opposite response and enhance histamine release. No therapeutic agents have yet been developed to exert a predictable response in the treatment of allergies.

PROSTAGLANDIN INHIBITORS

NONSTEROIDAL ANTIINFLAMMATORY DRUGS

Many therapeutic agents exert their effects through inhibition of the prostaglandin systems. These agents are referred to as **prostaglandin inhibitors,** or antiprostaglandins. Although the exact action of the prostaglandins in many areas of the body remains uncertain, it was found that prostaglandins figure prominently in the process of inflammation and are found in inflammatory exudates. The mechanism of action of many of the antiinflammatory agents is actually to prevent the synthesis of prostaglandins at the site of inflammation. These prostaglandin inhibitors are referred to as **nonsteroidal antiinflammatory drugs (NSAIDs).**

Many old and new agents are prostaglandin inhibitors.

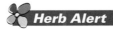 **Herb Alert**

White Willow

White willow is used in the treatment of rheumatism, inflammation, and fever. It reduces the effects of probenecid and enhances the antiplatelet action of NSAIDs and warfarin; thus it should not be taken with warfarin or NSAIDs. It also enhances the action of phenytoin and methotrexate. Its use should be avoided in patients with preexisting bleeding tendencies. See Chapter 35 for more information on white willow.

aspirin, USP; acetylsalicylic acid, BP. Although long used as an analgesic and an antiinflammatory agent, it is only recently that aspirin's true mechanism of action was found. It is now believed that aspirin inhibits the synthesis of prostaglandins.

Aspirin is used to relieve mild to moderate pain, treat headaches, act as an antiinflammatory medication in arthritic conditions, and reduce platelet aggregation, thus preventing blood clot formation. For this last use, low doses of aspirin are taken daily.

A relationship has been established in children between taking aspirin and the development of Reye's syndrome, an often fatal condition characterized by encephalopathy and liver damage. It is now recommended that aspirin not be given to children for minor febrile conditions. It is still used in inflammatory conditions such as juvenile rheumatoid arthritis, however.

Dosage:
   Adults: (Oral, Rectal) 325 to 650 mg every 4 hours.
   Children: (Oral) 65 mg/kg/day for inflammatory conditions only.

Considerations for Children

Aspirin

Avoid administering aspirin to children under age 18. Aspirin given to infants and young children is associated with the development of Reye's syndrome. Other nonsteroidal anti-inflammatory drugs, such as ibuprofen (Motrin), do not have this association.

indomethacin, USP, BP (Indocin). Used orally in the treatment of arthritis, this agent is also injected intravenously into newborns to induce closing of the ductus arteriosus. It should not be used in the elderly because the incidence of gastrointestinal bleeding is high.

> Dosage:
> Adults: (Oral) 25 mg three times daily.
> Newborns: (IV) 0.2 mg/kg; may be given up to six times.

tolmetin sodium, USP, BP (Tolectin). This agent is used for arthritis and more localized inflammatory conditions such as bursitis and tennis elbow.

> Dosage:
> Adults: (Oral) 400 mg three times daily, increased as necessary to 2 gm/day.
> Children: (Oral) 10 to 30 mg/kg/day in divided doses.

ibuprofen, USP, BP (Motrin). In addition to its use as an antiinflammatory drug, this agent is frequently used in the treatment of menstrual cramps and ovulation pain.

> Dosage:
> Adults: (Oral) 200 to 600 mg four times daily.
> Children: (Oral) 100 mg four times daily.

piroxicam, USP, BP (Feldene). The main advantage of this agent is that it has a prolonged half-life in the body and can be taken in a once-daily dose for the treatment of inflammatory conditions.

> Dosage:
> Adults: (Oral) 20 mg once daily.

ketorolac tromethamine (Toradol). This agent can be used intramuscularly for the relief of acute pain. In pain management studies, the overall analgesic effect of 30 mg Toradol was equivalent to 6 to 12 mg of morphine or 100 mg meperidine. Intramuscularly, it is very effective for postoperative pain, and the patient does not experience the sedation that accompanies narcotic analgesia. Orally, the agent is effective in mild to moderate pain and has been used for headaches, dental pain, and other chronic recurrent pain disorders.

> Dosage:
> (IM) 30 to 60 mg as a loading dose, then 15 to 30 mg IM every 4 to 6 hours; maximum daily dose, 150 mg. (Oral) 10 to 20 mg every 4 hours; maximum daily dose, 40 mg.

diflunisal, USP, BP (Dolobid)

> Dosage:
> Adults only: (Oral) 1000 mg initially, then 500 mg every 12 hours.

diclofenac (Voltaren)

> Dosage:
> Adults only: (Oral) 150 to 200 mg in two divided doses.

etodolac (Lodine, Lodine XL))

> Dosage:
> Adults only: (Oral) 200 to 400 mg every 6 to 8 hours, or, as the long-acting (XL) form, 400 to 1000 mg once daily.

fenoprofen calcium, USP, BP (Nalfon)

> Dosage:
> Adults only: (Oral) 600 mg four times daily.

flurbiprofen (Ansaid, Ocufen)

> Dosage:
> Adults only: (Oral) 200 to 300 mg daily in two to four divided doses.

ketoprofen (Orudis)

> Dosage:
> Adults only: (Oral) 150 to 300 mg daily in three to four divided doses.

leflunomide (Arava)

> Dosage:
> Adults only: (Oral) 100 mg daily for 3 days, then 20 mg daily.

meclofenamate (Meclomen)

> Dosage:
> Adults only: (Oral) 1200 to 2000 mg in three divided doses.

mefenamic acid (Ponstel)

> Dosage:
> Adults only: (Oral) 500 mg initially and then 250 mg every 6 hours.

naproxen, USP, BP (Naprosyn)

> Dosage:
> Adults: (Oral) 250 mg twice daily to a maximum of 740 mg daily.
> Children: (Oral) 5 to 10 mg/kg/day.

naproxen sodium (Anaprox)

> Dosage:
> Adults only: (Oral) 275 to 500 mg twice daily.

oxaprozin (Daypro)
Dosage:
Adults only: (Oral) 600 to 1200 mg once daily.

sulindac, USP, BP (Clinoril)
Dosage:
Adults only: (Oral) 400 mg daily in two divided doses.

CYCLOOXYGENASE-2 INHIBITORS

Cyclooxygenase-1 (COX-1) and **cyclooxygenase-2** (COX-2) are enzymes that are involved in the inflammatory process. The original NSAIDs inhibit both COX-1 and COX-2. The **COX-2 inhibitors** are a new class of NSAIDs that preferentially inhibit the COX-2 enzyme over COX-1. Knowledge of the particular function and differentiation of these enzymes is beyond the scope of this text. However, these agents are described as a class by this function, so it is necessary to recognize the term.

Special Considerations

NSAIDs

The simultaneous use of two NSAIDs, which includes the combination of a COX-2 inhibitor and low-dose daily aspirin, is a significant risk factor for gastrointestinal bleeds.

The main advantage of this group of NSAIDs is that they have considerably less antiplatelet effect, thus there are fewer bleeding tendencies as a side effect. The prolonged use of the original NSAIDs that is generally necessary for arthritic conditions causes a high percentage of severe gastrointestinal tract complaints, both abdominal pain and gastrointestinal bleeding. COX-2 inhibitors are effective as antiinflammatories, particularly for arthritis and other inflammatory conditions, but have a greatly reduced adverse effect on the gastrointestinal tract. These agents are used orally for adults only.

celecoxib (Celebrex)
Dosage:
100 to 200 mg twice daily.

valdecoxib (Bextra)
Dosage:
10 to 20 mg once daily.

CLINICAL IMPLICATIONS

1. Aspirin and other antiprostaglandin agents have as their main side effect gastric irritation. The patient should be observed for signs of gastric distress when these agents are administered.
2. Routine use of aspirin and similar drugs should be discontinued before surgical procedures, because bleeding disorders occur with prolonged use. Surgical patients should be questioned about self-administration of aspirin-containing drugs.
3. Patients allergic to aspirin should be cautioned about aspirin-containing drugs such as Darvon Compound, Fiorinal, Robaxisal, and many other such combinations, as well as commercial antihistamine-analgesic combinations.
4. The patient should be cautioned about signs of bleeding disorders, such as bleeding gums, black stools, and petechiae, which are side effects of these medications.
5. Fluid retention and visual problems occur as side effects of the prostaglandin inhibitors. The patient should be assessed for these problems.
6. NSAIDs are best taken about hour before meals to allow sufficient time for drug dissolution; the coating effect that food provides will then help to prevent gastric irritation.
7. Acetaminophen is generally preferred to aspirin in children because of the association of aspirin intake with the development of Reye's syndrome.
8. Certain of the prostaglandin inhibitors have a cross sensitivity with aspirin. These should be avoided in aspirin-sensitive persons.
9. In addition to the antiinflammatory medications, the application of warm compresses and physical therapy measures may increase joint mobility in the treatment of arthritic conditions.
10. Elevations in blood pressure may signify fluid retention, which may be observed as a side effect of these medications.
11. Parents should be advised to keep aspirin and other drugs safely out of the reach of children.
12. Prostaglandins given to affect one body system may have a series of untoward effects on other systems.
13. The COX-2 type of NSAID may be used if there is a history of abdominal distress with the nonselective NSAIDs.

Online Resources

For updated drug information and Web activities, go to http://evolve.elsevier.com/Asperheim.

❓CRITICAL THINKING QUESTIONS

1. The patient has been having considerable trouble with menstrual cramps. What agents may be prescribed to relieve her symptoms? She states she has used many over-the-counter preparations without relief.

2. The patient has been using acetaminophen (Tylenol) tablets without relief for her arthritis. The doctor told her to get ibuprofen (Motrin) at the drugstore, but she states that this irritates her stomach and she wants to take Tylenol instead. How could you explain the difference in these drugs to her?

3. The patient has a long history of peptic ulcers. He now has rheumatoid arthritis and must take an NSAID. Which agent may be best and why?

REVIEW QUESTIONS

1. Prostaglandins have been found to be:
   a. only located in the prostate gland.
   b. active in many bodily tissues.
   c. useful as an oral contraceptive.
   d. useful in opening the infant ductus arteriosus.

2. An agent that has a protective effect on the gastric mucosa is:
   a. ibuprofen.
   b. mefenamic acid.
   c. naproxen.
   d. misoprostol.

3. Which drug is contraindicated in pregnancy?
   a. misoprostol
   b. dinoprostone gel
   c. penicillin
   d. acetaminophen

4. The advantage of COX-2 inhibitors when used for arthritis is:
   a. increased secretion of acid in the stomach.
   b. more efficient reduction of joint swelling.
   c. reduced gastric irritation.
   d. less sedation.

5. Aspirin is contraindicated for use in young children because it is implicated in causing:
   a. birth defects.
   b. clotting disorders.
   c. Reye's syndrome.
   d. diarrhea.

6. An injectable agent that has analgesic properties similar to morphine is:
   a. ibuprofen.
   b. ketorolac.
   c. piroxicam.
   d. tolmetin.

7. An example of a COX-2 inhibitor is:
   a. meclofenamate.
   b. diclofenac.
   c. celecoxib.
   d. indomethacin.

8. Which agent may be used to induce an abortion?
   a. dinoprostone
   b. epoprostenol
   c. misoprostol
   d. alprostadil

9. An agent used for the treatment of pulmonary hypertension is:
   a. dinoprostone.
   b. ibuprofen.
   c. epoprostenol.
   d. alprostadil.

10. The main disadvantage of the COX-2 inhibitors as compared to ibuprofen is increased:
    a. gastric irritation.
    b. platelet aggregation.
    c. cost.
    d. side effects generally.

Drugs That Affect the Autonomic Nervous System

Objectives

After completing this chapter, you should be able to do the following:

1. Explain the major effects of drugs on the autonomic nervous system.
2. Define the effects of sympathetic stimulation.
3. Give an example of an adrenergic drug.
4. Give an example of an adrenergic blocking agent.
5. Define cholinergic effects and describe the effects.
6. Give an example of a cholinergic agent.
7. Give an example of a cholinergic blocking agent.
8. Become familiar with the different classes of antihypertensive agents.

Key Terms

Acetylcholine (ăs-ē-tĭl-KŌ-lēn), p. 136
Adrenergic (ĂD-rĭ-NŬR-jĭk), p. 136
Autonomic (ăw-tō-NŎM-ĭk) **nervous system**, p. 136
Cholinergic (KŌ-lĭn-ŬR-jĭk), p. 136
Epinephrine (norepinephrine), p. 136
Ganglion (GĂNG-glē-ŏn), p. 136
Neuron (NUR-on), p. 136
Parasympathetic (păr-ă-sĭm-pă-THĔT-ĭk) **nervous system**, p. 136
Sympathetic (sĭm-pă-THĔT-ĭk) **nervous system**, p. 136
Synapse (SIN-aps), p. 136

SYMPATHETIC AND PARASYMPATHETIC SYSTEMS

The **autonomic nervous system** is composed of nerves leading from the central nervous system that innervate and control smooth muscle, cardiac muscle, and glands (Figure 25–1). It controls many organ systems automatically; its actions are generally not under voluntary control.

The system is divided into two parts: the **sympathetic nervous system** and the **parasympathetic nervous system**. In general, if one system stimulates a function, the other inhibits it. The systems oppose one another in governing the functions of smooth muscle and glands in many parts of the body. Some of the major effects of the two systems are compared in Table 25–1.

From Table 25–1, it can be seen that the sympathetic nervous system is the body's defense mechanism for emergency situations. The release of the sympathetic hormones is increased at these times, enabling the body to run, fight, or meet the situation at hand (the "fight or flight" response). The sympathetic hormones may be given to relieve an asthmatic attack because of the relaxing effect on the smooth muscle of the bronchi. The parasympathetic system is more concerned with maintaining the normal "status quo" of body operations.

A **neuron,** or nerve cell, is the functional unit of the nervous system. Messages from the brain to various tissues and organs are transmitted as impulses along neurons. The junction (membrane-to-membrane contact) of any two neurons is called a **synapse;** a group of synapses is called a **ganglion** (Figure 25–2).

In both the sympathetic and parasympathetic nervous systems, two neurons function together to enable the central nervous system to control the muscles or glands. The first is a preganglionic (before the ganglion) neuron that leaves the central nervous system and travels toward the muscle or organ that is under autonomic nervous system control. At a certain point away from the central nervous system, this neuron joins (forms a synapse) with the second, postganglionic (after the ganglion) neuron that travels on to the muscle or organ in question. Because more than one neuron may travel to a given muscle or organ, several synapses will occur at the junctions, forming the ganglion.

There is evidence that the transfer of nerve impulses at the synapse is carried out by chemicals liberated at the junctions. A neurotransmitter agent called **acetylcholine** is liberated at the ganglia of both systems and at the postganglionic parasympathetic nerve endings; cells that release acetylcholine are termed **cholinergic. Epinephrine** and **norepinephrine,** also neurotransmitter agents, are liberated at the postganglionic sympathetic nerve endings; the cells that release epinephrine and norepinephrine are referred to as **adrenergic.** It is thought that these chemicals exist in the tissues and are activated or released by an impulse carried along the nerve.

The activity of these chemicals after they are liberated is short lived. Acetylcholine is rapidly inactivated by the enzyme acetylcholinesterase, and epinephrine is inactivated by the enzyme monoamine oxidase.

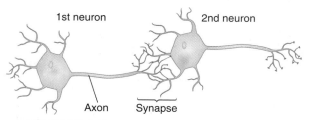

FIGURE 25-2 The junction of two neurons (nerve cells).

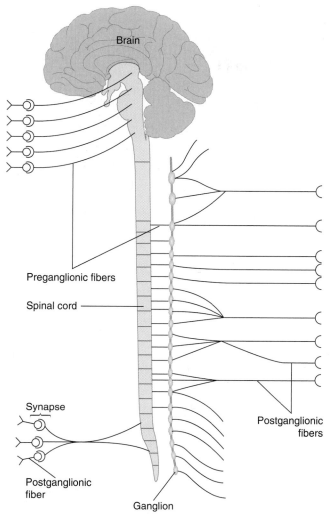

FIGURE 25-1 The autonomic nervous system.

Drugs can act in four ways upon the autonomic nervous system. They may either stimulate or inhibit the sympathetic system, or they may stimulate or inhibit the parasympathetic system. Because the two systems oppose each other in action, it can be seen that a drug that acts by inhibiting the action of one system (e.g., the parasympathetic system) would actu-

ally have the same net effect as stimulation of the other system (i.e., the sympathetic system in this case).

SYMPATHOMIMETIC (ADRENERGIC) AGENTS

Sympathomimetic agents produce or "mimic" the effects of stimulation of the sympathetic nervous system.

epinephrine hydrochloride, USP, BP (Adrenalin, Epi-Pen). Epinephrine, as well as norepinephrine, is naturally produced by the adrenal medulla and at most sympathetic nerve endings. In stress situations the adrenal medulla secretes an increased amount of epinephrine. The stress reaction, or the "fight or flight" response, consists of those sympathetic effects mentioned previously.

Therapeutically, epinephrine is used to constrict blood vessels in the eye and nasal mucosa and to treat acute bronchial asthma and severe allergic reactions. It is perhaps the best heart stimulant in cases of heart block or acute heart failure.

This is a very potent drug, and care should be taken to be very accurate in the dosage given. It is used in advanced cardiac life support procedures. When large dosages are given, cardiac dilation, pulmonary edema, and cerebrovascular accident may occur. Death may also result from ventricular fibrillation as a result of overstimulation of the myocardium.

Dosage:

Adults: (subQ) 0.3 mg every 20 minutes or as necessary.

Children: (subQ) 0.01 mg/kg every 20 minutes or as necessary.

Table 25-1 | *Major Effects of the Sympathetic and Parasympathetic Systems*

SYMPATHETIC EFFECTS	PARASYMPATHETIC EFFECTS
Increase in cardiac rate and output*	Decrease in cardiac rate and output
Constriction of blood vessels in skin and viscera*	Dilation of these blood vessels (not pronounced)
Elevation of blood pressure*	Lowering of blood pressure
Elevation of blood sugar*	No effect
Relaxation of smooth muscle in bronchi	Constriction of smooth muscle in bronchi
Decrease in peristalsis	Increase in peristalsis
Tightening of sphincters	Relaxation of sphincters
Promotion of urinary retention	Decrease in urinary retention
Dilation of pupils	Constriction of pupils

*These are emergency reactions of the body.

levarterenol bitartrate injection, USP, BP (Levophed). Chemically related to epinephrine, this agent acts as an over-all vasoconstrictor when given intravenously. It is used to treat hypotension and shock and may be given slowly in intra-venous solutions for as long as it is needed for this purpose.

Care must be taken to prevent infiltration of the solution into the skin of the surrounding areas, because the powerful vasoconstriction that is produced will cause sloughing of the tissues. The best antidote for infiltration is Regitine, a sym-patholytic agent that is injected directly into the area of infil-tration.

Dosage:
Adults: (IV) 1 to 2 mcg/minute diluted in 1000 mL solution.

metaraminol bitartrate, USP, BP (Aramine). Metaraminol is often preferred over levarterenol in the treatment of hypotension because it is not nearly as damaging to skin if it is accidentally extravasated into the surrounding tissues. If intravenous administration is not feasible in certain cases, it may even be given intramuscularly.

Dosage:
Adults: (IV, IM) 0.5 to 5 mg as necessary to control blood pressure.

phenylephrine hydrochloride, USP, BP (Neo-Synephrine). Although this agent may be used parenterally for the sympa-thomimetic effects, its chief use is in nasal sprays and drops to relieve nasal congestion.

Dosage:
Adults and children: (Nasal) 0.5% to 1% solution in spray or drops three to four times daily.

SYMPATHOLYTIC (ADRENERGIC BLOCKING) AGENTS

These drugs oppose or nullify the effect of stimulation of the sympathetic nervous system. The net result is similar to that obtained upon stimulation of the parasympathetic nervous system.

The adrenergic blocking agents are classified according to the receptor for which they are most specific. The two types, known as alpha and beta receptors, are found together in many types of tissue. For example, blood vessels have both alpha receptors, which cause vasoconstriction, and beta receptors, which cause vasodilation. In contrast, the heart has primarily beta receptors and almost no alpha receptors.

An *alpha-blocker,* then, would block the alpha receptors, and a *beta-blocker* the beta receptors. The therapeutic effects of the adrenergic blocking agents therefore vary greatly.

Many of these agents are discussed also in other chapters, because they have effects on the eye, the gastrointestinal tract, and the circulatory and other systems.

methyldopa, USP, BP (Aldomet). Methyldopa is an antihy-pertensive drug that acts by interfering with the formation of the pressor amines norepinephrine and serotonin. It is used for patients with sustained, moderately severe hypertension. It is not used in pheochromocytoma and is usually not used in the milder forms of hypertension that may be treated with sedatives and diuretics. It is administered by the oral route. Side effects include hemolytic anemia, drug fever, drowsi-ness, weakness, aggravation of angina pectoris, dryness of the mouth, and nasal stuffiness. It should be used with cau-tion in patients with a history of liver disease.

Dosage:
Adults: (Oral) 500 mg to 2 gm daily in two to four divided doses.

methyldopa plus hydrochlorothiazide (Aldoril). This antihypertensive compound is available in two dosage sizes: Aldoril-15, which contains 250 mg methyldopa and 15 mg hydrochlorothiazide in each tablet; and Aldoril-25, which contains 250 mg methyldopa and 25 mg hydrochloroth-iazide in each tablet. The combination of the antihyperten-sive and a thiazide diuretic provides potentiation of effect toward the lowering of blood pressure. Side effects are as described for the individual drugs.

Dosage:
Adults: (Oral) 2 to 4 of the combination tablets daily, based on individual requirements.

propranolol hydrochloride, USP, BP (Inderal). This adrenergic blocking agent blocks the beta receptors in the heart and within the smooth muscles of the bronchi and blood vessels. Through its action on the heart, it decreases heart rate, decreases cardiac output, and increases cardiac volume.

The effect on the kidneys results in an increase in salt retention; thus, dietary salt must be restricted, and a diuretic is often prescribed.

This agent is useful in the treatment of hypertension because it inhibits vasoconstriction and decreases cardiac output. It is used alone or with other antihypertensive agents to control moderate to severe hypertension. In some patients it is used to manage angina pectoris resulting from coronary atherosclerosis, particularly when the patient does not respond to nitroglycerin.

Although it is not the drug of choice in the treatment of cardiac arrhythmias, propranolol has been used in the man-agement of these patients. In some cases in which digitalis toxicity is present, this drug has been used to counteract the effects of digitalis excess.

The most common side effect is bradycardia, which may be accompanied by hypotension or shock. Severe bradycar-dia may be treated with atropine. Propranolol should be used with caution in patients with coronary disease, because congestive heart failure may be precipitated. Fluid retention, ataxia, dizziness, hearing loss, and visual distur-bances have been noted, as well as abdominal distress, rashes, and transient blood dyscrasias. It should be discon-tinued slowly when therapy is to be stopped, to avoid rebound effects.

Dosage:

Adults: (Oral) For hypertension—initially, 80 mg/day in divided doses, then slowly increased to a maximum of 640 mg/day. For angina pectoris—10 to 20 mg three to four times daily, increased as necessary. For arrhythmias—10 to 30 mg three to four times daily. (IV) For arrhythmias—0.5 to 3 mg at a rate not exceeding 1 mg/minute.

Children: (Oral) 0.2 to 4 mg/kg/day in divided doses. (IV) 10 to 20 mcg/kg infused over 10 minutes.

clonidine hydrochloride, USP, BP (Catapres). After initial stimulation of adrenergic receptors, this agent then produces inhibition. It reduces blood pressure in both the supine and standing positions; thus orthostatic hypotension upon arising is mild and infrequent. It is used in the treatment of hypertension either alone or with other agents, such as diuretics. Side effects include dry mouth, sedation, dizziness, headache, nightmares, and depression.

Dosage:

Adults: (Oral) 0.1 mg twice daily, increased as necessary to a maximum of 1.2 mg daily in divided doses.
Children: No standard dosage is established.

diazoxide, USP, BP (Hyperstat). By causing direct vasodilation of the peripheral blood vessels, diazoxide is extremely valuable in the treatment of malignant hypertension or hypertensive crisis. It does cause salt and water retention; thus, a diuretic should be administered as well, particularly if repeated doses are to be used.

Mild hyperglycemia, orthostatic hypotension, and anginal pain, as well as gastrointestinal symptoms, have been observed after administration. The patient should remain recumbent for 30 minutes after IV administration.

This agent is occasionally used orally for the treatment of hypoglycemia but is effective for hypertension in the intravenous form only.

Dosage:

Adults: (Oral) 3 mg/kg/day in three divided doses for treatment of hypoglycemia. (IV) 300 mg undiluted over 30 seconds for treatment of hypertension. Children: (Oral) 3 mg/kg/day in three divided doses for treatment of hypoglycemia. (IV) 5 mg/kg in one dose for treatment of hypertension.

prazosin hydrochloride, USP, BP (Minipress). This oral agent is often used along with a diuretic in the treatment of hypertension. It may also be combined with other antihypertensive agents. The most notable side effect of this drug is a sudden loss of consciousness or "drop attack." This may be minimized by administering low initial doses with subsequent gradual increases. Vomiting, diarrhea, nervousness, skin rashes, and insomnia have been reported.

Dosage:

Adults only: (Oral) 1 mg three times daily, gradually increased to a total of 15 mg/day in divided doses.

metoprolol tartrate, USP, BP (Lopressor). This blocking agent has a preferential effect on the beta receptors in the myocardium of the heart. It is given to reduce systolic blood pressure and has the effect of reducing the heart rate and cardiac output as well.

Dosage:

Adults only: (Oral) 100 mg daily in single or divided doses; may be increased to 450 mg daily.

nadolol, USP, BP (Corgard). This agent is used to treat hypertension and angina pectoris. It is a beta-blocking agent.

Dosage:

Adults only: (Oral) 40 mg daily; may be increased to 240 mg daily.

atenolol (Tenormin). This beta-blocker is used in the treatment of hypertension, alone or with other agents. It reduces cardiac output and both the systolic and diastolic blood pressures.

Dosage:

Adults only: (Oral) 50 mg daily in one dose; may be increased to 100 mg daily.

ERGOT ALKALOIDS

Although these agents do not lend themselves readily to classification as typical sympatholytic agents, they nevertheless do fall into this category. With the exception of ergotamine, the ergot alkaloids are used almost exclusively in obstetrics; thus they are discussed in Chapter 27. It is important to note that, because of the similarity in the names of the ergot alkaloids ergotamine (used to treat migranes) and ergonovine (used to stimulate contraction of the uterus), serious errors can occur if the drugs are confused.

ergotamine tartrate, USP, BP (Gynergen). Ergotamine is used to treat migraine headaches because of its ability to constrict the cerebral blood vessels. The periodic excruciating pain of migraine headaches is associated with factors such as stress and food allergies and is accompanied by dilation of the cerebral arterioles and later by edematous swelling of their walls. The pain is relieved by the vasoconstrictive effect of ergotamine.

Dangerous side effects can accompany too prolonged or too frequent use of this drug. Over a period of time the constriction of the blood vessels in the toes, fingers, hands, and feet causes gangrene, resulting in death of the tissues and loss of the affected body part. Constriction of the vessels in the retina of the eye may cause blindness.

Dosage:

Adults: (Oral) 2 mg at the onset of headache; may be repeated one or two times if necessary for relief. No more than 3 doses per day or 10 doses per week should be given.

methysergide maleate, USP, BP (Sansert). A synthetic drug, this agent is used to prevent migraine headaches. In this respect it differs from the other drugs used in the treatment of migraine headaches, because they are effective only during an attack.

Although the incidence of side effects is lower with methysergide maleate than with ergotamine, it should not be given when there is preexisting peripheral vascular disease or atherosclerosis.

The drug may be used for 6 months, followed by a drug-free period of 3 to 4 weeks.

Dosage:
Adults: (Oral) 2 mg three times daily.

PARASYMPATHOMIMETIC (CHOLINERGIC) AGENTS

Parasympathomimetic agents "mimic" the effect of stimulation of the parasympathetic nervous system.

Because acetylcholine is so rapidly inactivated by the enzyme acetylcholinesterase, it is not used therapeutically. Instead, synthetic analogs of acetylcholine have been developed that, although they produce the parasympathomimetic effects of the natural hormone, are more resistant to the inactivating influence of the enzyme. Some drugs directly mimic the effects of acetylcholine, whereas others act by inhibiting acetylcholinesterase and prolonging the action of natural acetylcholine.

pilocarpine nitrate, USP, BP; pilocarpine hydrochloride, USP. By stimulating the effector cells associated with the parasympathetic nerves, pilocarpine notably increases secretions, especially sweat, saliva, and nasal secretions. It is used mainly in the eye to produce miosis and to relieve pressure within the eye caused by glaucoma.

Dosage:
Adults and children: (Optic) 3 to 4 drops of a 1% to 2% solution every 3 to 4 hours.

bethanechol chloride, USP, BP (Urecholine). Bethanechol is similar in action to acetylcholine but is less active as well as less toxic. It is chiefly used in the treatment of postoperative abdominal distention, urinary retention, and retention of gastric contents.

Dosage:
Adults only: (Oral) 10 to 30 mg three to four times daily. (subQ) 2.5 to 5 mg at 15- to 30-minute intervals to a maximum of four doses.

neostigmine methylsulfate, USP, BP; neostigmine bromide, USP (Prostigmin). Like physostigmine, neostigmine inhibits acetylcholinesterase. It is not as potent as physostigmine but is often preferred when a drug to restore peristalsis or treat atony of the bladder is indicated. It may be used in the treatment of postoperative abdominal distention, urinary retention, and myasthenia gravis.

Dosage:
Adults: (Oral, IM, IV) Wide range 0.25 to 15 mg three times a day depending on indications.

Children: (Optic) 1 to 2 drops of a 5% solution.

edrophonium chloride, USP, BP (Tensilon). The main use of this acetylcholinesterase inhibitor is as an antidote for curare and similar drugs. It increases the tone of skeletal muscles; thus it overcomes the excessive relaxation produced by curariform agents. It has been used in the treatment of myasthenia gravis.

Dosage:
Adults: (IM, IV) 10 mg.
Children: (IM, IV) 1 to 5 mg; dose is individualized.

echothiophate iodide (phospholine iodide), USP, BP. This drug, a so-called irreversible anticholinesterase, has a much more prolonged effect than physostigmine or neostigmine. It is chiefly employed in the treatment of glaucoma.

Dosage:
Adults and children: (Optic) 1 to 2 drops of 0.06% to 0.25% solution one to three times daily.

PARASYMPATHOLYTIC (CHOLINERGIC BLOCKING) AGENTS

These drugs oppose or nullify the effect of stimulation of the parasympathetic nervous system; hence they have the same net effect as stimulation of the sympathetic nervous system.

BELLADONNA

Three alkaloids are obtained from this plant drug: atropine, hyoscyamine, and scopolamine. These drugs make tissues insensitive to acetylcholine, thus paralyzing the effects of the parasympathetic nerves. Atropine is the one most often used, although there is not a great deal of difference among the actions of the three drugs.

atropine sulfate, USP, BP. Perhaps the most important action of atropine is on the smooth muscles and the secretory glands. These drugs make tissues insensitive to acetylcholine, thus paralyzing the effects of the parasympathetic nerves. The gastrointestinal tract is relaxed and there is decreased peristalsis and muscle tone; hence atropine is used as an antispasmodic in many of the various "colics." The smooth muscle of the bronchi is also relaxed, and this is accompanied by a decreased amount of secretion from the nose, pharynx, and bronchi.

Dosage:
Adults: (subQ) Atropine—0.5 mg every 4 to 6 hours.
Also: Scopolamine—0.6 mg every 4 to 6 hours.
Hyoscyamine—0.5 mg every 4 to 6 hours.

Atropine Poisoning

Usually the first indications of atropine poisoning are headache, dryness of the throat and skin, dilated pupils, and dimness of vision. The skin is flushed and a rash may appear. The temperature rises because of decreased perspiration, and the pulse is rapid.

Antidote

Parasympathomimetic drugs such as pilocarpine, gastric lavage, or tannic acid (tea) are used to treat atropine poisoning. The patient should be catheterized to prevent reabsorption of the drug from the urine. The symptoms are then treated (e.g., cold sponging for fever, administration of respiratory stimulants).

OTHER PARASYMPATHOLYTIC AGENTS

clidinium bromide plus chlordiazepoxide (Librax). Each capsule of Librax contains 2.5 mg clidinium bromide and 5 mg chlordiazepoxide. This combination of the anticholinergic agent with chlordiazepoxide, a mild tranquilizer, is of benefit in the treatment of spastic colitis and as an adjunct in the treatment of peptic ulcer. It is contraindicated in patients with glaucoma or bladder neck obstruction. Drowsiness, blurred vision, nausea, constipation, and blood dyscrasias have been reported as side effects. This drug should not be combined with alcohol or other sedative agents.

Dosage:
Adults only: (Oral) 1 capsule four times daily.

propantheline bromide, USP, BP (Pro-Banthine)
Dosage:
Adults: (Oral) 15 mg four times daily.

prochlorperazine plus isopropamide (Combid). Each capsule of this combination drug contains 10 mg prochlorperazine maleate (Compazine) and 5 mg isopropamide iodide. Also a combination of a tranquilizer and an antispasmodic, this agent is used to treat spastic colitis and is quite effective in controlling hyperemesis.

Dosage:
Adults only: (Oral) 1 capsule every 12 hours.

GANGLIONIC BLOCKING AGENTS

These drugs prevent the transfer of impulses across the ganglia of the autonomic nervous system between the preganglionic and postganglionic neurons. They are used primarily to relieve severe hypertension.

mecamylamine hydrochloride, USP, BP (Inversine). This agent blocks the transmission of impulses at both sympathetic and parasympathetic ganglia. It produces vasodilation, increased peripheral blood flow, and decreased blood pressure. It is used in the treatment of severe hypertension when the patient is refractory to other drugs. Nausea, vomiting, dilated pupils, blurred vision, impotence, constipation, fatigue, and pulmonary edema have been observed.

Dosage:
Adults only: (Oral) 2.5 mg twice daily, increased gradually to a total daily dose of 25 mg in two to four divided doses.

NEUROMUSCULAR BLOCKING AGENTS

pancuronium bromide (Pavulon). This synthetic, nondepolarizing neuromuscular blocking agent is used to provide short-term skeletal muscle relaxation to facilitate procedures such as endotracheal intubation, endoscopic exams, ventilator therapy, or surgery.

Dosage:
Adults and children: (IV) 0.04 to 0.1 mg/kg given as needed. Repeat dose every 25 to 60 minutes.

vecuronium bromide (Norcuron). Pharmacologically this agent is similar to pancuronium bromide. Its indications for use are the same.

Dosage:
Adults and children: (IV) 0.08 to 0.1 mg/kg. Duration of effect is usually 25 to 30 minutes.

succinylcholine chloride (Anectine). This agent is used for the same indications as listed under pancuronium, and in addition it is generally considered to be the drug of choice for orthopedic manipulations as well as electroconvulsive therapy. The drug is very short acting. It is the drug of choice for procedures lasting under 3 minutes.

Dosage:
Adults and children: (IV) 0.1 mg/kg in diluted solution.

CLINICAL IMPLICATIONS

1. The drugs that affect the autonomic nervous system are not very specific, and side effects may be observed frequently, according to which segment of the system is affected.
2. Assess the pulse and blood pressure for changes or irregularity when autonomic drugs are administered.
3. Weakness, nausea, vomiting, diarrhea, and abdominal cramps are frequent side effects of these agents. The patient should be carefully observed for these effects, which should be duly reported.
4. Blurred vision is a frequent side effect of these agents because there are both adrenergic and cholinergic receptors in the eye.
5. Nursing procedures may be used to alleviate certain side effects (e.g., dry mouth can be treated by the use of gum, hard candy, or lemon-glycerin mouth swabs).
6. Constipation as a side effect of anticholinergic drugs should be carefully monitored, and laxatives should be requested as necessary.
7. Patients who have glaucoma generally may not take anticholinergic drugs.
8. Eye discomfort or pain should be immediately reported if a patient is on anticholinergic drugs, because there may be underlying and unsuspected glaucoma.
9. Flushing and elevated temperature should be observed and reported to the physician as possible untoward effects of these agents.

10. When beta-blockers are administered, bradycardia and congestive heart failure may occur as serious toxic effects.

11. Beta-blockers may increase blood sugar levels in diabetic patients on these medications.

12. When peripheral vasodilators are given for the treatment of peripheral vascular diseases, signs of improvement in the patient's condition may be seen as decreased blanching of the extremities, decreased paresthesia, and improved nailbed color.

13. Postural hypotension is a common side effect of antihypertensive medications. The patient should be out of bed with assistance only, particularly in the early days of treatment.

14. The patient should be observed carefully for any signs of urinary retention when on anticholinergic drugs.

15. Patients should be carefully observed for side effects of the autonomic drugs.

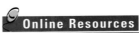
Online Resources

For updated drug information and Web activities, go to http://evolve.elsevier.com/Asperheim.

CRITICAL THINKING QUESTIONS

1. The patient has been feeling tired lately and having morning headaches. He has not been to a doctor for 10 years, works hard, drinks alcohol excessively at times, and is 30 pounds overweight, but otherwise has no significant medical history. His blood pressure is noted to be 160/110 mm Hg. As he leaves the office, he comments that he hopes his blood pressure gets cured fast because he surely doesn't want to be on medicine when he goes to Europe this fall. Would you have any suggestions as to how he should be counseled regarding his medication?

2. The patient has just been diagnosed as having a duodenal ulcer. Her doctor prescribed a bland diet, Maalox, and cimetidine (Tagamet). She expresses to you her annoyance with her uninteresting diet (she is a gourmet cook) and secretly worries that she will become a drug addict. How would you help her understand her treatment?

3. The patient has been taking propranolol hydrochloride for hypertension. She states that lately she has been feeling weak and listless. When taking her vital signs, you notice her pulse is 58. Is this related to her medication? Should the doctor be notified?

REVIEW QUESTIONS

1. A significant characteristic of the autonomic nervous system is that:
   a. it is tightly controlled by the central nervous system.
   b. it is ordinarily not under voluntary control.
   c. it controls voluntary muscles.
   d. it is overactive in depressive disorders.

2. All of the following are sympathetic effects except:
   a. lowering of blood pressure.
   b. decrease in peristalsis.
   c. tightening of sphincters.
   d. elevation of blood sugar.

3. All of the following are parasympathetic effects except:
   a. increase in peristalsis.
   b. constriction of pupils.
   c. hypertension.
   d. vasodilation.

4. Adrenergic agents have an effect that:
   a. counteracts the sympathetic nervous system.
   b. mimics the sympathetic nervous system.
   c. mimics the voluntary nervous system.
   d. mimics the parasympathetic nervous system.

5. The "fight or flight" response is a function of the:
   a. parasympathetic nervous system.
   b. musculoskeletal system.
   c. sympathetic nervous system.
   d. anticholinergic system.

6. Which agent is an adrenergic blocking agent?
   a. metaraminol
   b. phenylephrine
   c. levarterenol
   d. propranolol

7. Malignant hypertension may be treated in the emergency room with:
   a. epinephrine.
   b. levarterenol.
   c. diazoxide.
   d. diazepam.

8. A beta-blocker commonly used in the treatment of hypertension is:
   a. atenolol.
   b. ergot.
   c. bethanechol.
   d. edrophonium.

REVIEW QUESTIONS—cont'd

9. What untoward effect may occur after a large dose of epinephrine?
   a. Pulmonary edema
   b. Slowing of the heart
   c. Hypotension
   d. Bronchial constriction

10. Beta-blockers are often used in the treatment of:
   a. hypotension.
   b. irritable bowel disease.
   c. hypertension.
   d. duodenal ulcers.

26 Drugs That Affect the Digestive System

Objectives

After completing this chapter, you should be able to do the following:

1. Have a general understanding of the function of the gastrointestinal system and the drugs that affect it in various ways.
2. Identify the drug groups that affect the digestive system.
3. Become familiar with specific disorders of the intestinal tract, such as peptic ulcer disease and irritable bowel syndrome, and recognize the drugs used for these conditions.
4. Become familiar with the way the antisecretory agents and the antacids each reduce the acidity of the stomach.
5. List the various types of cathartics, and give an example of each one.
6. List the antiemetics and become familiar with their uses.
7. Explain how fecal softeners achieve their effects.
8. Discuss nursing responsibilities related to use of antacids and laxatives.

Key Terms

Antacids (ănt-ĂS-ĭds), p. 146
Antiemetics (ăn-tī-ē-MĔ-tĭks), p. 148
Cathartics (kă-THĂR-tĭks), p. 149
Constipation (cŏn-stĭ-PĀ-shŭn), p. 149
Diarrhea (dī-ăh-RĒ-ă), p. 151
Digestants (dĭ-JĔS-těnts), p. 147
Digestion (dĭ-JĔST-yŭn), p. 144
Emetics (ē-MĔ-tĭk), p. 148
Laxatives (LĂK-să-tĭvs), p. 149
Ulcers, p. 145

The digestive system is composed of organs or structures that enable food to be ingested (introduced into the system), digested (broken down into the basic components of the food), and absorbed (passed into the bloodstream). **Digestion** is a mechanical, chemical, and enzymatic process whereby food is converted to material suitable for use in the body. The bloodstream then transports the nutrients to various sites for utilization in growing tissue or producing energy.

Very simply stated, the digestive system consists of a tube within the head and trunk of the body with two external openings (Figure 26–1). Only after food is digested and has left this tube and its components have passed through a membrane into the bloodstream may it actually be considered to have entered the body.

The tube is not of one size throughout. There are enlargements and constrictions in some areas as well as characteristic qualities at different places. From the cells of its glands come enzymes and various chemical reagents that transform crude masses of food into simpler compounds suited for use by the body.

The intestinal part of the tract is in almost continual movement and carries on its functions without the knowledge of the individual, except in terms of the appreciation of the strength and well-being gained from food or the periodic removal of residue from the tract.

When food is taken into the mouth, it is cut and ground by the teeth and thoroughly mixed with saliva. The saliva performs three functions: it acts as a solvent (thus making taste possible), it initiates digestion, and it lubricates the food so that it can be swallowed. Saliva contains the enzyme ptyalin, which reduces the more complex carbohydrates to simpler forms. In some cases saliva also contains maltase, which breaks maltose down into glucose.

The gastric juice normally contains mucin, hydrochloric acid, and the enzymes pepsin, rennin, and lipase. Mucin is a thick, sticky fluid that tends to cling to the surface of the mucosa, serving to protect it from injury by coarse particles of food and, to a certain extent, from the action of the enzymes and hydrochloric acid. The enzymes pepsin and lipase act on protein and fat, respectively, to break these molecules into smaller, usable fractions. Rennin coagulates milk, producing a clumped mass that is wool-like in appearance and is called *curd* and a clear fluid called *whey*. (Rennin obtained from calves' stomachs is used in making cheese because of its ability to coagulate milk.) Hydrochloric acid is necessary to provide an acid environment for the action of pepsin as well as to kill or inhibit many of the microorganisms that find their way into the stomach via food or other ingested materials.

Sometimes, however, the acid becomes so strong that it can actually wear down an area of the stomach lining by its dissolving action. Ordinarily, the stomach is peculiarly resistant to this digestive action because of a protective coat of mucus, but under certain conditions, such as excessive or

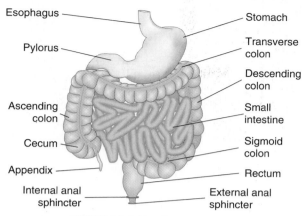

Esophagus — **Stomach** — **Transverse colon** — **Descending colon** — **Small intestine** — **Sigmoid colon** — **Rectum** — **External anal sphincter** — **Pylorus** — **Ascending colon** — **Cecum** — **Appendix** — **Internal anal sphincter**

FIGURE 26-1 The digestive system.

prolonged secretion of hydrochloric acid during periods of worry or stress, a small area of the surface membrane breaks down. The underlying connective tissue of the wall of the stomach is not nearly as resistant to acid as the lining membrane. The gastric juice may then eat away at the tissue and cause a lesion through skin or mucous membrane, usually accompanied by inflammation. These lesions are known as **ulcers,** and those that occur in the gastric system are often called *peptic ulcers.*

It is necessary to neutralize the hydrochloric acid over a period of weeks to allow the ulcer to heal. The goal of this therapy is the reestablishment of the completely intact lining membrane with its natural resistance to the action of the acid.

HELICOBACTER PYLORI AND PEPTIC ULCER DISEASE

Peptic ulcer disease has long been believed to be caused by a high level of gastric secretion, in some cases aggravated by stress or drug therapy with gastric irritants such as nonsteroidal antiinflammatory drugs (NSAIDs).

An infectious agent, *Helicobacter pylori,* has been found in 75% of duodenal ulcers. The majority of the remaining 25% of ulcers are caused by NSAIDs. Research has shown that many people are actually infected with *H. pylori,* but most do not develop an ulcer.

In chronic peptic ulcer disease, it has been found that treatment to kill the microorganism prevents ulcer relapse in about 95% of cases. In addition, there is increasing evidence

Herb Alert

Comfrey

Comfrey is used for the treatment of gastritis and peptic ulcers, as well as for inflammatory conditions. However, this herb is hepatotoxic. Therefore, long-term oral use is not advisable, and it should not be used by patients with preexisting liver disease. See Chapter 35 for more information on comfrey.

of a relationship between *Helicobacter* infection and adenocarcinoma of the stomach. In some cases, eradication of the microorganism has apparently cured some malignancies.

Treatment for *Helicobacter* includes the following options.

Prev-Pak. This is a prepackaged dosage form that provides the patient with the following combination of drugs, to be taken twice daily for 10 to 14 days. Each twice-daily dose contains:

1 gm amoxicillin (Amoxil)
500 mg clarithromycin
30 mg lansoprazole

An alternative would be a 14- or 21-day treatment with the following:

tetracycline, 500 mg three times daily
metronidazole (Flagyl), 250 mg three times daily
bismuth (Pepto-Bismol), 2 tablets four times daily

ANTISECRETORY AGENTS

Although most of the anticholinergic agents currently used as adjuncts in the treatment of peptic ulcer inhibit gastric secretion indirectly, direct inhibition of gastric secretion, particularly secretion of hydrochloric acid, is now possible.

cimetidine, USP, BP (Tagamet). This agent inhibits the effect of histamine on the parietal cells that produce hydrochloric acid; thus it greatly reduces acid output in the stomach. It is used in the treatment of peptic ulcers and in Zollinger-Ellison syndrome (a combination of peptic ulcer and pancreatic tumors). Antacids may be used as well to reduce pain. Treatment with this agent is usually continued for 4 to 6 weeks. It is usually administered orally; however, intravenous therapy may be used in certain instances.

Cimetidine is not the drug of choice for elderly patients because they show an increased susceptibility to the mental disturbances that may occur with this agent.

Many side effects of this drug are caused by its inhibition of some microsomal enzyme systems in the liver. As a result, it interferes with the metabolism of certain drugs by the liver. This causes the drugs to have an enhanced or prolonged effect on the body, and inadvertently can then cause toxic effects as well. This effect is more pronounced in the elderly.

Drugs whose effects may be enhanced or prolonged by their concurrent use with cimetidine include coumarin, phenytoin, propranolol, alprazolam, and diazepam. Current drug interaction information should always be checked when giving cimetidine with any other drug.

Dosage:

Adults and children older than 12 years: (Oral) 300 mg four times daily with meals and at bedtime. (IV) 300 mg in diluted solution every 6 hours.

Considerations for Older Adults

Cimetidine (Tagamet)

Older adults are more susceptible to the central nervous system effects of cimetidine (Tagamet) than are younger adults. Advise older adults to select other antisecretory agents. Mental confusion, agitation, psychosis, and hallucinations have been reported in older adults and seriously ill patients taking cimetidine.

---

ranitidine, USP, BP (Zantac). The primary use of this agent is to inhibit gastric acid secretion. It is used to assist in the healing of peptic ulcers and associated conditions. Ulcers are generally healed in 2 weeks. Ranitidine only minimally inhibits the liver metabolism of drugs, so it does not share the drug interactions of cimetidine. It is better tolerated by elderly patients.

> **Dosage:**
> Adults and children older than 12 years: (Oral) 150 mg twice daily for 2 to 4 weeks.

pantoprazole (Protonix). This antisecretory agent is used to treat erosive gastritis, erosive esophagitis, and gastroesophageal reflux disease.

> **Dosage:**
> Adults: (Oral) 10 to 40 mg daily.

omeprazole (Prilosec). Omeprazole is indicated for the short-term treatment of active duodenal ulcers. It may be used in combination with other agents for the treatment of *Helicobacter* infections.

> **Dosage:**
> Adults: (Oral) 20 mg once daily.

nizatidine (Axid). Nizatidine is an antisecretory agent used to inhibit the acid secretion of the parietal cells. It is indicated for treatment of active duodenal ulcer for up to 8 weeks and may be used for maintenance therapy at a reduced dose. Sweating, urticaria, and somnolence are infrequent side effects.

> **Dosage:**
> Adults: (Oral) 300 mg daily in one or two divided doses; 150 mg orally may be taken at bedtime or as a maintenance dose.

misoprostol (Cytotec). This agent, which is also discussed in Chapter 24 with the prostaglandins, has both antisecretory and mucosal protective properties. It is particularly effective in counteracting the erosive effects of NSAIDs on the gastrointestinal tract. The NSAIDs are antiprostaglandin agents, and as such, they diminish bicarbonate and mucus secretion in the intestine, contributing to mucosal damage. Misoprostol counteracts these effects. The most frequent side effects are diarrhea and abdominal pain. Misoprostol is a prostaglandin abortifacient, and thus it is contraindicated in pregnant women.

> **Dosage:**
> Adults: (Oral) 200 mcg four times daily with food.

ANTACIDS

Antacids destroy the gastric acid, either wholly or in part, by neutralizing or adsorbing it and rendering it inactive.

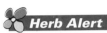
Herb Alert

Ginger

Ginger has been used for centuries for heartburn, as an antiemetic, as an antiinflammatory, and as a laxative. It has also been used to treat motion sickness and for morning sickness in pregnancy. Ginger enhances the antiplatelet action of the nonsteroidal antiinflammatory drugs and warfarin, and it enhances the effects of digitalis. Its use should be avoided in patients with gallstones or bleeding disorders. See Chapter 35 for more information on ginger.

---

sodium bicarbonate, USP, BP (baking soda). This is the home remedy used most often for gastric hyperacidity and heartburn. Heartburn is a burning sensation caused when some of the acid from the stomach is regurgitated into the esophagus.

Sodium bicarbonate has been greatly overused by the general public, and far too many people feel justified in using it for any number of ailments. There are many disadvantages to the use of sodium bicarbonate as an antacid. Because of its solubility, it rapidly neutralizes all the acid present in the stomach and, just as rapidly, passes out of the stomach into the intestines. This frequently results in "acid rebound," or a very high level of secretion of stomach acid after the rapid neutralization of stomach acid results in alkalinization of the stomach. This may cause considerable distress shortly after the administration of the antacid. Unknowing, and thinking this distress is a recurrence of the indigestion, the individual may consume more sodium bicarbonate, thus causing the whole cycle to repeat itself. The alkaline reaction produced in the stomach also inhibits the action of pepsin because hydrochloric acid is needed to activate this enzyme.

Another undesirable effect is caused by the absorption of sodium bicarbonate from the intestine, which produces a disturbance in the acid-base balance in the blood known as alkalosis. Alkalosis results in stress on the kidneys as they attempt to maintain the blood in stable acid-base balance. Renal failure may occur if the disturbance is prolonged.

A further disadvantage is the production of gas in the stomach as a result of the neutralization reaction:

$$HCl + NaHCO_3 \rightarrow NaCl + H_2O + CO_2$$

The carbon dioxide thus produced causes distention of the stomach, a symptom that is quite uncomfortable and may be quite dangerous, particularly if the patient has an ulcer near the perforation point. Oral use of sodium bicarbonate is not recommended. It is used intravenously to correct acidosis in cardiac emergencies and other conditions.

Dosage:

> Adults: (IV) 1 mEq/kg, then titrated as necessary. Repeated doses of 0.5 mEq/kg may be used as necessary. Children: (IV) 1 to 5 mEq/kg, then titrated as necessary.

aluminum hydroxide gel, USP, BP (Amphojel, Creamalin). This gel is formed when aluminum oxide is added to water. It is insoluble and contains colloidal particles that will not precipitate out of the gel; therefore, it does not have some of the undesirable effects of sodium bicarbonate. Because it is insoluble and therefore not absorbed, it does not interfere with the acid-base balance of the blood. Because of its insolubility, its neutralization reaction is slower; thus the acid rebound caused by the faster acting baking soda is eliminated. Carbon dioxide is not produced; therefore, no abdominal distention is observed.

The colloidal particles possess absorptive properties. Hydrochloric acid adheres to the surface of these particles and is inactivated in this way in addition to the chemical neutralization that takes place.

Aluminum hydroxide gel is a mild astringent and demulcent. These qualities are helpful for local action in protecting and soothing the ulcer.

The main disadvantage of this drug is the constipation produced, and it may actually produce a bowel obstruction in persons prone to constipation.

Dosage:

> Adults: (Oral) 8 mL three to six times daily.

magnesium oxide, USP, BP. This is used quite frequently in powder form for its protective and antacid properties. In small doses it is an antacid; in large doses it is a laxative.

Dosage:

> Adults: (Oral) As an antacid—250 mg three to four times daily; as a laxative—500 mg to 1 gm daily.

sucralfate (Carafate). This complex of sucrose and aluminum hydroxide is used to aid in the healing of ulcers by its topical, soothing effect. It adheres to the ulcer itself, thus acting as a mechanical protectant against the action of acid and digestive enzymes.

Dosage:

> Adults only: (Oral) 1 gm four times daily.

DIGESTANTS

Digestants are drugs that promote the process of digestion in the gastrointestinal tract and constitute a type of replacement therapy in deficiency states.

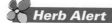

Herb Alert

Cayenne (Capsicum)

Cayenne is taken orally as a digestive aid. It stimulates the production of gastric juices and helps relieve gas. In addition, various antimicrobial effects have been shown after administration of cayenne pepper. Capsaicin, the active ingredient of the pepper, can be applied topically to relieve the pain of diabetic neuropathy, and for the topical treatment of muscle and joint disorders. Cayenne reduces the effect of antihypertensive medications. See Chapter 35 for more information on cayenne.

hydrochloric acid, USP, BP (diluted). A deficiency of hydrochloric acid in the stomach can result from (1) deficient secretion of the acid; (2) excess secretion of mucus, which neutralizes the acid; (3) regurgitation of alkaline substances from the intestine; (4) pernicious anemia; or (5) carcinoma of the stomach. If there is decreased secretion of hydrochloric acid from the stomach gland, the condition is known as *hypochlorhydria*. If there is no secretion, it is known as *achlorhydria*. Achlorhydria is common in carcinoma and is also observed in pernicious anemia, infections, renal disease, and diabetes. Occasionally, it occurs in individuals apparently otherwise normal in every respect. Dilute hydrochloric acid may be given to combat these conditions. It is taken in water through a glass straw to protect the enamel of the teeth.

Dosage:

> Adults: (Oral) 4 mL of the dilute acid.

pancreatin, USP, BP (Viokase). This commercial preparation of the pancreas tissue of hogs and oxen contains all the pancreatic digestive enzymes. It is used to replace pancreatic enzymes in such conditions as cystic fibrosis and various malabsorption syndromes.

Dosage:

> Adults and children: (Oral) 500 mg three times daily with meals.

pancrelipase, USP, BP (Cotazym, Pancrease, Ku-Zyme, Creon, Ultrase, Zymase). This standardized pancreas enzyme replacement is made from hog pancreas. It has more digestive enzymes on a weight basis than does the cruder product pancreatin. It is used in cystic fibrosis and other disorders of pancreatic dysfunction.

Dosage:

> Adults: (Oral) 900 mg with each meal and 300 mg with each snack.

lactase enzyme (Lactaid). Lactase is the enzyme that digests lactose, or milk sugar. It may be given to milk-intolerant individuals to enable them to consume milk and milk products. It is supplied in caplets and chewable tablets and in the form of drops to be added directly to milk.

Dosage:

> Adults and children: (Oral) Drops: 5 to 15 drops per quart of milk. Caplets: 1 to 3 caplets (3000 units each) with milk product.

APPETITE STIMULANT

megestrol acetate (Megace). This agent is a synthetic derivative of the female hormone progesterone. It enhances the appetite and is used in the treatment of cachexia from serious illnesses, as well as anorexia. Its use as an antineoplastic agent is discussed in Chapter 29. Some adrenal suppression has been observed following use of this agent, as has exacerbation of diabetes. Other side effects include vomiting, diarrhea, rash, and headache.

Dosage:
> Adults: (Oral) 800 mg once daily.

ABSORPTION INHIBITOR

orlistat (Xenical). Orlistat is a lipase inhibitor for obesity management. It acts by blocking absorption of dietary fats. When present in the lumen of the stomach, it forms a covalent bond with gastric and pancreatic lipases. The inactivated enzymes are then unable to digest fat. It should be used with a reduced-calorie diet and exercise plan. Side effects include weight loss and vitamin deficiencies, abdominal discomfort, and diarrhea.

Dosage:
> Adults: (Oral) 120 mg three times daily with each meal.

Considerations for Pregnant and Nursing Women

Orlistat (Xenical)
Orlistat (Xenical) is not recommended for pregnant or nursing women. The drug may reduce gastric absorption of fat-soluble vitamins and beta-carotene. It is not known whether orlistat is distributed in breast milk, but it is not recommended for nursing mothers.

EMETICS

Emetics produce vomiting. They are used today primarily as a first aid measure when prompt emptying of the stomach is essential. Large amounts of tepid water will distend the stomach and produce this effect, and 2 teaspoonfuls of salt or mustard in the tepid water will hasten emesis. Mild soapsuds solution is also used.

The use of emetics should be avoided in cases of poisoning with a corrosive or caustic substance (a strong acid or alkali that can cause burns and tissue damage), because damage to the mouth, pharynx, and esophagus is increased by the second passage of the material over these structures.

The use of emetics at present is limited because to a great extent they have been replaced by gastric lavage using a stomach tube.

ipecac syrup, USP, BP. This syrup is administered orally to produce vomiting when indicated in the management of acute poisonings. After oral administration almost all patients will vomit within 30 minutes. It is important to give additional fluids after the dose of ipecac to increase the effectiveness of the drug. This should be ideally 200 to 300 mL of a clear liquid. Milk inhibits the effect of ipecac.

Emesis should not be produced when caustic substances, such as lye, have been ingested or for ingestion of petroleum distillates, such as gasoline, fuel oil, or paint thinners. If the second dose does not produce emesis within 30 minutes, gastric lavage should be performed. No more than two doses should be given.

Ipecac syrup is available without a prescription.

Dosage:
> Adults and children older than 12 years: (Oral) 30 mL.
> Children 1 to 11 years: (Oral) 15 mL.
> Children 6 months to 1 year: (Oral) 5 mL.

ANTIEMETICS

Antiemetics relieve nausea and vomiting. Numerous preparations have been used, but ordinarily the most effective treatment must be chosen after consideration of the cause of the nausea. Vomiting may be attributed to irritation of the gastric mucosa, stimulation of the vomiting center in the brain, or possibly a combination of both.

Antiemetics readily available for home use are carbonated drinks and hot tea.

Herb Alert

Chamomile
Chamomile is a popular remedy for nervous stomach and is known for its calming effect on the smooth muscle of the intestinal tract. Used externally, it relieves skin irritations and hemorrhoids. Used as a mouthwash, it may relieve the pain of toothache. Chamomile enhances the effects of sedatives and warfarin, as well as the antiplatelet effects of nonsteroidal antiinflammatory drugs. See Chapter 35 for more information on chamomile.

Certain types of vomiting are relieved by administering central depressants such as the bromides or barbiturates. Other agents used include the following.

dimenhydrinate, USP, BP (Dramamine). This agent inhibits vomiting and causes sedation. It is frequently used to relieve motion sickness and control the nausea, vomiting, and vertigo associated with other conditions, such as electroconvulsive therapy, radiation sickness, and hypertension.

Dosage:
> Adults: (Oral) 50 mg three times daily.

Children older than 8 years: (Oral, IM) 25 mg three times daily.

meclizine hydrochloride, USP, BP (Bonine, Antivert). This drug prevents the nausea and vomiting of motion sickness and the morning sickness of the first months of pregnancy, and it is used to treat the vertigo of labyrinthitis.

Dosage:

Adults: (Oral) 25 mg three times daily.
Children: Not recommended.

prochlorperazine maleate, USP, BP (Compazine). In addition to its tranquilizing effect, this agent is very effective in controlling vomiting. It is used postoperatively for this purpose, and it may also be given orally in tablet or liquid form.

Dosage:

Adults: (Oral, Rectal, IM, IV) 5 to 10 mg three to four times daily.
Children: (Oral) 2.5 to 5 mg two times daily.

trimethobenzamide hydrochloride, USP, BP (Tigan). Effective orally, rectally, or parenterally, this agent is closely related to the antihistamines. It acts centrally on the vomiting center to decrease nausea and vomiting.

Dosage:

Adults: (Oral, IM, Rectal) 100 to 250 mg one to four times daily.
Children: (Oral) 100 mg three times daily. (Rectal) 100 mg every 8 hours.

ondansetron hydrochloride (Zofran). The antiemetic activity of this agent is believed to be mediated by the central nervous system. It is administered IV and is effective in controlling the nausea and vomiting caused by chemotherapy, as well as postoperative nausea and vomiting. It should not be used for routine prophylaxis.

Dosage:

Adults (IV) 32 mg infused over 15 minutes.
Children older than 3 years: (IV) 0.15 mg/kg infused over 15 minutes.

granisetron hydrochloride (Kytril). This centrally acting antiemetic is used to prevent the nausea and vomiting associated with chemotherapy. It may be administered orally or IV.

Dosage:

Adults and children older than 2 years: (IV) 10 mcg/kg as 5-minute infusion.
Adults only: (Oral) 1 mg twice daily.

CATHARTICS

Cathartics relieve **constipation,** the condition in which bowel movements are infrequent or incomplete. Constipation occurs when fecal material remains too long in the large intestine and too much water is absorbed from it. It becomes hardened, and the lower bowel becomes dis-

tended. Constipation usually results from one or more of the following causes: (1) an improper diet that leaves too little residue in the intestinal tract, (2) insufficient fluid intake, (3) nervous tension and worry, (4) lack of exercise (an important factor in hospitalized patients), or (5) failure to respond to the normal defecation impulses. In most cases correction of one or more of these simple health problems will take care of the constipation problem. In other cases, however, cathartics should be given as an adjunct.

It is important to remember that there is no set time limit between bowel movements. Many parents become extremely upset when a child does not develop a regular habit of moving the bowels once every 24 hours. Continually lecturing the child about regularity can create an emotional problem in the child as well as constipation. As long as the stool is of normal consistency and as long as there is no discomfort resulting from distention after elimination, there is no constipation. Many perfectly healthy individuals may have normal eliminations no more often than every 3 or 4 days.

The administration of laxatives or cathartics of any kind must be absolutely avoided in the presence of abdominal pain, nausea, vomiting, or similar symptoms that may indicate the presence of appendicitis.

BULK-INCREASING LAXATIVES

Laxatives are cathartics that evacuate the bowel by a mild action. Bulk-increasing laxatives act by swelling when in the presence of water and mechanically stimulate the intestine to contract because of the increased volume. They usually take 24 to 48 hours for action.

Bulk-increasing laxatives generally substitute for fiber that should be part of a good diet. Information on natural fiber is presented in Chapter 15 (Vitamins, Minerals, and General Nutrition).

agar. This is a hydrophilic colloid obtained from seaweed. In water it swells to form a mucilaginous (moist and sticky) mass that is soothing to the gastric mucosa. It increases the bulk and keeps the intestinal contents moist and soft. It is contained in the commercial preparation Agoral.

Dosage:

Adults: (Oral) 4 gm once daily.

psyllium seed. The powdered mucilaginous portion of these seeds swells in water to form a gel. It has a soothing effect on the mucosa and produces a soft, moist stool. It can be found in the commercial preparation Metamucil. [AU3]

methylcellulose, USP, BP (Citrucel). This compound is made synthetically from cellulose. In water it swells to form a gel. It is available in tablet or liquid form and is found in the commercial preparations Cellothyl, Cologel, and Hydrolose.

Dosage:

Adults: (Oral) 1 gm once daily.

LUBRICANT LAXATIVES

These laxatives act by mixing with and softening the fecal mass but do not increase the bulk. They take 12 to 18 hours for action.

mineral oil, USP, BP. A mixture of hydrocarbons obtained from petroleum, mineral oil is indigestible and not absorbed. It is purely a mechanical lubricant. One disadvantage to its continued use, however, is that it prevents absorption of the fat-soluble vitamins and carries them through the intestinal tract. If mineral oil is aspirated when swallowing, a lipid pneumonia may result. This may be a problem particularly in the elderly.

Dosage:
Adults: (Oral) 15 mL once daily.

SALINE CATHARTICS

These are highly water-soluble substances that are poorly absorbed from the gastrointestinal tract. Because of their high osmotic pressure, they hold water in the tract and cause more water to be absorbed into the tract from other tissues. This greatly increases the bulk in the intestine and promotes contraction of the smooth muscle.

In addition to their use as laxatives, these agents may also be used to treat edematous conditions as well as food poisoning in which the most rapid evacuation possible is desired. They act in 1 to 4 hours, but considerable gripping (severe spasms of pain in the abdomen) may be produced.

Osmosis is the passage of water through a semipermeable membrane from a less concentrated to a higher concentrated area; this tends to dilute the more highly concentrated solution and to equalize the concentrations of the solutions on either side of the semipermeable membrane.

Osmotic pressure may be best explained by an example. An aqueous solution of sugar or salt is placed in a small, closed semipermeable (permeable to water; impermeable to the dissolved molecules) sac made of cellophane, parchment, or sausage skin and immersed in a container of water. Water from the container is drawn into the sac by osmosis, but the sugar or salt solution does not pass out. The pressure within the sac increases because of the increased volume of water; the walls of the sac become distended and may rupture. The force created in this way is spoken of as the osmotic pressure.

magnesia magma, USP, BP (milk of magnesia). The mildest of the saline cathartics, this is the agent preferred for children. In addition to its use as a laxative, if it is given in smaller doses it is an effective antacid.

Dosage:
Adults and children: (Oral) As an antacid—4 mL every few hours; as a laxative—15 mL at bedtime.

magnesium citrate solution, USP, BP (citrate of magnesia). This is a fast-acting saline cathartic in liquid form. Because the solution contains a considerable amount of sugar, it should not be given to a diabetic unless this sugar is taken into consideration.

Dosage:
Adults: (Oral) 6 to 12 ounces.

electrolytes for oral solution (NuLYTELY, GoLYTELY). Polyethylene glycol combined with sodium chloride, sodium bicarbonate, and potassium chloride is reconstituted in a 4-L jug for bowel cleansing prior to colonoscopy or barium enema examinations. It induces diarrhea, which rapidly cleanses the bowel, usually within 4 hours. Side effects include nausea, abdominal distention, and pain, although these effects are generally mild.

Dosage:
Adults: (Oral) 4 L at a rate of 8 ounces every 10 to 15 minutes.
Children: (Oral) 25 mL/kg/hr until rectal effluent is clear.

sodium phosphate monobasic monohydrate (Visicol). This combination of salts is used in a tablet form as a bowel evacuant prior to colonoscopy or barium enema examination. It should be used with caution in patients with impaired renal function. Side effects include abdominal distention and pain.

Dosage:
Adults only: (Oral) 2 doses of 30 gm approximately 12 hours apart.

IRRITANT CATHARTICS

These agents act by irritating the mucosa of the intestinal tract; thus they produce contraction of the muscle and elimination.

castor oil, USP, BP. This oil is broken down in the intestine (hydrolyzed), like any other digestible fat, to glycerin and a fatty acid. It is this fatty acid that is responsible for the irritation and the laxative effect of the oil. It is given in larger doses than are strictly needed for the laxative effect (laxation) because, as soon as enough oil is hydrolyzed, laxation is produced, and the remainder of the unhydrolyzed oil gives a soothing effect to the mucosa as the mass moves through the tract.

Dosage:
Adults: (Oral) 15 mL.

senna, USP, BP (Senokot). Senna consists of the dried leaf of *Cassia acutifolia*. It contains glucosides, which are stimulant cathartics. It is only slightly absorbed from the small intestine and produces a bowel movement generally in 6 to 12 hours after the dose.

Dosage:
Adults and children older than 12 years: (Oral) 0.5 to 2 gm. (Rectal) 30 mg one to two times daily.
Children 6 to 12 years: (Oral) 0.25 to 1 gm.

bisacodyl (Dulcolax). This commercial irritant laxative is used either in tablet or suppository form.

Dosage:
Adults: (Oral, Rectal) 10 mg once daily.

FECAL SOFTENERS

Fecal softeners are surface-active agents (surfactants) or detergents. This means that their action is accomplished by mixing with the fecal material, causing it to be "wetted" by the water in the gastrointestinal tract, thereby emulsifying and softening it for easier elimination. These agents gain the desired effect without irritating the gastric mucosa and without increasing the bulk content of the intestine. For these reasons they are the agents of choice for cardiac patients.

The fecal softeners take 1 to 3 days for action; thus they cannot be used when a faster elimination is desired.

Occasionally, the surface-active agent is combined with one or more of the other laxatives for a faster effect.

Fecal Softeners Used as Single Agents

docusate calcium (Dioctal, Surfak)
   Dosage:
      (Oral) 240 mg/day.

docusate sodium (Colace, Correctol, Modane)
   Dosage:
      (Oral) 100 to 200 mg/day.

Fecal Softeners in Combination

docusate sodium, 100 mg, plus casanthrol, 30 mg (Peri-Colace, Doxidan)
   Dosage:
      1 to 2 capsules daily.

OTHER LAXATIVES

tegaserod maleate (Zelnorm) Tegaserod is used to treat the constipation phase of irritable bowel syndrome. At this time it is recommended for women; it has not been sufficiently evaluated in men. The treatment course generally runs for 4 to 6 weeks, but this can be repeated for a second course of treatment if indicated. Side effects include abdominal pain, headache, dizziness, and back pain.
   Dosage:
      Adults: (Oral) 6 mg twice daily before meals.

ANTIDIARRHEALS

These agents are used to treat **diarrhea**, a disorder associated with too rapid passage of intestinal content, gripping action, and abnormally frequent, watery stools. Some of the causes of diarrhea are (1) contaminated or partially decomposed food, (2) intestinal infection, (3) nervous disorders, (4) circulatory disturbances, and (5) inflammatory conditions of the adjacent viscera. In view of these numerous causes, the treatment of diarrhea varies greatly. In some cases even a cathartic that brings about emptying of the entire bowel may be a means of relieving the diarrhea because it removes the irritating material. If the condition is caused by an infection, the treatment must be directed toward killing the invading organism.

AGENTS USED FOR SIMPLE DIARRHEA
Demulcents

These agents have a soothing effect on the irritated membrane of the gastrointestinal tract. Boiled starch and boiled milk are convenient home remedies of this type. Others are acacia, glycyrrhiza, and glycerin.

Adsorbents

These agents act by adsorbing the irritating material on the surface of the gastrointestinal tract and thereby removing it. Examples of this type are activated charcoal, kaolin, and kaolin-pectin mixture (Kaopectate). This last mixture combines the adsorbing properties of kaolin with the demulcent effect of pectin. Sometimes an agent that decreases peristalsis is added to these preparations, such as paregoric or belladonna alkaloids. Antibiotics may be combined with the adsorbents also.

AGENTS USED FOR SEVERE DIARRHEA

diphenoxylate hydrochloride plus atropine sulfate (Lomotil). Diphenoxylate acts on the smooth muscle of the intestinal tract in a manner similar to morphine, inhibiting gastrointestinal motility. Although this drug in standard dosages has essentially no analgesic effect, the administration of opioid antagonists may precipitate a withdrawal syndrome in patients who take it regularly.

Atropine is added to diphenoxylate as a deterrent to overdose. In higher doses the side effects of atropine produces an unpleasant tachycardia along with the other symptoms of atropine overdose (see the discussion of atropine in Chapter 25, Drugs That Affect the Autonomic Nervous System.)

Each tablet or 5 mL of the liquid contains diphenoxylate hydrochloride 2.5 mg with atropine sulfate 0.025 mg. The dosages below are those of diphenoxylate only.
   Dosage:
      Adults: (Oral) 5 mg four times daily.
      Children 2 to 12 years: 0.3 to 0.4 mg/kg/day.

loperamide hydrochloride (Imodium). Loperamide slows intestinal motility by exerting a direct effect on the nerve endings of the intestinal wall. It prolongs the transit time of the intestinal contents and thus reduces fecal volume, diminishing loss of fluid and electrolytes.
   Dosage:
      Adults: (Oral) 4 mg initially, then 2 mg after each unformed stool.
      Children: (Oral) 0.08 to 0.24 mg/kg/day in two to three divided doses.

alosetron hydrochloride (Lotronex). Alosetron is indicated *only* for women with severe, diarrhea-prominent irritable bowel syndrome. It should not be used in patients with constipation. Side effects include abdominal discomfort, nausea, abdominal distention, hemorrhoids, and tachycardia.

Dosage:
Adults: (Oral) 1 mg daily for 4 weeks, then 1 mg twice daily.

CLINICAL IMPLICATIONS

1. Antacids interfere with the absorption of many drugs, particularly antibiotics. The ideal time for administration of antacids is 2 hours after a meal when the acid rebound that follows the completion of digestion of food occurs. [AU6] They should be given alone, not at the time when other drugs are administered.
2. Many drugs that affect the gastrointestinal tract are liquids. They should be shaken well before administration.
3. Observe the patient for symptomatic relief when gastrointestinal drugs are being administered. This is generally noted as reduced gastric pain and abdominal distention.
4. Dietary habits should be discussed with the patient. A bland diet that eliminates fried or spicy foods and any beverages that contain alcohol or caffeine should be encouraged.
5. Liquid antacids may cause either constipation or diarrhea, depending on their composition. The patient should be observed for these effects.
6. Antiemetic drugs have as their usual side effects dry mouth, blurred vision, and urinary retention. The patient should be observed for these effects.
7. Injectable antiemetics should be administered into a large muscle mass because they are often irritating to tissues.
8. The primary side effect of antiemetic agents is central nervous system depression. The patient should be cautioned about this effect. Concurrent administration with other depressants such as alcohol and sedative or hypnotic agents should be avoided if possible.
9. The nurse can often instruct the patient in changes in dietary habits to include substances such as bran and fiber to eliminate the need for routine laxative therapy.
10. Laxatives are often necessary in hospitalized patients because inactivity and bed rest alter normal bowel function.
11. Laxatives are generally given to hospitalized patients at bedtime to promote effects the following morning.
12. Antidiarrheal preparations may be habit forming. The patient should be instructed not to overuse these agents.
13. Laxatives may be overused by the patient to have a "normal" bowel movement every morning. The nurse should discuss the range of "normal" with regard to bowel habits.
14. Hyperemesis may be associated with eating disorders.
15. Peptic ulcer disease often has an infectious cause and can be treated specifically.

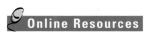

Online Resources

For updated drug information and Web activities, go to http://evolve.elsevier.com/Asperheim.

CRITICAL THINKING QUESTIONS

1. The patient, 12 years old, is brought to the physician by her mother, who reports that, in spite of every laxative and food program she could think of, the child is "constantly constipated," having a bowel movement only every 3 or 4 days. There never seems to be any problem or pain associated with the stools, but the mother is concerned that her daughter become "regulated." What is your advice?

2. The patient had a heart attack 2 months ago but is now doing well except that he is constipated. He calls the office to speak to you because he doesn't want to bother the doctor. He is just about to take a big dose of Epsom salts to "flush out his system," but his wife made him call to check with you first. What is your advice?

3. The patient calls the physician's office nearly frantic because her 2-year-old has eaten half a bottle of baby aspirin. The doctor is not back from lunch yet. What would you advise?

REVIEW QUESTIONS

1. A frequent cause of peptic ulcer disease is:
   a. infection with *Escherichia coli.*
   b. infection with *Pseudomonas* organisms.
   c. hypertension.
   d. *Helicobacter pylori* infection.

2. A drug that is often implicated in peptic ulcer disease is:
   a. penicillin.
   b. misoprostol.
   c. ibuprofen.
   d. clarithromycin.

3. A drug that inhibits the secretion of gastric hydrochloric acid is:
   a. ibuprofen.
   b. cimetidine.
   c. pancreatin.
   d. magnesium oxide.

4. A digestant is intended to:
   a. directly digest food.
   b. counteract stomach acid.
   c. replace deficient enzymes of the gastrointestinal tract.
   d. heal peptic ulcers.

REVIEW QUESTIONS

5. An agent used to promote weight loss is:
   a. dimenhydrinate.
   b. orlistat.
   c. pancrelipase.
   d. omeprazole.

6. An agent that prevents vomiting associated with chemotherapy is:
   a. dimenhydrinate.
   b. meclizine.
   c. trimethobenzamide.
   d. granisetron.

7. A cathartic may be necessary if:
   a. there has been no bowel movement for 24 hours.
   b. the stool is of normal consistency.
   c. there is discomfort associated with elimination.
   d. the stools are too loose.

8. An example of a fecal softener is:
   a. magnesium sulfate.
   b. docusate.
   c. tegaserod.
   d. loperamide.

9. An agent that slows intestinal motility is:
   a. docusate.
   b. loperamide.
   c. castor oil.
   d. mineral oil.

10. All of the following are causes of diarrhea except:
    a. emesis.
    b. food poisoning.
    c. nervous disorders.
    d. bowel inflammation.

The Endocrine Glands and Hormones

Objectives

After completing this chapter, you should be able to do the following:

1. Name the glands that are included in the endocrine system.
2. State the function of each endocrine gland.
3. Identify conditions caused by abnormal functioning of each endocrine gland.
4. Identify contraceptives, how they function, and some contraindications for their use.
5. Identify the agents used to promote ovulation.
6. Identify oxytocic agents and discuss precautions to be observed when these are administered.
7. Become familiar with the different types of diabetes and the agents used to treat it.
8. Understand replacement therapy for gonadal dysfunction.

Key Terms

cortisone (KŎR-tǐ-sōn), p. 156
endocrine (ĔN-dō-krěn) **gland,** p. 154
estrogen (ĔS-trō-jěn), p. 151
follicle-stimulating hormone (FSH), p. 160
hormones (HŌR-mōns), p. 154
hydrocortisone (hī-drō-KŎR-tǐ-sōn), p. 156
insulin (ĬN-sū-lǐn), p. 157
luteinizing (LŪ-tē-ǐn-Ī-zǐng) **hormone (LH),** p. 160
oxytocic agents (ŏk-sē-TŌ-sǐk), p. 164
progesterone (prō-JĔS-tě-rōn), p. 161
testosterone (tĕs-TŎS-tě-rōn), p. 165

The **endocrine glands** do not possess ducts or any openings to the exterior but rather secrete internally. Their secretions, called **hormones,** are chemical substances that pass into the bloodstream and are carried to the various tissues of the body, upon which they exert their action—altering the function or activity of that target organ.

A hormone may be defined as any substance formed by a tissue of the body and carried in the blood to some tissue or organ upon which it acts.

The organs of the endocrine system, although separated physically, are unified and well integrated (Figure 27–1). The main organs belonging to this group of structures that furnish internal secretions to the body are the pituitary, the thy-

roid, the parathyroids, the adrenals, the gonads, and the pancreatic islets of Langerhans. The endocrine glands as well as the mammary glands and the growth of the body's skeletal system are under the control of the anterior lobe of the pituitary gland, sometimes called the "master gland."

PITUITARY GLAND

The anterior lobe of the pituitary, a small gland located at the base of the brain, secretes regulating hormones that control the action of other endocrine glands of the body. These regulating hormones are called the tropic hormones and are named according to the gland they affect (e.g., the thyrotropic hormone affects the thyroid gland, the adrenocorticotropic hormone affects the cortex of the adrenal glands). These regulating hormones cause the endocrine glands to secrete their respective hormones into the bloodstream.

THYROID GLAND

The thyroid gland is composed of two lobes located on either side of the larynx. The thyrotropic hormone from the anterior pituitary stimulates the thyroid gland to secrete the thyroid hormone. The exact mechanism of action of this hormone, thyroxine (T_4), is not known, but it apparently causes all cells to accelerate their rate of metabolism.

Hypothyroidism means a reduced activity of the thyroid gland. If the thyroid gland of a growing child does not function adequately, the child fails to develop normally. The child has pronounced mental retardation and slow sexual development, and the skin is thickened, dry, and wrinkled. The tongue is thick and protrudes from the mouth, the abdomen protrudes, the legs are short, the hands and feet are poorly developed, and the body musculature is weak. Such a child is called a cretin; the disorder is called cretinism.

Cretinism develops whenever the thyroid gland fails to function properly during the formative years of a child's development. For the most part, it occurs in regions having a deficiency of iodine in the drinking water and food. Cretinism may be corrected if thyroid hormone therapy is given in early infancy. If therapy is not begun until later, permanent mental retardation results.

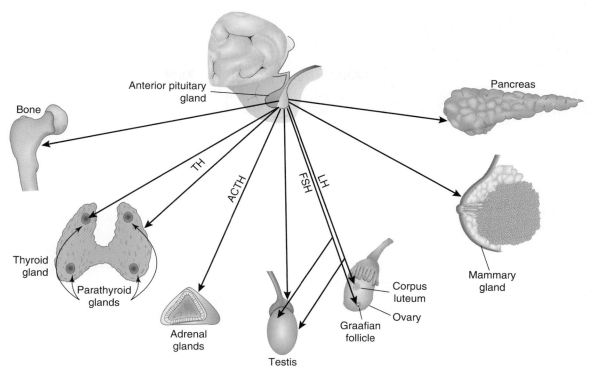

FIGURE 27-1 The endocrine system.

Hypothyroidism in the adult, called myxedema, is characterized by a gradual slowing of mental and physical functions. The hands and feet are puffy, the skin is thick and leathery, and the patient is hypersensitive to cold. Good results are usually obtained by treatment with thyroid hormone, because full mental and physical development has already been achieved.

Hyperthyroidism, the condition caused by an overproduction of the thyroid hormone, is characterized by an enlargement of the thyroid gland, protruding eyes, elevation of the basal metabolic rate, disturbance of carbohydrate metabolism, nervousness, and hyperactivity. The condition is also known as Graves' disease. Hyperthyroidism may be treated with an antithyroid drug such as propylthiouracil (dose: 100 mg), methimazole (dose: 10 mg), or radioactive iodine, or else part of the gland may be removed surgically.

Hashimoto's disease, also known as chronic lymphocytic thyroiditis, is considered to be caused by an autoimmune process. The serum of these patients contains antibodies to one or more of the thyroid antigens, and it is presumed that the destruction of the thyroid is caused by the antigen-antibody process. Thyroid treatment should be started based on the thyroid studies as soon as the disease is diagnosed. The prognosis is excellent.

Goiter is the term applied to an enlarged thyroid gland. This increase in size may be caused by hyperthyroidism (overactivity of the gland), or it may be caused by hypothyroidism, the growth resulting then from a body "reflex" to compensate for the inefficiency of the gland. It is, therefore, impossible to predict which thyroid abnormality is causing the enlarged appearance of the gland.

 Considerations for Pregnant and Nursing Women

Thyroid Agents

Thyroid agents do not readily cross the placenta and can be administered during pregnancy. However, thyroxine levels are lower than normal during pregnancy, and monitoring generally includes a measurement of serum thyrotropin, to ensure accurate dosing. Although only minimal amounts of thyroid agents are secreted in breast milk, breast-feeding is generally discouraged for women taking thyroid products.

THYROID PREPARATIONS

Thyroid drugs are either natural or synthetic preparations containing hormones that would be naturally produced in the thyroid gland. The synthetic products permit a greater accuracy and predictability when treating thyroid dysfunction.

thyroid, USP, BP. Thyroid is the cleaned and dried thyroid gland obtained primarily from hogs. It may be used in varied dosages as necessary to attain thyroid function in the normal range.

The T_4 level is often used to evaluate thyroid function and therapy. The normal range is 5 to 12 mcg/dL, with the most effective range from 7 to 10 mcg/dL.

Full thyroid replacement of normal function is 180 mg/day. Partial hypothyroidism requires smaller doses.

Table 27-1 | *Thyroid Equivalent Dosage*

THYROID AGENT	EQUIVALENT DOSE
thyroid	60 mg
levothyroxine (Levoxine,	
Levothyroid, Synthroid, T4)	100 mcg
liothyronine (Cytomel, T3)	25 mcg

Dosage:
Adults and children: (Oral) 30 to 60 mg daily, up to 180 mg daily. Dosage is individualized.

Synthetic Thyroid Preparations

There is obvious natural variability in the amount of thyroid in pulverized crude gland when used for therapy; a more accurate form of thyroid replacement can be achieved with synthetic preparations. They have various potencies; a comparative dosage scale is shown in Table 27–1.

It should be remembered that direct substitution is not possible between the thyroid preparations. Patients may metabolize or excrete one thyroid agent differently than they metabolize another. There have even been some untoward reactions when substituting a generic drug for a formerly used brand-name drug.

ANTITHYROID AGENTS

Hyperthyroidism, or Graves' disease, is a condition resulting from an overproduction of thyroid hormone. It is also a condition that must be treated medically or surgically. The symptoms of hyperthyroidism include protruding eyes, weight loss, increased appetite, tachycardia and palpitations, nervousness, diarrhea, abdominal cramps, increased pulse and blood pressure, headache, intolerance to heat, fever, and menstrual irregularities.

 Considerations for Pregnant and Nursing Women

Antithyroid Agents
Antithyroid agents such as propylthiouracil and methimazole (Tapazole) should not be taken by pregnant women because these drugs can induce goiter and hypothyroidism in the developing fetus.

methimazole, USP, BP (Tapazole). Methimazole inhibits the synthesis of thyroid hormones by preventing the incorporation of iodine into the hormone. It is used for palliative treatment of hyperthyroidism and preoperatively before surgical or radiation procedures.
Dosage:
Adults: (Oral) 15 to 60 mg daily.
Children: (Oral) 0.4 mg/kg initially, then decreased.

propylthiouracil, USP, BP. Propylthiouracil also interferes with the incorporation of iodine into the thyroid hormone molecule. It is used both to suppress the thyroid

gland prior to surgical procedures and for medical suppression.
Dosage:
Adults: (Oral) 300 to 1200 mg daily in divided doses.
Children 6 to 10 years: (Oral) 50 to 150 mg/m² daily.

ADRENAL GLANDS

The adrenal glands are located directly above the kidneys and are composed of two parts: an outer portion, the cortex, and an inner part, the medulla. The medullary portion secretes epinephrine and norepinephrine. The cortex secretes a number of hormones that are essential to life. Death results when this cortex is removed or severely impaired.

Some of the hormones secreted by the adrenal cortex are **cortisone, hydrocortisone,** aldosterone, and deoxycorticosterone. These hormones are secreted when the gland is activated by the adrenocorticotropic hormone from the anterior pituitary. The most important functions of these hormones in the body are (1) regulation of water and salt metabolism, (2) regulation of carbohydrate metabolism, and (3) production of antiinflammatory effects.

A destructive disease of the adrenal cortex in humans is known as Addison's disease. If untreated, it is gradually progressive, and death occurs within 2 or 3 years. This condition is characterized by weight loss, weakness, and disturbed carbohydrate and mineral metabolism; in addition, there is increased bronzing pigmentation of the skin. The skin may be mottled, with areas of depigmentation adjacent to areas of overpigmentation. Addison's disease may be treated by administering deoxycorticosterone along with a diet high in sodium and low in potassium.

Cortisone and hydrocortisone are potent antiinflammatory drugs. When irritation or inflammation is present anywhere in the body, there is an increase in the production of these hormones by the adrenal cortex. If the inflammation is very severe, the adrenals may be unable to secrete an adequate supply to overcome the effects. Additional hormones may be administered to the patient from another source, thus increasing their levels in the circulation and affording relief from the symptoms. Cortisone and hydrocortisone are useful in the suppression of the symptoms of rheumatoid arthritis, bursitis, and various types of skin diseases. The antiinflammatory properties of these agents have made them useful in the treatment of multiple sclerosis. They can shorten the duration of a relapse and accelerate recovery. The effect on the long-term course of the disease remains questionable. Neither cortisone nor hydrocortisone nor any of their derivatives cures the disease or causes any real improvement. They merely suppress the symptoms; upon withdrawal of the drug symptoms recur.

With continued use of these adrenocorticoid agents many side effects will occur. These are primarily salt and water retention, "moon facies," muscular weakness, hirsutism, acne, and occasionally mental disturbances. Because their action is to suppress the inflammatory response of the body, this suppression occurs also when it is not desired; hence ulcers may be perforated before the patient is aware of them and tuberculosis may advance at an alarming rate. These drugs should be used with caution in patients with peptic ulcers, and they are contraindicated for individuals suffering from tuberculosis or other severe infectious diseases.

The newer synthetic compounds are similar in action to cortisone and hydrocortisone, but to a great extent they have lessened the number and severity of the side effects produced.

cortisone acetate, USP, BP (Cortogen, Cortone)
  Dosage:
    Adults: (Oral) 25 to 300 mg/day. (IM) 20 to 300 mg/day.

hydrocortisone, USP, BP (Hydrocortone, Cortef, Solu-Cortef)
  Dosage:
    Adults: (Oral) 25 mg to 300 mg/day. (IM, IV, Intrathecal) 100 to 500 mg per dose over 4-6 hours or as ordered.

prednisone, USP, BP (Deltasone, Sterapred)
  Dosage:
    Adults: (Oral) 5 to 60 mg/day.

prednisolone, USP, BP (Prelone, Cotolone)
  Dosage:
    Adults: (Oral) 5 to 60 mg/day.

methylprednisolone, USP, BP (Medrol, Solu-Medrol)
  Dosage:
    Adults: (Oral) 4 to 60 mg/day. (IM, IV) 10 mg to 1.5 gm daily.

triamcinolone acetonide, USP, BP (Aristocort, Kenalog)
  Dosage:
    Adults: (Oral) 4 to 48 mg/day. (Intralesional, Intraarticular) 2 to 20 mg per dose as ordered.

dexamethasone, USP, BP (Decadron)
  Dosage:
    Adults: (Oral) 0.75 mg/day. (IM, IV, Intraarticular) 0.5 to 24 mg/day.

betamethasone, USP, BP (Celestone)
  Dosage:
    Adults: (Oral) 0.6 to 7.2 mg/day. (IM, IV, Intraarticular) 0.5 to 9 mg/day.

fludrocortisone acetate (Florinef)
  Dosage:
    Adults: (Oral) 0.1 to 0.2 mg/day.

fluocinolone A, USP, BP (Synalar)
  Dosage:
    Adults: (Topical) 0.025% once or twice daily.

flurandrenolide ointment, USP, BP (Cordran)
  Dosage:
    Adults: (Topical) 0.05% once or twice daily.

PANCREAS

Clusters of cells known as the islets of Langerhans are found on the pancreas and are the sources of the hormone known as **insulin.** In a healthy individual, insulin serves three purposes: (1) it aids in the utilization of glucose as energy, (2) it stores excess glucose as glycogen in the liver, and (3) it is responsible for the conversion of glucose to fat. However, when the pancreas does not secrete sufficient insulin to carry out these reactions, the glucose level in the blood becomes quite high after the ingestion of carbohydrates. This condition is known as diabetes mellitus.

If diabetes is not treated, sugar spills over into the urine, and acidosis and ketosis occur as a result of the metabolism of fat for energy, resulting in the creation of ketones as by-products. If untreated, the patient in ketosis eventually becomes comatose and dies.

INSULIN THERAPY

The dose of insulin required to treat this condition varies from individual to individual. It is determined by four factors: (1) the weight of the patient, (2) the metabolic rate, (3) physical activity, and (4) any residual function of the pancreas. It is obviously very important to be accurate in the dosage of insulin because an overdose can lead to insulin shock, and too small a dose can result in diabetic coma (Table 27–2). For mild cases, diet therapy alone may be sufficient, along with regulated exercises to maintain the blood sugar level. In more severe cases the oral hypoglycemics or insulin must be given.

The insulin that is used for therapy is structurally the same as human insulin, but it is not extracted from humans. It is prepared biosynthetically using recombinant DNA technology and special laboratory strains of microorganisms, usually *Escherichia coli.* Insulin from pork is still available, but rarely used. A comparison of the different types of insulin is seen in Table 27–3.

New technology continues to change the way diabetes is treated. The transplantation of new islet cells from human organ donors has achieved limited but encouraging success thus far. It appears to offer promise for the future.

Insulin requirements vary based on individual needs. Many diabetic patients are treated successfully on 40 to 60 units of insulin per day. In certain cases, however, insulin resistance occurs and very high doses are requi-red, in some cases up to 100 units/day. This resistance may be due to cirrhosis of the liver, hemochromatosis, allergy, or infection. In many cases, however, the cause of the insulin resistance is unknown. The U-500 dosage form is used for those with

Table 27-2 | *Symptoms of Hyperglycemic and Hypoglycemic Reactions*

DIABETIC COMA	REGULAR INSULIN REACTION	PROTAMINE ZINC OR NPH INSULIN REACTION
ONSET		
Slow (days) in adults	Sudden, rapid (minutes)	Insidious, slow (hours)
Fairly rapid in children	Reaction occurs in daytime	Reaction occurs in evening
SYMPTOMS		
Weakness, mental dullness	Trembling, mental confusion, weakness, drowsiness, nervousness	Weakness, drowsiness, nervousness, trembling, irritability
Frequently	**Frequently**	**Occasionally**
Nausea, vomiting	*No* nausea	Nausea, vomiting
No appetite	Hunger	**Frequently**
Thirst	*No* abdominal pain	Headache
Hot, dry skin	Cold, clammy skin	Hunger
Abdominal pain	Double vision	*No* abdominal pain
Dim vision	Normal or shallow breathing	Cold, clammy skin
Deep, labored breathing	Loss of consciousness	Double vision
Air hunger		Normal or shallow breathing
Loss of consciousness		Loss of consciousness
Fruity odor on breath		
Treatment		
Check urine—high sugar	Check urine—will contain sugar	Check urine—most likely will be sugar-free
Call doctor, who will prescribe regular insulin	Keep awake: give sugar or orange juice	Give sugar or orange juice for fast effect, and milk, crackers, or bread for prolonged effect
	Call doctor	Call doctor

Table 27-3 | *A Comparison of the Types of Insulin*

INSULIN TYPE	ONSET (HR)	PEAK (HR)	DURATION (HR)
RAPID-ACTING			
regular insulin (Humulin R)	½–1	2–3	4–8
insulin lispro	½–1	2–3	4–8
INTERMEDIATE-ACTING			
isophane insulin (Humulin N)	1½	4–12	Up to 24
lente insulin zinc (Humulin L)	2½	7–15	Up to 24
LONG-ACTING			
ultralente insulin (Humulin U)	4–8	12–18	Up to 28
insulin glargine (Lantus)	4	Steady	24

high insulin requirements. Most patients will use the U-100 strength, which means 100 units/mL.

Angiotensin-converting enzyme inhibitors (ACE inhibitors), when added to the diabetic regimen, have been shown to reduce the cardiovascular complications of diabetes. The risk of myocardial infarction and strokes as well as renal pathology seems to be reduced significantly in completed studies. ACE inhibitors are discussed more fully in Chapter 21.

Individual Insulin Products

human insulin, USP, BP. This biosynthetic insulin can be prepared in various forms to lower blood sugar rapidly or over a prolonged time. Dosages vary widely based on individual needs.

The family of human insulins is structurally identical to the insulin produced by the human. It is synthesized by a special non–disease-producing strain of *E. coli* that has been genetically altered by the addition of the gene for human insulin production.

human insulin injection, regular (Humulin R, Novolin R). This product consists of zinc-insulin crystals that are dissolved in a clear fluid. Nothing has been added to change the speed or duration of its activity. It takes effect rapidly and generally lasts 4 to 6 hours. It is given by subcutaneous (subQ) injection. It may not be used IM, but may be given IV.

Regular insulin is the only insulin form that may be given IV. The effect of regular insulin, regardless of the mode of administration, lasts only a few hours.

The Novolin R PenFill and Humulin R cartridges contain 100 units of regular insulin and are easily carried for self-administration of regular insulin.

human insulin injection, isophane (Humulin N, Novolin N). Also known as isophane insulin, or NPH, this is an intermediate-acting insulin containing a suspension of zinc-insulin crystals and protamine sulfate. The onset of action is in 1 1/2 hours, peak activity is expected from 4 to 12 hours, and the duration of action will be up to 24 hours. It is given subQ only; it may not be given IM or IV. The Novolin N PenFill and Humulin N Pen contain 100 units of isophane insulin for self-administration.

lente human insulin zinc injection (Humulin L, Novolin L). This intermediate-acting product is a mixture of crystalline and amorphous insulin in a ratio of 7:3. Onset of action is within 2 1/2 hours, peak hours are from 7 to 15 hours, and duration of action is up to 24 hours. It is given subQ only, not IM or IV.

ultralente human insulin injection (Humulin U). This long-acting insulin is a crystalline suspension of human insulin with zinc that provides a slower onset of action and a longer duration of activity. Onset of activity may be expected in 4 to 8 hours, with peak activity from 12 to 18 hours and duration of action up to 28 hours. It is only given subQ, not IM or IV.

Insulin Analog

insulin lispro (Humalog). This analog of human insulin has undergone a slight change from the human insulin molecule. It has a slightly more rapid onset of action when given subQ or IV, but for all practical purposes it is interchangeable with regular insulin. There is also a Humalog Pen for self-injection that contains 100 units of insulin.

Combination Insulin Products

Humulin 50/50—a combination of 50% regular and 50% isophane insulin

Humulin 70/30 and Novolin 70/30—combinations of 70% isophane and 30% regular insulin

Insulin Pump Therapy

Insulin pump therapy, or continuous subcutaneous insulin infusion, is designed to simulate normal pancreatic beta-cell function and deliver both basal and bolus insulin doses in patients with type 1 diabetes.

The use of insulin pumps for diabetics was first reported in the late 1970s, and demonstrated the possibility of achiev-ing strict glucose control in a select group of individuals. Since then pumps have become dramatically smaller, safer, and easier to use. Current models have electronic memory, multiple basal rates, several bolus options, and a remote control. They are worn on the belt, and are now about the size of a pager, as compared to the large backpack required with the earliest models.

Several factors are key to successful treatment with insulin pumps. The most important is the frequency of blood glucose monitoring. Monitoring blood glucose three or more times a day gives better control. Other important factors in the success of the pump include the logbook recording of insulin doses and blood glucose results, counting carbohydrates, and the use of the long-acting insulin lispro with regular insulin. These pumps are being used for pediatric patients with great success in controlled studies.

Some pumps are waterproof and immersible to a depth of 8 feet, allowing patients to swim while wearing the pump. It can be disconnected during exercise if desired.

The most serious adverse effect of intensive insulin therapy is severe hypoglycemia. Patients who have had type 1 diabetes for more than 5 years often lose their counterregulatory mechanism for identifying and reversing hypoglycemia. They commonly develop a condition known as hypoglycemic unawareness, and so no longer recognize the symptoms of low blood glucose levels, such as fatigue, sweating, dizziness, palpitations, and impaired cognition.

One strategy for preventing hypoglycemia is to set a higher target blood glucose level, using a lower basal insulin delivery rate and eliminating the wide glycemic swings.

Available insulin pumps are the Medronic MiniMed, the Disetronic, and the Animus. Deltec pumps will be available shortly.

ORAL HYPOGLYCEMIC AGENTS

More recent developments in diabetes research have produced oral hypoglycemic agents. These are not insulin derivatives but agents that lower the glucose level in the blood by a variety of actions.

chlorpropamide, USP, BP (Diabinese). Although a potent oral hypoglycemic agent, this is not a routine insulin substitute. It acts on the pancreatic cells to cause them to release residual insulin. Not all patients with diabetes are suitable candidates for chlorpropamide therapy. It is essential that the patients be carefully selected by the physician because the drug would be of little value if the pancreatic cells contained little or no residual insulin to release. This drug should not be used alone in the juvenile type of diabetes (type 1) or when the disease is complicated by acidosis, coma, infection, surgical procedures, or severe trauma. In these cases insulin is indispensable. Any physician using chlorpropamide should insist that the patient report at least once weekly for the first month of therapy because the initial test period should be carefully controlled. The main indication for the use of this agent is uncomplicated diabetes of the stable, mild, or moderately severe maturity-onset or adult type

(type 2). It may, however, be used in other types of the disease to decrease insulin requirements.

Dosage:

Adults: (Oral) 100 mg/day.

tolbutamide, USP, BP (Orinase). Because of suspected cardiovascular difficulties with tolbutamide dosage, its recommended use has been restricted to those cases in which diet and insulin are ineffective. Its effect is similar to that of chlorpropamide.

Dosage:

Adults: (Oral) 500 mg to 1 gm/day.

glipizide (Glucotrol). Like the other sulfonylurea agents, glipizide lowers blood glucose levels in diabetic and nondiabetic patients. On a weight basis, it is the most potent drug in this class. It is used as an adjunct to dietary control in the management of non–insulin-dependent (type 2) diabetes.

Dosage:

Adults only: (Oral) 2.5 to 40 mg daily in divided doses.

glyburide (Diabeta, Micronase, Glynase). In addition to lowering blood sugar, this agent produces a mild diuresis. It is used along with dietary management to control non–insulin-dependent diabetes.

Dosage:

Adults only: (Oral) 1.25 to 20 mg daily in divided doses.

acarbose (Precose). This agent inhibits enzymes known as the alpha-glucosidase enzymes that break down complex carbohydrates into glucose and other monosaccharides. In the diabetic patient, inhibition of these enzymes results in delayed carbohydrate breakdown, delayed glucose absorption, and a resultant reduction in postprandial hyperglycemia. It may be used singly or in combination with other agents for the management of type 2 diabetes.

Dosage:

Adults: (Oral) 25 mg with the first bite of each meal three times daily.

metformin hydrochloride (Glucophage). Metformin is ineffective in the absence of some endogenous insulin. It is believed to improve sensitivity to insulin at the receptor sites. It may be used alone or with another agent.

Dosage:

Adults: (Oral) 500 to 850 mg/day.

Other Oral Hypoglycemics

All dosages are adult (only) and oral.

glimepiride (Amaryl), 1 to 4 mg once daily
pioglitazone (Actos), 15 to 30 mg/day
repaglinide (Prandin), 0.5 to 16 mg three times daily, before meals
miglitol (Glyset), 25 to 300 mg three times daily, before meals

rosiglitazone maleate (Avandia), 4 to 12 mg/day
nateglinide (Starlix), 60 to 120 mg three times daily, before meals

Combination Oral Hypoglycemics

metformin plus glyburide (Glucovance). This combination comes in two strengths, 1.25/250 and 2.5/500, indicating the strength in milligrams of metformin and glyburide, respectively.

Dosage:

Taken before meals; dosage is individualized, not to exceed a daily dose of 20 mg glyburide/2000 mg metformin.

rosiglitazone plus metformin (Avandamet). This combination is available in three strengths, 1/500, 2/500, and 4/500, indicating the strength in milligrams of rosiglitazone and metformin, respectively.

Dosage:

Usual maximum dose is 8 mg rosiglitazone/200 mg metformin.

glipizide plus metformin (Metaglip). This combination is available in three strengths, 2.5/250, 2.5/500, and 5/500, indicating the strength in milligrams of glipizide and metformin, respectively.

Dosage:

Usual maximum dose is 20 mg glipizide and 2000 mg metformin daily.

GONADS

The gonads (sex glands) of the female are the ovaries and those of the male are the testes. These gonads, under the stimulation of the gonadotropic hormones from the anterior pituitary gland, release the sex hormones. The same gonadotropic hormones are produced in both the male and the female, but they naturally act on different organs, and the sex hormones released by the respective glands are different. The gonadotropic hormones from the anterior pituitary are the **follicle-stimulating hormone (FSH)** and the **luteinizing hormone (LH)**.

FEMALE HORMONES

Figure 27–2 is a cross section of the female reproductive organs. At maturity, FSH stimulates the maturation of the graafian follicles in the ovaries. These follicles are developed from the germinal epithelial cells that cover the surface of the ovary. Small groups of cells separate from the columns and become arranged with a large cell in the center and others in a single layer around it. These primary graafian follicles are found in great numbers in fetal ovaries and in the ovaries of children. The central, somewhat large, cell is called a primitive ovum. Under the influence of FSH, the cells around the ovum produce the female hormone estradiol, which is responsible for (1) the changes in the acces-

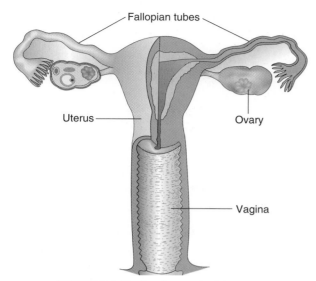

FIGURE 27-2 The female reproductive organs.

sory organs of reproduction during the first part of the menstrual cycle, and (2) the development of the secondary sex characteristics.

The removal of the ovaries of a young female animal prevents it from becoming sexually mature. The accessory organs fail to develop, menstruation does not occur, secondary sex characteristics do not appear, and the sex instinct is never manifested. Injection of the female sex hormone into such an animal corrects all the effects of ovariectomy.

As the follicle matures or ripens, it becomes distended by the accumulation of fluid and moves outward to the surface of the ovary. It projects from the surface of the ovary as a small cystlike swelling that eventually bursts and discharges the ovum. In women this process is known as ovulation and occurs about every 28 days (Figure 27–3).

The cavity of the ruptured follicle becomes filled with a clot of blood that is soon replaced by a mass of cells filled with a yellow, fatlike material called lutein. The structure is now called the corpus luteum, and under the developmental

stimulation of LH, the corpus luteum produces **progesterone,** a hormone that prepares the uterus for the reception of the ovum.

Progesterone is responsible for (1) the uterine changes characteristic of the first half of the menstrual cycle (e.g., thickening of the uterine wall, increased supply of blood vessels); (2) the development of the placenta (the organ that enables the embryo to receive nourishment from the mother during pregnancy; after the birth of a child, the placenta is expelled from the uterus as the "afterbirth"); (3) the maturation of the mammary glands during pregnancy; (4) the multiplication of the uterine muscle fibers; and (5) the inhibition of uterine contraction. In short, progesterone induces favorable conditions for the growth and development of the fetus.

If fertilization occurs, the corpus luteum continues to increase in size until the later months of pregnancy, and its hormone continues to exert an influence on the growth and functional integrity of the placenta and uterus.

As the conclusion of pregnancy approaches, the corpus luteum disintegrates, the uterus contracts because the inhibiting influence of progesterone is no longer present, and parturition (birth) occurs.

Progesterone may be given parenterally in cases of threatened abortion. If the corpus luteum disintegrates early or if progesterone is not produced naturally, full-term pregnancy can be brought about by administration of the deficient hormone.

If fertilization does not occur, the corpus luteum disintegrates, and the unfertilized ovum as well as the thickened uterine lining passes off in the menstrual flow. Figure 27–4 is a diagrammatic illustration of the menstrual cycle, showing the fluctuations in hormone concentrations in the blood, the growth of the follicle and corpus luteum, and the changes in the uterine lining during the menstrual cycle.

Estradiol is the naturally occurring female hormone in humans and other mammals. The term **estrogen** is a generic term referring to natural and synthetic agents that exert the biologic effect of estradiol.

If fertilization occurs, the placenta produces hormones that are similar to the gonadotropins produced by the

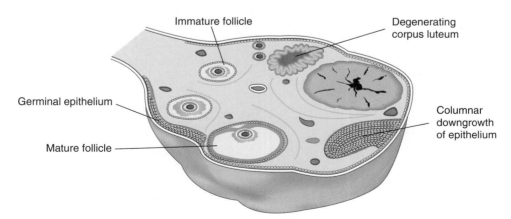

FIGURE 27-3 Ovulation.

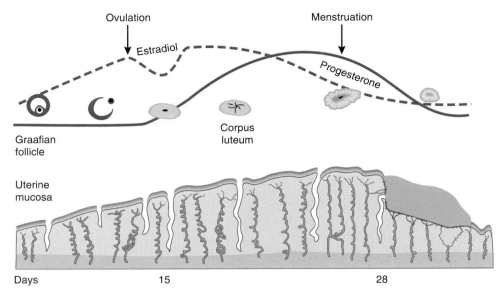

FIGURE 27-4 The menstrual cycle.

anterior pituitary gland. These hormones are called the anterior pituitary–like hormones or the chorionic gonadotropins, named after the chorion, which is the part of the placenta that develops around the fetus. The presence of these hormones in the urine is the basis for the pregnancy test.

It is necessary to provide female sex hormone therapy in cases in which a known deficiency of this hormone is present, because therapy brings about a normal physiologic state. Estrogen is used to treat conditions such as sexual infantilism and in senile vaginitis in perimenopausal women to provide a smooth transition during perimenopause.

Contrary to popular opinion, 85% of women have almost no symptoms at perimenopause. Only one third of the remaining 15% have symptoms that are severe enough to warrant treatment. Although formerly hormones were used during this transition phase only, now longer term hormone therapy appears to have benefit in preventing osteoporosis and other tissue changes in postmenopausal women and so is often routinely prescribed both during perimenopause and after the menopause. An increased risk of uterine cancer has been observed after continued hormone use, however.

It has also been found that estrogens in high concentration in the blood tend to inhibit the female organs; thus estrogenic preparations may be given postpartum to inhibit lactation if the mother does not choose to nurse the infant. Commercial preparations used to suppress lactation include the following.

estradiol suspension, USP, BP
  Dosage:
    Adults: (IM) 1.66 mg daily until symptoms are controlled.

estrone, USP, BP (Theelin)
  Dosage:
    Adults: (IM) 4.5 mg every 4 hours for five doses.

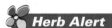
Herb Alert

Black Cohosh

Black cohosh is an herbal remedy used to treat the hot flashes of menopause, premenstrual tension, and dysmenorrhea (painful menstruation). Black cohosh must not be used during pregnancy because it is associated with an increased risk of spontaneous abortion (miscarriage). Black cohosh enhances the effects of antihypertensives and diuretics and the antiplatelet action of warfarin and the nonsteroidal antiinflammatory drugs. See Chapter 35 for more information on black cohosh.

Hormone Replacement Therapy
Estrogen replacement therapy (ERT) has been used for the treatment of menopausal symptoms, urogenital dryness, and the prevention and treatment of osteoporosis. Recent studies have shown some increase in breast cancer and cardiovascular complications with the use of replacement therapy. Studies are still ongoing, however.

estrogens, conjugated, USP, BP (Premarin)
  Dosage:
    Adults: (Oral) 0.625 to 2.5 mg daily. (IV) 25 mg daily. (Vaginal) As cream once daily.

esterified estrogens tablets, USP (Estratab)
  Dosage:
    Adults: (Oral) 0.3 to 0.625 mg daily.

Estrogen Agonist-Antagonists

raloxifene hydrochloride (Evista). Raloxifene is an estrogen agonist-antagonist. It is used as an alternative to cyclic estrogen/progestogen treatment in postmenopausal women. It is believed that this agent has a lower incidence of breast cancer as a side effect than the cyclic estrogen replacement.

Dosage:
Adults: (Oral) 60 mg/day.

Oral Contraceptives

Oral contraceptives are agents that prevent pregnancy by virtue of their estrogen content. Estrogens act to prevent ovulation by suppressing the release of FSH from the anterior pituitary. The estrogens are administered in combination with progesterone to prevent the side effects of estrogen administration (i.e., breakthrough bleeding and prolonged menses).

Side effects of oral contraceptives include breast changes, loss of scalp hair, dermatoses, headache, nervousness, thromboembolic disorders, and emotional instability. Oral contraceptives accelerate the growth of preexisting uterine fibroids and cervical polyps and will accelerate the growth of preexisting breast and uterine carcinomas. They are contraindicated in patients with a history of breast or genital cancer or thrombophlebitis, myocardial infarction or coronary artery disease, or preexisting liver, kidney, or heart dysfunction. They should be used with extreme caution in patients with epilepsy. An important side effect to remember when oral contraceptives are used is that they become LESS effective in preventing ovulation when the patient is also taking antibiotics.

levonorgestrel plus ethinyl estradiol (Triphasil). This oral contraceptive consists of three different drug combinations to be taken at appropriate times during the month. It more nearly replicates the natural hormone variations.

Phase 1 (6 tablets): Each tablet contains 0.05 mg levonorgestrel and 30 mcg ethinyl estradiol.

Phase 2 (5 tablets): Each tablet contains 0.075 mg levonorgestrel and 40 mcg ethinyl estradiol.

Phase 3 (10 tablets): Each tablet contains 0.125 mg levonorgestrel and 30 mcg ethinyl estradiol.

levonorgestrel plus ethinyl estradiol (Seasonale). This is an extended-cycle oral contraceptive consisting of 84 active tablets and 7 inert tablets per cycle. It is based on a 91-day regimen that reduces the number of menstrual periods from 12 to 13 per year to 4 per year. Because there are fewer menstrual cycles with this product, pregnancy should be ruled out before it is started. The side effects are those of the general oral contraceptives. Active ingredients are 0.15 mg levonorgestrel and 30 mcg ethinyl estradiol per tablet.

For other oral contraceptives, see Table 27–4.

Injectable and Transdermal Contraceptives

medroxyprogesterone acetate, USP, BP (Depo-Provera). Medroxyprogesterone is administered intramuscularly every 3 months for contraception. The level of this progesterone-like hormone is sufficient to prevent ovulation.

Menses may cease entirely or become irregular with the administration of this agent.

Statistically, it is 99% effective in preventing pregnancies and is useful for women who do not wish to take oral contraceptives for any reason.

Dosage:
(IM) 150 mg every 3 months.

norelgestromin plus ethinyl estradiol (Ortho Evra). This contraceptive transdermal patch is placed on weekly for 3 weeks, then left off for a week.

Table 27-4 | *Oral Contraceptives*

BRAND NAME	COMPONENT DRUGS	DOSE		
Enovid	norethynodrel	5 mg		
	mestranol	0.075 mg		
Enovid-E	norethynodrel	2.5 mg		
	mestranol	0.1 mg		
Ortho Novum (three strengths)	norethindrone	2 mg	1/50	1/80
	mestranol	2 mg	1 mg	1 mg
	ethynodiol diacetate	0.1 mg	0.05 mg	0.08 mg
Ovulen	mestranol	1 mg		
	ethinyl estradiol	0.1 mg		
Demulen	ethynodiol diacetate	50 mcg		
	ethinyl estradiol	1 mg		
Norlestrin (two strengths)	norethindrone acetate	50 mcg	*or*	50 mcg
	ethinyl estradiol	1 mg		2.5 mg
Ovral	norgestrel	50 mcg		
	ethinyl estradiol	500 mcg		
Lo/Ovral	norgestrel	0.03 mg		
		0.3 mg		

Each patch contains 6 mg norelgestromin and 0.75 mg ethinyl estradiol. It releases 150 mcg of norelgestromin and 20 mcg of ethinyl estradiol into the bloodstream per 24 hours.

Although there is an obvious advantage to not having to remember an oral contraceptive daily, the transdermal patch has its disadvantages also. About 2% to 6% of the patches reportedly completely detached. They are less satisfactory in warm, humid climates.

Emergency Contraception

Immediate use of an emergency contraceptive agent will reduce the woman's risk of pregnancy to 1% to 2%. Various methods are used. Because these agents are available by prescription only and not yet available over the counter, they would need to be prescribed in advance of need.

High Doses of a Combination Oral Contraceptive. The first dose should be taken within 72 hours of unprotected intercourse.

ethinyl estradiol plus levonorgestrel (Preven). Each tablet contains 100 mcg of ethinyl estradiol and 0.5 mg of levonorgestrel.

> **Dosage:**
> 2 tablets within 72 hours of unprotected intercourse and 2 tablets 12 hours later.

levonorgestrel plus ethinyl estradiol (Ovral). Two of the standard Ovral contraceptive tablets will equal the dose of Preven.

> **Dosage:**
> 2 tablets within 72 hours of unprotected intercourse and 2 tablets 12 hours later.

Progestin-Only Regimen.
levonorgestrel (Plan B). Single tablets containing 0.75 mg levonorgestrel.

> **Dosage:**
> 2 tablets once, or 1 tablet within 72 hours of unprotected intercourse and 1 tablet 12 hours later.

Agents to Promote Ovulation

Agents to promote ovulation are occasionally used as a last resort in an attempt to promote pregnancy in a woman previously unable to conceive. Only one agent is approved for use in the United States at this time.

clomiphene citrate, USP, BP (Clomid). Clomiphene is a synthetic, nonsteroidal compound that may be administered orally to promote ovulation in women who have been anovulatory. It is believed to act by promoting the release of pituitary gonadotropins, which in turn promote ovulation. Multiple conceptions (including triplets, quadruplets, quintuplets, and sextuplets) increase 10-fold when this drug is used. Infant mortality is very high in the multiple conceptions,

often because of premature delivery. This drug is contraindicated in patients with a history of liver disease and those with abnormal uterine bleeding. Side effects include blurred vision, hot flashes, abdominal discomfort, nausea, vomiting, breast engorgement, headache, dizziness, and skin reactions.

> **Dosage:**
> Adults: (Oral) 50 mg daily for 5 days, then individualize.

Oxytocic Agents

Although many drugs may be used during the course of pregnancy and delivery and immediately postpartum, the drugs specifically related to uterine function are the **oxytocic agents**, which are uterine stimulants. Oxytocic drugs are so named because they resemble the action of oxytocin, a hormone secreted from the posterior pituitary gland.

oxytocin injection, USP, BP (Pitocin, Syntocinon). Oxytocin stimulates the uterine muscles and produces rhythmical contractions. Sensitivity to this drug increases as the pregnancy progresses. It is contraindicated in the first stage of labor because, if used when the cervix is undilated and rigid, severe laceration and trauma are likely.

Overdose of oxytocin may produce uterine tetany. The drug must be given with great caution to patients with a cardiovascular disease or a previous cesarean section, or when there is a malpresentation of the fetus or threatened rupture of the uterus for any reason.

This drug is administered in small doses as an intravenous drip to induce labor, but this procedure must be carried out under close medical supervision. An infusion pump is necessary for precise control of this medication when given intravenously.

> **Dosage:**
> Adults: (IM) 3 to 10 units. (IV) 10 units diluted in 1000 mL using infusion pump.

ergonovine maleate, USP, BP (Ergotrate). The dangerous similarity in names between this ergot alkaloid and ergotamine, a drug used to treat migraine headaches, is discussed in Chapter 25.

Like oxytocin, this drug has a constricting effect on uterine muscles, although it appears to have a greater selective action on the uterus, causing less peripheral vasoconstriction, and it acts more quickly than oxytocin. It is used for the treatment of postpartum and postabortion hemorrhage.

Chronic use of this drug may produce ergotism, a prolonged constriction of the blood vessels in other parts of the body that may lead to gangrene and loss of the affected parts of the body.

> **Dosage:**
> Adults: (IM, IV, Oral) 0.2 mg every 2 to 4 hours for a total of five doses.

methylergonovine maleate, USP, BP (Methergine). This synthetic drug may be administered orally or parenterally to cause constriction of the uterus. Its action is similar to that of ergonovine, but it is more potent and has a more prolonged duration of action. In addition, it has less tendency to cause an elevation in blood pressure; thus it is preferred for patients with threatened eclampsia.

Dosage:

Adults: (IM, IV, Oral) 0.2 mg every 2 to 4 hours for a total of five doses..

sodium chloride 20% injection. Injected directly into the amniotic fluid, this concentrated sodium chloride solution is useful in the induction of second trimester abortions. When injection is performed correctly, there is little sodium chloride is absorbed by the mother. However, it is recommended that at least 2 L of water be given to the mother before the abortion is induced.

Side effects include a sensation of heat, thirst, and mental confusion, and there have been reported maternal deaths as a result of hypernatremia.

Dosage:

Adults: (IV) 200 to 250 mL by transabdominal intraamniotic catheter.

urea 40% to 50% injection (carbamide). Hypertonic urea, especially in conjunction with intravenous oxytocin, induces fetal death and abortion. When the procedure is performed correctly, there is little risk. However, the patient should take fluids during the procedure to facilitate urea excretion. Monitoring for signs of fluid and electrolyte imbalance should be performed throughout the procedure.

Dosage:

Adults: (IV) 200 to 250 mL by transabdominal intraamniotic catheter.

dinoprostone (Prostin E$_2$). This naturally occurring prostaglandin is prepared synthetically for commercial use. It is used intravaginally to induce abortion during the second trimester of pregnancy. Abortion generally occurs within 12 to 14 hours following intravaginal administration.

Dosage:

Adult: (Intravaginal) 20 mg every 3 to 5 hours until abortion occurs.

dinoprostone cervical gel (Prepidil). This gel is administered endocervically. Its purpose it to stimulate the myometrium of the gravid uterus to contract. It also has a softening or effacement effect on the cervix, enhancing dilation. It is used in pregnant women at or near term with a medical or obstetrical need for labor induction.

Dosage:

0.5 mg endocervically via catheter. May be repeated once in 6 hours.

mifepristone (RU-486, Mifeprex). This oral abortifacient was used for some time in Europe before being approved in the United States. It may be taken orally anytime before the eighth week of pregnancy. When the tablets are absorbed, they block receptors of progesterone, a hormone needed to maintain pregnancy.

Dosage:

Adults: (Oral) 3 tablets (200 mg each) taken on day 1, and 2 tablets of misoprostol (200 mcg each) taken on day 3. Posttreatment examination is necessary on day 14.

MALE HORMONES

In the human male, as already stated, the same two gonadotropic hormones are produced by the anterior pituitary as are found in the female. In the male, however, FSH causes production of spermatozoa, whereas LH causes development of the interstitial cells that produce **testosterone,** the male hormone.

Testosterone is responsible for normal development of the male reproductive tract and maintains the secondary sex characteristics. It plays a role in the development of the penis, the seminal vesicles, and the prostate gland and in the descent of the testes from the abdominal cavity.

The accessory sexual characteristics affected by testosterone are the depth of the voice, the distribution of facial and body hair, and the development of the masculine skeletal muscles. Muscular strength and endurance are increased immeasurably by the administration of the male hormone.

Testosterone confers a sense of "well-being" and restores mental equilibrium and energy. It can also increase the resistance of the central nervous system to fatigue. It may be used therapeutically in the following instances: (1) when a deficiency of the hormone is known, (2) in females to treat certain ovarian dysfunctions such as menorrhagia and dysmenorrhea, and (3) in females to treat breast engorgement and suppress lactation. (Some commercial preparations contain a combination of estrogen and androgen for this purpose.)

testosterone gel (Androgel) This clear gel provides a continuous transdermal delivery of testosterone after a single application to clean, dry skin. It is used for testosterone replacement therapy in males.

Dosage:

5 gm gel delivering 5 mg testosterone applied to clean, dry skin once daily.

testosterone transdermal system (Androderm). This patch is applied once every 24 hours and delivers testosterone for the 24-hour period. It is used as replacement therapy in males.

Dosage:

Transdermal patch, 2.5 or 5 mg, applied daily.

Agents that treat erectile dysfunction are covered in Chapter 28 (Diuretics and Other Drugs That Affect the Urinary System).

CLINICAL IMPLICATIONS

1. When preparing the vial of insulin before giving an injection, rotate the bottle between the palms. Vigorous shaking produces bubbles, which interfere with accurate dosage.
2. Carefully measure the exact dose of insulin to be administered using a calibrated insulin syringe or a tuberculin syringe.
3. The sites of injection are to be rotated. Chart the site of injection for effective rotation.
4. Finger stick blood samples for blood sugar levels should be used to determine the patient's status and response to insulin.
5. It is necessary for a diabetic to follow his or her diet closely. The nurse should be familiar with dietary requirements and be available to answer any questions that the patient may have regarding the diet.
6. Vigorous exercise alters the diabetic's requirements for insulin and dietary requirements.
7. The patient who is vomiting or who has missed a meal should have the insulin dosage reduced to prevent insulin shock.
8. Infection, surgery, and physical and emotional stresses alter the requirements for insulin.
9. The diabetic patient should become familiar with the MedicAlert tags and wear them at all times.
10. Thyroid tablets deteriorate with excessive exposure to light and moisture. The patient should be instructed in their proper storage.
11. Excessive thyroid medication produces symptoms of hyperthyroidism, including hypertension, tachycardia, chest pain, and heat intolerance.
12. The symptoms of Cushing's syndrome are similar to the side effects experienced when adrenocorticoid drugs are administered to a patient.
13. Patients should be instructed about taking oral contraceptives daily as prescribed. Pregnancy can result if pills are missed during the month. If a period does not occur at the end of the cycle, the patient should be instructed not to resume the oral contraceptive and to consult her physician.
14. Symptoms of breakthrough bleeding midcycle are seen with some of the oral contraceptives. This can often be corrected by increasing the strength of the contraceptive.

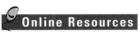

Online Resources

For updated drug information and Web activities, go to http://evolve.elsevier.com/Asperheim.

CRITICAL THINKING QUESTIONS

1. The patient is brought to the office for a checkup by her daughter. She is afraid of doctors and has not seen one since her last child was born 25 years ago. She is noted to speak slowly, and has dry hair that is thinning in the central scalp, and skin that has a puffy appearance. What may be her problem?

2. The patient has received dexamethasone for his rheumatoid arthritis for the last 6 months. He is noted to have a rounder face than previously and has gained 8 pounds, although he claims he has not changed his eating habits. His arthritis is improved, but he is afraid the doctor will stop the medication because of his "side effects." What would you tell him?

3. The pediatric patient was diagnosed as having diabetes mellitus 1 year ago. Since yesterday he has been vomiting and is unable to eat. This morning his mother gave him his regular insulin dose. Now, 3 hours later, the mother calls to say he is sweaty, trembling, and nervous. What is the most likely diagnosis? What should the mother do before she brings her son to the office?

   After the boy has recovered, the mother wants to know if his medication can be changed to the diabetic "pills" that she has heard about so he won't have all this trouble with insulin anymore. What is your answer?

4. The patient has been married 1 month and comes to the office with her husband, who states that she cries all the time, although they are "deliriously happy." She has been on oral contraceptives for 4 months now and takes no other medication. She also states she doesn't know why she acts this way and wants a mood elevator. What other steps might be taken?

5. The patient has had recurrent problems with varicose veins for 8 years. Her surgeon is now speaking about vein stripping in the near future. She wants to know if she can be placed on oral contraceptives because a pregnancy would be inconvenient now that surgery is a possibility. May she?

REVIEW QUESTIONS

1. The master gland of the body is the:
   a. anterior pituitary.
   b. posterior pituitary.
   c. adrenal cortex.
   d. adrenal medulla.

2. All of the following are symptoms of hypothyroidism except:
   a. enlarged thyroid gland.
   b. hypersensitivity to heat.
   c. slowing of mental functions.
   d. slowing of physical functions.

3. Insulin is secreted in the body by the:
   a. islets of Langerhans.
   b. adrenal medulla.
   c. sympathetic nervous system.
   d. anterior pituitary.

4. If not treated with insulin, a diabetic will have the inability to:
   a. metabolize sugar.
   b. metabolize fat.
   c. metabolize cholesterol.
   d. digest fiber.

5. A side effect of the oral contraceptives is:
   a. ovulation.
   b. thromboembolic disorders.
   c. increased fertility.
   d. hirsutism.

6. Which of the following is an estrogen agonist-antagonist?
   a. Estradiol
   b. Conjugated estrogens
   c. Raloxifene
   d. Ortho Evra

7. An agent that promotes ovulation is:
   a. conjugated estrogens.
   b. testosterone.
   c. clomiphene.
   d. medroxyprogesterone.

8. An agent that stimulates the uterine muscles and promotes rhythmical contractions of the uterus is:
   a. esterified estrogens.
   b. acarbose.
   c. OxyContin.
   d. oxytocin.

9. A hormone that is given via transdermal patch is:
   a. testosterone.
   b. conjugated estrogens.
   c. pancrelipase.
   d. oxytocin.

10. Which of the following may be used to treat diabetes?
    a. liothyronine
    b. medroxyprogesterone
    c. clomiphene
    d. glimepiride

Diuretics and Other Drugs That Affect the Urinary System

After completing this chapter, you should be able to do the following:

1. Understand the function of the kidney.
2. Understand the role of the kidney in selectively regulating output and its importance in drug excretion.
3. Explain the importance of antidiuretic hormone in regulating urine output.
4. Become familiar with the different classes of diuretics and how they are used.
5. Identify drugs used to treat urinary tract infections.
6. Identify drugs used to treat enuresis.
7. Become familiar with the action of drugs that treat prostate hypertrophy and erectile dysfunction.
8. Discuss nursing responsibilities in the administration of diuretics.

Key Terms

antihypertensive (ăn-tĭ-hī-pĕr-TĔN-sĭv) **drugs,** p. 170
diuresis (dī-ū-RĒ-sĭs), p. 168
enuresis (ĕn-ū-RĒ-sĭs), p. 172
incontinence (ĭn-KŎN-tĭ-nĕns), p. 172
steroid (STĬR-ōyd) **antagonists,** p. 170
thiazide diuretics, p. 168

The kidney is the principal organ of the body involved with water balance. If the output of water from the body exceeds the water intake, the body is said to be in a negative water balance. This imbalance leads to dehydration of the body. At the other extreme, a positive water balance occurs when the intake of water exceeds the output. Ordinarily, however, the body maintains a balance between the water ingested and the water excreted.

In addition to excretion via the kidney, water may also be lost through perspiration. Perspiration may occur by diffusion through the skin, termed *insensible perspiration* because it is not perceived as happening. Or, perspiration may involve the sweat glands, producing "sensible perspiration" that is recognized as sweat. Sweat consists of a weak solution of sodium chloride and a few other substances. It is possible to lose 3000 mL of water through the skin in 24 hours when both sensible and insensible perspiration routes are active.

The kidney has the ability to regulate its output according to the amount of fluid ingested and the amounts lost by other routes from the body. Thus, in very warm weather when perspiration is greater, the output from the kidneys is considerably less than it is in cool weather.

The kidney consists of more than 1 million functional units, or nephrons (Figure 28–1). The nephron is composed of a tuft of capillaries, called a glomerulus, which is encapsulated in a cuplike structure known as Bowman's capsule. Water, salts, and waste products can filter through the thin walls of the capillaries into Bowman's capsule and through the series of collecting tubules to the pelvis of the kidney. The renal pelvis opens into the ureter, the ureter leads to the bladder, and excretion from the bladder is accomplished via the urethra.

A great deal more fluid is filtered into Bowman's capsule than is excreted in the urine, however. This is because much of the fluid is reabsorbed where the collecting tubule from Bowman's capsule circles back through another capillary bed on its way to the renal pelvis. It is estimated that, for every 125 mL of fluid filtered through the glomerulus, only 1 mL is eventually secreted.

Reabsorption of the filtered fluid is largely due to the influence of the antidiuretic hormone from the posterior pituitary gland. Diabetes insipidus is a disease in which this hormone is missing or present in inadequate amounts. This disease is characterized by diuresis (the formation and excretion of increased amounts of urine); in this case, copious amounts of urine are produced—sometimes 10 to 12 L a day. Diabetes insipidus is treated by the administration of posterior pituitary hormone.

DIURETICS

A diuretic is a drug that increases the flow of urine. If sodium and fluids are retained in excessive amounts, there is edema, particularly of the extremities. Fluid accumulation in the lungs results in pulmonary edema.

There are several classes of diuretics; all work in different areas of the urinary tract.

THIAZIDE (BENZOTHIADIAZINE) DIURETICS

Thiazide diuretics, although they act in part by inhibiting the enzyme carbonic anhydrase, also exert action directly

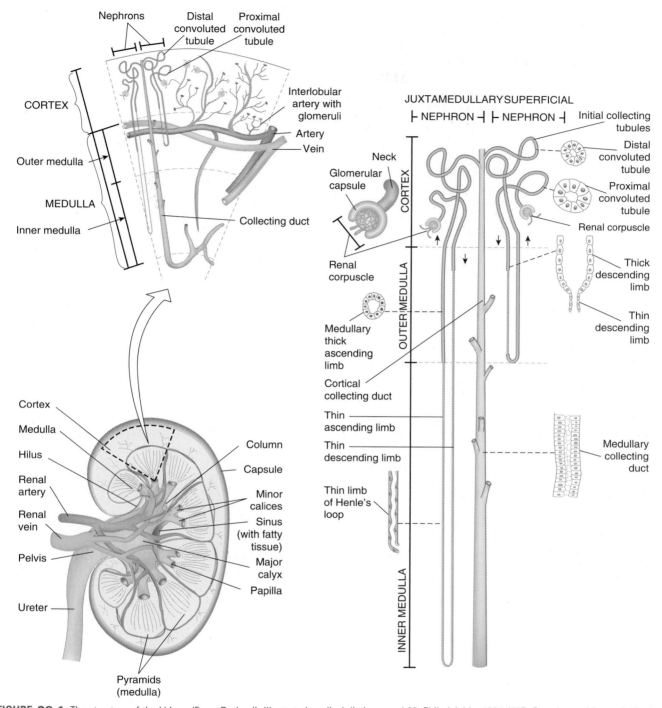

FIGURE 28-1 The structure of the kidney. (From *Dorland's illustrated medical dictionary*, ed 28, Philadelphia, 1994, W.B. Saunders, with permission.)

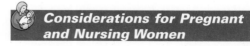

Considerations for Pregnant and Nursing Women

Thiazide Diuretics

Thiazide diuretics are generally contraindicated in pregnant women. These agents cross the placental barrier and appear in cord blood. Thrombocytopenia and jaundice are among the effects in the newborn that have been attributed to the use of thiazide diuretics during pregnancy.

on the collecting tubules of the kidney and promote the excretion of sodium, potassium, chloride, and bicarbonate along with the necessary excretion of water. Potassium depletion often is a problem when the thiazide diuretics are used over a prolonged period of time; thus a potassium supplement or foods high in potassium, such as oranges and bananas, are often added to the diet.

In addition to their activity as diuretics, the thiazides have an additional effect as antihypertensive drugs (that is, they lower high blood pressure). This action is separate from their effect on diuresis, but it is not completely understood as yet. When used by themselves, their action in lowering the blood pressure is mild; when combined with other drugs, however, they are a useful adjunct in the treatment of hypertensive patients because they greatly increase the activity of these drugs.

Side effects of these drugs include alterations in the body chemistry, such as hypokalemia, hypochloremic alkalosis, hypotension, tachycardia, aplastic anemia, jaundice, hyperuricemia, glycosuria, muscle cramps, and weakness. They should be used with caution in patients known to have gout or liver or kidney disorders. Potassium supplements are recommended when these agents are prescribed.

chlorothiazide, USP, BP (Diuril). Chlorothiazide was the first diuretic to be synthesized in the thiazide group. It is used as a diuretic in heart failure, during pregnancy, and in premenstrual fluid retention, or as an adjunct in the treatment of hypertension.

Dosage:
Adults: (Oral) 500 mg one to two times daily.
Children: (Oral) 10 mg/kg two times daily.

hydrochlorothiazide, USP, BP (HydroDIURIL). A small alteration in the chemical structure of chlorothiazide greatly increases the potency of this compound. Greatly decreased doses of this drug provide diuretic effects comparable to those of chlorothiazide.

Dosage:
Adults: (Oral) 25 to 100 mg one to two times daily.
Children: (Oral) 1 mg/kg twice daily.

polythiazide, USP, BP (Renese, Minizide). Polythiazide is said to conserve more serum potassium than other drugs while still promoting excretion of an effective amount of sodium. Its uses and diuretic effects are comparable to those of the other diuretics in this class.

Dosage:
Adults: (Oral) 1 to 4 mg daily.
Children: (Oral) 20 to 80 mcg/kg once daily.

STEROID ANTAGONISTS

The steroid antagonists are diuretics that act by inhibiting aldosterone, an adrenal hormone that promotes the retention of sodium and the excretion of potassium. The excretion of sodium and chloride caused by steroid antagonists is accompanied by an appropriate amount of water.

spironolactone, USP, BP (Aldactone). Spironolactone is useful in the treatment of edema associated with congestive heart failure, hepatic cirrhosis with ascites and nephritis, and edema of unknown origin. @dt:Side effects observed with the use of this drug include mild headache, confusion, dermatitis, drowsiness, ataxia, and mild abdominal pain.

Dosage:
Adults: (Oral) 50 to 400 mg daily.
Children: (Oral) 3.3 mg/kg daily in divided doses.

hydrochlorothiazide plus spironolactone (Aldactazide). Aldactazide is a combination of 25 mg hydrochlorothiazide and 25 mg spironolactone per tablet. The combined form of the two drugs is more effective as a diuretic than either of the two used singly, because the reabsorption of fluids and electrolytes in the kidney is blocked by two methods.

Dosage:
Adults: (Oral) 1 tablet four times daily (25 mg of each drug).
Children: (Oral) 1.65 to 3.3 mg/kg of each drug daily in divided doses.

MISCELLANEOUS DIURETICS

triamterene, USP, BP (Dyrenium). This drug is often combined with hydrochlorothiazide because the diuretic and hypotensive effects are increased by the combination. Nausea, vomiting, headache, and weakness occur occasionally with the use of this drug.

Dosage:
Adults: (Oral) 100 mg one to two times daily.
Children: (Oral) 4 mg/kg/day in two divided doses.

triamterene plus hydrochlorothiazide (Dyazide). Dyazide is commercial preparation containing a combination of 37.5 mg triamterene and 25 mg hydrochlorothiazide per capsule.

Dosage:
Adults: (Oral) 1 capsule daily.

furosemide, USP, BP (Lasix). Furosemide is a diuretic that has been shown to act throughout the collecting tubules of the nephron, particularly on the ascending limb of the loop of Henle, to prevent the reabsorption of, and hence cause the excretion of, sodium and chloride. Although usually administered orally, it may be administered intramuscularly or intravenously.

It may be used in congestive heart failure associated with liver or kidney disease. It is of particular value when other less potent diuretics have failed to decrease edema.

Side effects are electrolyte depletion, dizziness, weakness, jaundice, leg cramps, vomiting, and confusion.

Dosage:
Adults: (Oral) 20 to 80 mg once daily. (IM, IV) 20 mg to 1 gm daily.
Children: No standard dosage is established.

ethacrynic acid, USP, BP (Edecrin). Like furosemide, this agent works throughout the nephron tubules to prevent the reabsorption of sodium and water. The potency of the two drugs is approximately equal. Ethacrynic acid is available in oral form only.

Dosage:
Adults: (Oral) 50 to 400 mg daily.

Children: (Oral) Initially 25 mg, then stepwise increments until results are achieved.

metolazone (Zaroxolyn, Mykrox). This drug is structurally similar to the thiazide diuretics and generally has the same side effects. Hyperuricemia and gout, fluid depletion, nausea, and headaches have been described.

Dosage:
  Adults only: (Oral) 5 to 20 mg daily.

amiloride hydrochloride (Midamor). Structurally unrelated to the other drugs that are used as diuretics, this agent differs also in its action in that it is potassium sparing. It does not cause potassium depletion when used as a diuretic. Side effects include nausea, flatulence, and mild rash. Generally it is well tolerated.

Dosage:
  Adults: (Oral) 5 to 20 mg/day.
  Children: (Oral) 0.625 mg/kg/day.

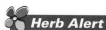

Herb Alert

Juniper

Juniper is used as a diuretic when administered orally. Juniper also has an antihypertensive effect and enhances the effects of lithium. However, prolonged oral administration may result in nephrotoxicity, and it should be avoided in patients with preexisting liver disease. See Chapter 35 for more information on juniper.

URINARY ANTISEPTICS

Bacterial infections of the urinary tract are the causative agents of various symptomatic conditions that may be described as cystitis, pyelitis, or pyelonephritis. These terms merely refer to the location of the infection or the source of the symptoms indicating an infection in the urinary tract.

Many patients who have had a single urinary tract infection have recurrences after asymptomatic periods. For this reason, they are often placed on long-term drug therapy.

Most of the sulfonamides, as well as antibiotics such as the tetracyclines, chloramphenicol, erythromycin, streptomycin, kanamycin, and cephalothin, may be used to treat these conditions. Because these drugs have previously been discussed in other chapters, this section is reserved for drugs used more exclusively as urinary antiseptics.

nitrofurantoin, USP, BP (Furadantin). This synthetic drug has a spectrum of activity that encompasses the majority of urinary tract infective agents. After oral administration, approximately 45% of the dose is excreted in the urine—imparting to it a brown color. The administration of the drug should be continued for at least 3 days after sterility of the urine has been achieved to minimize the possibility of recurrent infections. Nausea, vomiting, or sensitivity reactions may occur with administration of this drug. The gastrointestinal symptoms may be minimized if the dose is given with food or milk.

Dosage:
  Adults and children older than 12 years: (Oral) 50 to 100 mg four times daily.
  Children 6 to 12 years: (Oral) 500 mg four times daily.

methenamine mandelate, USP, BP (Mandelamine). This combination of methenamine and mandelic acid is a well-tolerated urinary antiseptic and is particularly useful for chronic, resistant, or recurrent infections. It is effective against almost all strains of microorganisms that are causative agents in urinary infections and may be effective even against strains resistant to antibiotics or sulfonamides. It may be given alone or in combination with other drugs. Sensitization in the form of allergic reactions rarely occurs with this drug, but it is contraindicated in patients with severe hepatitis or renal insufficiency.

Dosage:
  Adults: (Oral) 1 gm four times daily.
  Children older than 6 years: (Oral) 34 mg/kg four times daily.
  Children younger than 6 years: (Oral) 18 mg/kg four times daily.

Urised. Each tablet of this preparation contains:
  atropine sulfate 0.03 mg
  hyoscyamine 0.03 mg
  methenamine 40.8 mg
  methylene blue 5.4 mg
  phenyl salicylate 18.1 mg
  benzoic acid 4.5 mg

The action of the urinary antiseptics methenamine and methylene blue, along with the antispasmodic effects of atropine and hyoscyamine, makes this preparation relatively effective in treating mild urinary infections. Patients should be warned that the methylene blue in the tablet will turn the urine blue. Dryness of the mouth, dizziness, rapid pulse, and blurring of the vision occur occasionally. It is contraindicated in myasthenia gravis and glaucoma.

Dosage:
  Adults: (Oral) 2 tablets four times daily.
Children older than 6 years: Dosage reduced in proportion to body weight.

phenazopyridine hydrochloride, USP, BP (Pyridium). This drug acts promptly to produce an analgesic effect on the urinary tract mucosa. It usually acts within 30 minutes to relieve the symptoms of pain, burning, urgency, and frequency associated with urinary tract infections. This drug is compatible with any antibacterial or with other corrective therapy for infections of this nature. The patient should be informed that the urine will turn a reddish color.

Dosage:
Adults: (Oral) 200 mg three times daily.
Children: No standard dosage is established.

co-trimoxazole (trimethoprim-sulfamethoxazole; TMP/SMX) (Bactrim, Septra). The commercial preparations of Bactrim and Septra contain identical formulations, with tablets consisting of a combination of 80 mg trimethoprim and 400 mg sulfamethoxazole. Each company also produces a double-strength tablet labeled DS (Bactrim DS, Septra DS).

The combination of a sulfonamide with the synthetic antibacterial compound trimethoprim has been shown to be very effective against chronic urinary tract infections, primarily pyelonephritis, pyelitis, and cystitis. Its use should be reserved for chronic infections, however, because untoward effects do occur from this drug. The use of these agents in upper respiratory infections is discussed in Chapter 19, and their use for other indications is discussed in Chapter 16.

The patient should be warned to report sore throat, fever, pallor, purpura, or jaundice to the physician immediately because these may be early signs of blood dyscrasias that may occur with this drug. Adequate fluid intake should be maintained during therapy to prevent the formation of renal calculi. The drug should be used with caution in patients with impaired renal or liver function. It is contraindicated in pregnant women.

Dosage:
Adults: (Oral) 1 to 2 tablets every 12 hours for 10 to 14 days (or 1 tablet of the double-strength form every 12 hours).
Children: (Oral) 8 mg/kg trimethoprim and 40 mg/kg sulfamethoxazole daily in two divided doses.

DRUGS USED FOR THE TREATMENT OF ENURESIS

Enuresis is the involuntary discharge of urine and generally occurs at night; hence it is often referred to as "nighttime bedwetting." Enuresis is a fairly common problem in children. Without treatment, the percentage of bedwetters gradually decreases to the age of 21 years, but a small percentage are still wetting at that age.

It is well established that withholding fluids in the evening, many nightly awakenings by the parent, and other behavioral techniques may give temporary improvement, but 100% relapse occurs as soon as these interventions cease. Various alarms and early warnings of wetting have been devised, again without real improvement.

The problem seems to be a small or spastic bladder that is stimulated to empty automatically when a certain volume of urine is present, much as an infant's bladder will empty. Various drugs are in use for this problem.

imipramine hydrochloride (Tofranil). This agent, which acts as an antidepressant as well, may improve the symptoms of enuresis in some children. The mechanism of action in the improvement of enuresis is thought to be separate from its antidepressant effect.

Dosage:
Children older than 12 years: (Oral) 75 mg at bedtime.
Children 6 to 12 years: (Oral) 25 mg at bedtime.

oxybutynin chloride (Ditropan). This agent has a direct antispasmodic effect on the smooth muscle and relaxes bladder smooth muscle in patients with involuntary bladder symptoms. It may be used for day and night wetting. Side effects include drowsiness, decreased tearing, dry mouth, constipation, and palpitations.

Dosage:
Adults and children older than 12 years: (Oral) 5 mg three times daily.
Children 5 to 12 years: (Oral) 5 mg twice daily.

desmopressin acetate (DDAVP Nasal Spray). This is an antidiuretic agent that affects renal water conservation. It is an analog of vasopressin (antidiuretic hormone) that is used as a nasal spray. Side effects include headache, rise in blood pressure, nosebleed, and sore throat.

Dosage:
Children 6 years and older: 10 to 40 mcg by nasal spray pump at bedtime.

DRUGS USED FOR THE TREATMENT OF INCONTINENCE

The inability to control the discharge of excretions, either urine or feces, is referred to as incontinence. Urinary incontinence affects 10% to 35% of community-dwelling adults and 50% to 70% of the nursing home population. It is twice as common in women as in men. Certain age-related physiologic and anatomic factors increase the risk of incontinence, including:
- Nocturia, or excessive urination during the night
- Decline in bladder capacity
- Decrease in urethral closure pressure
- Increase in postvoiding residual volume
- Loss of elasticity or stiffening of the bladder tissue, such as produced after radiotherapy
- Benign prostatic hypertrophy
- In females, decreased pelvic muscle tone after childbirth

Although supportive treatment may help, incontinence is generally treated medically with the anticholinergic drugs.

oxybutynin chloride (Ditropan XL). This agent exerts a direct antispasmodic effect on smooth muscle, relaxing the bladder smooth muscle. Side effects include dry mouth, dry eyes, somnolence, and constipation.

Dosage:
> Adults: (Oral) 5 to 15 mg once daily.

tolterodine tartrate (Detrol, Detrol LA). By relaxing the smooth muscle of the bladder, this agent increases bladder capacity and decreases urge urinary incontinence. Side effects are the same as for oxybutynin.

Dosage:
> Adult: (Oral) 2 mg twice daily, or, for the long-acting form (Detrol LA), 2 to 4 mg once daily.

DRUGS USED FOR THE TREATMENT OF BENIGN PROSTATIC HYPERTROPHY

Benign prostatic hypertrophy (BPH), or hyperplasia (an increase in the number of cells), is an abnormal enlargement of the prostate gland that occurs in most men 55 years of age or older. It produces symptoms such as weakened urinary stream, difficulty in initiation of urination, urinary frequency, and urgency.

Surgery in the form of a transurethral resection of the prostate remains the treatment of choice, but if surgery is not an option, some cases respond to drug therapy as well. The potential coexistence of carcinoma of the prostate makes a careful differential diagnosis necessary.

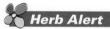
Herb Alert

Saw Palmetto

Saw palmetto has been used to suppress the symptoms of benign prostatic hypertrophy (BPH), including urinary hesitancy, nocturia, and urinary frequency. However, its use may mask coexisting prostate cancer, which should always be ruled out when symptoms of prostate obstruction are present. Saw palmetto reduces the effects of estrogens, androgens, adrenergic drugs, and oral contraceptives. Although it is used primarily by men, its use should be avoided by women during pregnancy and lactation. See Chapter 35 for more information on saw palmetto.

finasteride (Proscar). Finasteride is used to reduce prostate size and the associated symptoms of urinary obstruction. It is generally well tolerated. Side effects include impotence, decreased volume of ejaculate, abdominal pain, diarrhea, and flatulence.

Dosage:
> Adults only: (Oral) 5 mg once daily.

tamsulosin hydrochloride (Flomax). This agent is used to relieve mild to moderate obstructive manifestations of prostatic hypertrophy. Side effects include rash, urticaria, and angioedema of the tongue, lips, and face.

Dosage:
> Adults only: (Oral) 1 mg daily.

DRUGS USED FOR THE TREATMENT OF ERECTILE DYSFUNCTION

Erectile dysfunction remains a somewhat subjective diagnosis. It is defined as the persistent or repeated inability to maintain an erection sufficient for satisfactory sexual performance.

Prior to prescribing a drug for problems of this type, it is important to rule out other causes of erectile dysfunction such as hypertension and antihypertensive drugs, thyroid disease, cardiovascular disease, and psychological disorders.

sildenafil citrate (Viagra). Sildenafil is an oral agent that is effective in the temporary treatment of erectile dysfunction. It acts as a vasodilator and increases the tumescence and duration of the penile erection. Before this agent is used, it is important to obtain a careful medical history. If the patient has cardiac decompensation, this agent may have serious or even fatal effects. It potentiates the vasodilating effects of nitrites, producing potentially life-threatening hypotension. It is contraindicated in patients taking organic nitrates or nitrites such as nitroglycerin.

Dosage:
> Adults only: (Oral) 50 mg 1 hour prior to sexual activity.

vardenafil HCl (Levitra) This agent also prolongs the duration of penile erections. It should be avoided in patients with unstable angina, hypotension, recent history of stroke, arrhythmia, or myocardial infarction. Many drugs are incompatible with this agent, and current information should be obtained if the patient is on other medications. A partial list of incompatible drugs includes alpha blockers, nitrates, quinidine, procainamide, amiodarone, nifedipine, and many antiviral agents.

Dosage:
> (Oral) 10 mg 1 hour before sexual activity. May increase to 20 mg. Take up to once daily.

tadalafil (Cialis) The advantage of this agent is that it has a duration of action of up to 36 hours. The precautions and contraindications are similar to those for vardenafil. Priapism may occur. Current drug interaction information should be obtained if the patient is on other medications because there are many interactions.

Dosage:
> (Oral) 10 mg once daily before sexual activity. Dosage range 5-20 mg.

CLINICAL IMPLICATIONS

1. Diuretics are generally administered in the morning so that diuresis does not interfere with sleep.
2. The patient should be observed for the intended effects of diuretic medication. This will be seen in the increased urine volume, lessening of edema about the face and extremities, and weight loss.

3. The patient receiving a diuretic should be instructed in the importance of a low-sodium diet. Sodium promotes fluid retention and counteracts the desired effect of the diuretic.

4. Potassium loss is an untoward effect of many diuretics. The patient may receive potassium supplements or be instructed to consume foods that are high in potassium, such as raisins, oranges, and bananas.

5. Fluid and electrolyte changes that occur with diuretics may cause postural hypotension. The patient should be instructed to be observant if he or she experiences dizziness on arising or in ambulation.

6. Diuretics are often given to aid in the management of hypertension and to diminish the fluid and sodium content of the body.

7. Diuretics are of great value in the treatment of congestive heart failure when the weakened heart cannot mobilize excessive bodily fluids.

8. When a patient is receiving urinary antiseptics, it is often advisable to maintain an acid urine to aid the drug in its intended effect. Large doses of vitamin C and cranberries and prunes promote an acid urine. Carbonated beverages and citrus fruits produce an alkaline urine as a result of the metabolic by-products of sodium citrate and sodium bicarbonate.

9. Certain agents given for urinary tract infections, such as Urised and Pyridium, cause discolorations of the urine. The patient should be counseled to expect this effect.

10. An adequate fluid volume intake should be encouraged when the patient is being treated for a urinary tract infection.

11. The most common side effect of the urinary tract antiseptics is a skin rash. The patient should be observed for this effect. Other untoward reactions include headache, nervousness, and drug fever. An elevation of temperature may be a drug reaction, not a worsening of the infection.

12. The patient should be observed for signs of improvement of the urinary tract infection (i.e., less dysuria, frequency, and hesitancy on urination). The urine volume often increases as the infection is eradicated.

13. Withholding fluids before bedtime is not effective in treating enuresis.

14. All male patients over 55 years should be questioned about symptoms of prostate hypertrophy (i.e., difficulty in starting the urine flow and frequent nocturia).

15. Elderly patients should be questioned about symptoms of incontinence and advised that effective treatments are available.

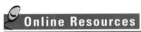

Online Resources

For updated drug information and Web activities, go to http://evolve.elsevier.com/Asperheim.

CRITICAL THINKING QUESTIONS

1. After taking hydrochlorothiazide (HydroDIURIL) for hypertension for 1 year, the patient now comes to the office with complaints of fatigue and weakness and many somatic complaints that include nonspecific malaise. Her blood pressure is 130/80 mm Hg. The doctor orders serum electrolyte determinations. The results are sodium, 145 mEq/L; potassium, 2.8 mEq/L; chloride, 110 mEq/L; and carbon dioxide, 28 mEq/L. What may be her problem? How can it be helped?

2. The patient has noted nausea and vomiting since he has been taking nitrofurantoin (Furadantin) for a urinary tract infection. He is now concerned that he is coming down with an intestinal virus and asks you to see if the doctor will give him some trimethobenzamide hydrochloride (Tigan), which he says usually works for him. Would you have any other recommendations?

3. The patient wants to see if the doctor will give him a prescription for sildenafil citrate (Viagra). What questions should be asked about his medical history?

4. A patient is brought to the office by his mother. She expresses a great deal of annoyance with the child because no matter "what she does" he continues to wet the bed. The mother has been withholding fluids after 5 PM, waking him up three times a night, setting alarm clocks for him to wake up, and so on. Nothing seems to work. What discussion would be appropriate with this mother?

5. The patient presents with pitting edema of the lower extremities that has slowly worsened over the last 3 days. He is worried because he can't take "water pills"; his potassium goes down too low. Which of the diuretics may be of use this time?

REVIEW QUESTIONS

1. The functional unit of the kidney is the:
   a. nephron.
   b. renal artery.
   c. ureter.
   d. posterior pituitary hormone.

2. An example of a thiazide diuretic is:
   a. spironolactone.
   b. amiloride.
   c. hydrochlorothiazide.
   d. aldactazide.

3. Spironolactone functions as a diuretic by:
   a. causing potassium depletion.
   b. increasing output of Bowman's capsule.
   c. inhibiting aldosterone.
   d. inhibiting corticosteroids.

4. The most common side effect of the thiazide diuretics is:
   a. hypertension.
   b. cirrhosis of the liver.
   c. hypokalemia.
   d. sodium retention.

5. An example of a urinary antiseptic is:
   a. metolazone.
   b. furosemide.
   c. spironolactone.
   d. nitrofurantoin.

6. A drug that will turn the urine a reddish color is:
   a. phenazopyridine.
   b. co-trimoxazole.
   c. sulfamethoxazole.
   d. pyribenzamine.

7. A drug used for the treatment of urinary incontinence is:
   a. sulfamethoxazole.
   b. oxybutynin.
   c. diazepam.
   d. sildenafil.

8. A drug used for the treatment of erectile dysfunction is:
   a. desmopressin.
   b. oxybutynin.
   c. imipramine.
   d. sildenafil.

9. Desmopressin acetate is useful in the treatment of:
   a. urinary tract infections.
   b. prostatic hypertrophy.
   c. enuresis.
   d. erectile dysfunction.

10. Reabsorption of filtered urine is under the influence of:
    a. the diuretic hormone from the anterior pituitary.
    b. the antidiuretic hormone from the posterior pituitary.
    c. the glomerular stimulating hormone.
    d. thiazide diuretics.

29 Antineoplastic Drugs

After completing this chapter, you should be able to do the following:

1. Identify antineoplastic drugs and understand their different modes of action.
2. Explain the use of antineoplastic drugs in immunosuppressive therapy.
3. Understand the use of hormones in the treatment of certain tumors.
4. Understand and anticipate the toxic effects of the antineoplastic agents.
5. Discuss nursing measures that provide supportive therapy for cancer patients.

Key Terms

Alkylating (ĂL-kĭ-LĀ-tǐng) **agents,** p. 176
Androgens (ĂN-drĕ-jǐns), p. 179
Antimetabolite (ăn-tĭ-mĕ-TĂB-ĕ-līt), p. 178
Antineoplastic drugs, p. 176
Carcinoma (KĂR-sĭ-NŌ-mĕ), p. 176
Corticosteroid (KŌR-tĭ-kō-STĬR-ŏyd), p. 179
Estrogens (ĔS-trŏ-jǐns), p. 179
Neoplasm (NĒ-ō-PLĂZ-ĕm), p. 176
Recombinant (rē-KŌM-bĭ-nĕnt), p. 182

Neoplastic diseases, or cancer, are caused by abnormal tissues known as **neoplasms** that grow by excessive cellular proliferation. Neoplasms that invade both surrounding and distant healthy tissues or organs, interfering with function and capable of causing the death of the entire organism, are referred to as **carcinomas.**

Surgery and radiation are still the primary tools in the fight against such malignant diseases, but **antineoplastic drugs** (that is, drugs used to treat cancer) have a very important role in the therapy of certain tumors, and for prophy-

Special Considerations

Immunity

A patient receiving an antineoplastic agent has reduced immunity to infections. She or he should avoid contact with infected persons and anyone who has recently received a live virus vaccine.

lactic treatment after a surgical procedure. Systemic drug treatment is important also when cancer is widespread or when the organ or tissue involved cannot be removed.

Because the malignant cell is dividing more rapidly than normal cells, it has a higher metabolic rate; thus it is more sensitive than normal cells to antineoplastic agents, which interfere with cell growth or metabolism. This difference in metabolic rate is not great enough to clearly separate malignant cells from normal cells, however, and the main disadvantage of the cancer drugs is that they are often toxic to normal cells as well. The more rapidly dividing healthy tissues (such as the gastrointestinal epithelium, oral mucosa, bone marrow, lymphoid tissue, and gonads) are the first to be affected by the antineoplastic drugs, and too much tissue destruction in these areas often requires withdrawal of the antineoplastic drug before the disease is brought under control.

Antineoplastic drugs may be classified as follows:

1. *Alkylating agents,* which attach "alkyl groups," or organic side chains, to the proteins within the cancer cell, thus interfering with its function.
2. *Antimetabolites,* which interfere with some phase of normal cellular metabolism. Antimetabolites are substances that compete with, replace, or antagonize a metabolic or bodily function.
3. *Hormones,* which may antagonize certain tumors of the reproductive tract and accessory sex organs by altering normal hormonal balance.
4. *Antitumor antibiotics,* which act usually by interfering with DNA or RNA synthesis.
5. *Enzyme inhibitors,* which interfere with tumor enzymes.
6. *Immunomodulating agents,* which enhance the body's own defense mechanisms to attack the cancer cells.
7. *Molecular medicine and gene therapy,* which treat cancer at the cellular level with agents that are developed to arrest cancer at that level.
8. *Miscellaneous drugs,* which are a heterogeneous group of drugs having various mechanisms of action.

ALKYLATING AGENTS

As previously stated, **alkylating agents** alter the chemical composition of proteins, probably the nucleoproteins, of the cell. The cell cannot function normally in the presence of these abnormal molecules. The alkylating agents were one of the first forms of antineoplastic therapy and have remained in use because of their undisputed effectiveness in the palliation of certain types of cancer. They are all highly toxic compounds, however, and produce many unpleasant as well as dangerous side effects upon continued use.

mechlorethamine hydrochloride, USP, BP (nitrogen mustard, Mustargen). This drug was produced as a result of experiments with the poisonous mustard gas used in World War I. It is particularly useful for lymphosarcoma, Hodgkin's disease, polycythemia vera, and mycosis fungoides. Nitrogen mustard is very irritating to the skin; thus extreme caution should be used when the drug is mixed. It may be administered intravenously, intraarterially, or as an intracavitary instillation. Side effects include nausea, vomiting, diarrhea, bone marrow suppression, and dermatitis. Chlorpromazine or a similar antiemetic may be given 1 hour before administration of this drug to minimize vomiting.

Dosage:
Adults and children: (IV) 0.1 to 0.4 mg/kg daily.

carboplatin (Paraplatin). This agent is used parenterally only for the treatment of ovarian and cervical cancer, small cell lung cancer, Wilms' tumor, and testicular neoplasms. Side effects include bone marrow suppression, nausea, vomiting, ototoxicity, and liver toxicity.

Dosage:
Adults only: (IV) 300 mg/m^2 once every 4 weeks.

cisplatin (Platinol-AQ). Cisplatin is used in the treatment of metastatic testicular tumors, in advanced ovarian and bladder cancers, and in a wide variety of other neoplasms. Side effects include bone marrow suppression, nausea, vomiting, ototoxicity, and liver toxicity.

Dosage:
Adults only: (IV) 20 mg/m^2 daily for 5 days.

chlorambucil, USP, BP (Leukeran). Chlorambucil has its greatest effect on the blood-forming tissues; thus it is used primarily in the treatment of leukemias and malignancies of the lymphatic system. It has an advantage over mechlorethamine in that it can be administered orally. Side effects are similar to those of mechlorethamine.

Dosage:
Adults and children: (Oral) 0.1 to 0.2 mg/kg daily.

busulfan, USP, BP (Myleran). Like chlorambucil, this drug is administered orally and is used primarily for malignancies of the blood-forming organs.

Dosage:
Adults: (Oral) 4 to 8 mg daily.
Children: (Oral) 0.06 mg/kg daily.

cyclophosphamide, USP, BP (Cytoxan). Cyclophosphamide may be administered orally, intramuscularly, intravenously, or as an intracavitary infusion. It is used occasionally in leukemias when the patient has become resistant to other drugs. In addition, it has been useful in the treatment of Hodgkin's disease, multiple myeloma, and carcinoma of the reproductive tract, and as an immunosuppressive agent. Side effects are similar to those of nitrogen mustard, with the exception that cyclophosphamide is not as irritating to tissues.

Dosage:
Adults: (Oral) 1 to 5 mg/kg daily. (IV) 10 to 20 mg/kg daily for 2 to 5 days, then 10 to 15 mg/kg every 7 to 10 days.
Children: (Oral) 2 to 8 mg/kg daily. (IV) 2 to 8 mg/kg daily.

thiotepa, USP, BP (Thioplex). Thiotepa is administered topically or as an intracavitary infusion as well as intravenously, intraarterially, or intramuscularly. It is primarily used in the treatment of cancer of the reproductive tract, lymphomas, leukemias, and cancer of the bladder. It is often instilled into the pleural space to decrease pulmonary effusions that occur with local neoplastic diseases. It is occasionally instilled into the bladder to aid in the treatment of small bladder tumors by topical action. Side effects are similar to those of the other drugs within this group.

Dosage:
Adults and children: (IV, IM, Intraarterial) Up to 200 mcg/kg daily for 5 days, then once weekly. (Topical) 15 mg diluted with a small amount of water.

carmustine (BiCNU). This alkylating agent is a derivative of nitrosourea. It is used in the treatment of malignant brain tumors and in combination with other agents for the treatment of multiple myeloma and Hodgkin's disease. The most serious and frequent side effect is a cumulative and delayed bone marrow toxicity that usually occurs 4 to 6 weeks after therapy. Nausea, vomiting, and renal and hepatic toxicity occur, as well as skin rashes.

Dosage:
Adults: (IV) 200 mg/m^2 body surface every 6 weeks.

dacarbazine, USP, BP (DTIC-Dome). The exact mechanism of action of this agent is not known, but it is presumed to be an alkylating agent. It is used in the treatment of malignant melanoma and with other agents in the treatment of Hodgkin's disease, soft tissue sarcomas, and neuroblastomas. Bone marrow suppression, nausea, vomiting, and a flulike syndrome of fever, myalgia, and malaise frequently occur with therapy.

Dosage:
Adults: (IV) 2.5 to 4.5 mg/kg daily for 10 days. This regimen may be repeated at 4-week intervals.

lomustine (CCNU, CeeNU). This agent is well absorbed from the gastrointestinal tract and is generally administered orally, although it may be used as a topical application in certain cases. It is used in the treatment of brain tumors and tumors of the gastrointestinal tract and kidney. It has been used topically in the treatment of mycosis fungoides and psoriasis. Delayed bone marrow toxicity, nausea, vomiting, alopecia, liver and kidney toxicity, and skin reactions occur with therapy.

Dosage:

Adults and children: (Oral) 130 mg/m^2 body surface as a single dose. It is given at intervals of at least 6 weeks.

melphalan, USP, BP (Alkeran). Melphalan is used alone and in combination with other antineoplastic agents for the treatment of multiple myeloma and nonresectable ovarian cancer, amyloidosis, and polycythemia vera. Side effects include bone marrow toxicity, nausea, vomiting, alopecia, and liver and kidney toxicity.

Dosage:

Adults: (Oral, IV) 6 mg initially, then 2 mg daily. Dose varies widely.

Children: No standard dosage is established.

ifosfamide (Ifex). This agent is structurally related to cyclophosphamide. It is particularly useful in the treatment of germ cell testicular neoplasms. Side effects resemble those of cyclophosphamide.

Dosage:

Adults only: (IV) 1.2 gm/m^2 daily for 3 to 5 consecutive days.

temozolomide (Temodar). Temozolomide is used in the treatment of refractory astrocytoma in adults. Thrombocytopenia and neutropenia are dose-limiting toxicities. Also seen are nausea, vomiting, and headache.

Dosage:

Adults only: (Oral) 150 mg/m^2 daily for 5 consecutive days.

ANTIMETABOLITES

Antimetabolites are a group of antineoplastic drugs that act by interfering in a specific phase of cell metabolism. Because neoplastic cells grow more rapidly than normal cells, theoretically they are affected by these drugs at dosage levels that cause only minimal interruption in the metabolism of normal cells. Unfortunately, this does not always prove to be true, and severe bone marrow suppression in particular will occur very often, requiring withdrawal of the drug. Loss of the gastrointestinal epithelium and ulcers of the oral mucosa are also frequent side effects of the antimetabolites.

methotrexate, USP, BP (Amethopterin). Methotrexate is a folic acid antagonist that exerts its action by interfering with the formation of the reduced, or active, form of folic acid in the body. It is administered orally and is particularly useful in the treatment of acute lymphocytic leukemias of childhood. The disease eventually becomes resistant to this compound, but often remissions lasting months or even years

may be obtained. In addition, it has been used effectively to treat uterine choriocarcinoma and in lymphosarcoma, as well as in the treatment of psoriasis, psoriatic arthritis, and rheumatoid arthritis.

It is also available in a parenteral form that may be given intramuscularly, intravenously, intraarterially, or intrathecally (within the spinal cord). Because the oral form is highly effective, parenteral administration is largely limited, with the exception of the intrathecal route, which is used in the treatment of leukemic meningitis. Other forms of administration do not allow sufficient concentrations of the drug to cross the blood-brain barrier.

The dosage of this drug varies widely because of its many uses.

Dosage:

Adults: (Oral, IV, IM) As an antineoplastic—2.5 to 30 mg daily. (Oral) As an antipsoriatic—10 to 25 mg once a week. (Oral) For rheumatoid arthritis—7 to 5 mg once weekly.

Children: (Oral, IV, IM) As an antineoplastic—0.12 mg/kg daily.

mercaptopurine, USP (Purinethol, 6-MP). Mercaptopurine is an antimetabolite that inhibits the synthesis of purines (components of DNA). It is administered orally with some effectiveness in the treatment of acute lymphocytic leukemias, Hodgkin's disease, and other tumors of the lymphatic system.

Dosage:

Adults and children: (Oral) 2.5 mg/kg daily.

fluorouracil, USP (5-FU). Fluorouracil is a chemical analog of uracil, a component of DNA. When incorporated into the DNA molecule, it interferes with normal growth and metabolism of the cell. It is administered intravenously or intraarterially for the treatment of carcinomas of the reproductive tract, liver, pancreas, and gastrointestinal tract. It may also be applied topically to treat actinic keratoses.

Dosage:

Adults: (IV) 12 mg/kg once daily for 4 days, then 6 mg/kg every other day for four doses. Maintenance dosage ranges from 10 to 15 mg/kg once a week. (Topical) 1% to 5% cream, applied twice daily to the lesion.

cladribine (Leustatin). Cladribine is indicated for the treatment of hairy cell leukemia. Side effects include nephrotoxicity, bone marrow suppression, nausea, vomiting, headache, and edema.

Dosage:

Adults only: (IV) 0.09 mg/kg/day for 7 days.

thioguanine. This agent is used to treat acute nonlymphocytic leukemia, Hodgkin's lymphoma, multiple myeloma, and solid tumors. There is usually cross-resistance between mercaptopurine and thioguanine. Side effects include myelosuppression, pancytopenia, hyperuricemia, nausea, vomiting, intestinal necrosis, and perforations.

Dosage:
> Adults and children: (Oral) 2 mg/kg/day for 4 weeks.

capecitabine (Xeloda). Capecitabine is used orally to treat metastatic breast cancer that is resistant to other agents. Side effects include nausea, vomiting, diarrhea, abdominal pain, stomatitis, edema, paresthesias, and hyperbilirubinemia. It is contraindicated in patients allergic to fluorouracil.

Dosage:
> Adults only: (Oral) 2500 mg/m² daily in divided doses for 2 weeks.

cytarabine, USP, BP (Cytosar, DepoCyt). The antimetabolic effect of this drug appears to occur by interference with DNA formation. It is used primarily in the treatment of acute myelocytic leukemia in adults, although it has been used in the treatment of other adult and childhood leukemias. It may be used intrathecally for the treatment of lymphomatous meningitis. The primary side effects are suppression of bone marrow and gastrointestinal symptoms. Fever, rash, cellulitis, pain at the injection site, sore throat, conjunctivitis, and alopecia also occur frequently. When used intrathecally, arachnoiditis is a common side effect.

Dosage:
> Adults only: (IV) 100 to 200 mg/m² daily. (Intrathecal) 5 to 75 mg/m² or 30 to 100 mg once every 2 to 7 days.

floxuridine, USP, BP (FUDR). By interfering with the synthesis of DNA, floxuridine has been found to be beneficial in certain malignancies. It is recommended only for intraarterial infusion and is used primarily for treatment of tumors of the head, neck, brain, liver, gallbladder, and bile ducts. Side effects are generally related to the area where the drug was infused and include oral stomatitis, esophagopharyngitis, duodenal ulcer, and gastrointestinal bleeding. Localized erythema, ataxia, blurred vision, and vertigo have also been noted.

Dosage:
> Adults: (Intraarterial) 100 to 600 mcg/kg in diluted solution daily. Therapy is generally continued until toxicity occurs.

dacarbazine (DTIC-Dome). This agent has many uses, including treatment of melanoma and Hodgkin's disease. Side effects include adverse hematologic, hepatic, and gastrointestinal symptoms.

Dosage:
> Adults only: (IV) Wide dosage range from 2 mg/kg/day for 10 days, to 375 mg/m²/day repeated every 15 days.

fludarabine phosphate (Fludara). Many tumors are treated with fludarabine, including chronic lymphocytic leukemia and non-Hodgkin's lymphoma. Side effects are dose related and include neurotoxicity and myelosuppression.

Dosage:
> Adults only: (IV) 25 mg/m² daily for 5 days.

gemcitabine hydrochloride (Gemzar). Gemcitabine's uses include treatment of adenocarcinoma of the pancreas and lung and bladder cancer. Side effects include hematologic toxicity, and gemcitabine should be given with caution to patients with renal and hepatic impairment.

Dosage:
> Adults only: (IV) 1 gm/m² once weekly.

HORMONES

Hormones have varied uses in the treatment of malignant diseases.

Corticosteroids (hormones produced by the adrenal cortex, and their synthetic forms) have long been shown to be of value in producing remissions of certain malignancies, notably acute lymphocytic leukemia of childhood, and they are used either alone or in combination with other drugs. The mechanism of action here is not fully understood. They have been used with less effectiveness in the treatment of Hodgkin's disease and lymphosarcoma. Side effects are those of excessive administration of corticosteroids (i.e., salt and water retention, moon facies, edema, and striae). In many cases dietary salt may have to be strictly curtailed during administration. Prednisone is the corticosteroid that is used perhaps more than any other in treating malignancies, but other compounds would be similarly effective.

Sex hormones have been used to palliate carcinomas of the reproductive tract. **Estrogens,** steroids responsible for feminine characteristics, may be administered to men with carcinoma of the prostate and have also been found to be of value in the treatment of postmenopausal women with breast cancer. **Androgens,** substances causing masculinization, are administered to premenopausal women with breast cancer. These agents are only palliative, not curative. Side effects are as expected: virilization (masculinization) when androgens are given to a woman and feminization when estrogens are given to a man.

ANDROGENS

testolactone suspension, USP, BP (Teslac). This analog of testosterone is a hormone derivative that is used exclusively in the treatment of malignancies. It has been used as palliative therapy for metastatic breast carcinoma in premenopausal women when surgery is not feasible. There are definite advantages to the use of this compound for the treatment of carcinoma in preference to the regularly used testosterone preparations, but the mechanism of action of this drug is not yet fully understood. It is administered intramuscularly or orally. Side effects include neurologic symptoms, nausea, vomiting, and alopecia.

Dosage:
> Adults: (Oral) 50 mg three times daily.

methyltestosterone (Android, Testred). This agent is used to treat women with advanced and inoperable metastatic breast cancer. The primary goal of therapy is ablation of the ovaries. It may also be used for androgen replacement therapy. Side effects include virilization, deepening of the voice, hirsutism, acne, clitoromegaly, and amenorrhea.

> **Dosage:**
> Adults only: (Oral) 50 to 200 mg daily.

ANTIANDROGENS

nilutamide (Nilandron). Nilutamide is a nonsteroidal, orally active antiandrogen. It is used to treat metastatic prostate cancer. Side effects include hepatic impairment, respiratory insufficiency, and interstitial pneumonia.

> **Dosage:**
> Adults only: (Oral) 6 tablets (50 mg each), once daily for 30 days.

flutamide (Eulexin). This agent is an orally active antiandrogen used to treat metastatic cancer of the prostate. Side effects include gynecomastia, impotence, drowsiness, anemia, and edema.

> **Dosage:**
> Adults only: (Oral) 60 mg once daily.

bicalutamide (Casodex). Generally this agent is used in combination therapy for the treatment of metastatic cancer of the prostate. Side effects include hepatic impairment, back pain, headaches, flulike symptoms, anorexia, and vomiting.

> **Dosage:**
> Adults only: (Oral) 50 to 200 mg daily.

ESTROGENS

megestrol acetate (Megace). Chemically related to progesterone, megestrol is used in the treatment of endometrial carcinoma, breast cancer, endometriosis, and prostatic hypertrophy. It is also used as an appetite stimulant (see Chapter 26). Very few side effects occur with this agent. It should be used with caution in patients with a history of thrombophlebitis.

> **Dosage:**
> Adults: (Oral) 40 mg daily in divided doses.

estramustine phosphate sodium (Emcyt). Estramustine is a combination of 17-beta-estradiol and nornitrogen mustard. It is used for the treatment of metastatic prostate cancer. Absorption is significantly decreased when it is given with dairy products or other calcium-rich foods. Side effects include angioedema, thromboembolic disorders, and cardiovascular and hepatic effects.

> **Dosage:**
> Adults only: (Oral) 14 mg/kg daily in three or four divided doses.

ANTIESTROGENS

fulvestrant (Faslodex). Fulvestrant is used to treat metastatic breast cancer in women who have had a recurrence following tamoxifen therapy. Side effects include hematologic disorders as well as gastrointestinal effects of nausea, vomiting, diarrhea, and abdominal pain.

> **Dosage:**
> Adults only: (IM) 250 mg monthly.

Selective Estrogen Receptor Modulators

Within the antiestrogens is a group called the selective estrogen receptor modulators, or SERMs. The SERMs exert selective agonist or antagonist effects on various estrogen target tissues. These agents are chemically diverse, but possess a tertiary structure that allows them to bind to the estrogen receptor.

Because of their estrogen receptor–activating properties, SERMS can be used to prevent or treat diseases caused by estrogen deficiency, such as osteoporosis. Because of their estrogen receptor–blocking properties, they can also be used to prevent or treat diseases such as breast cancer. Currently available SERMS have two major limitations: they are only weak estrogen agonists, and they aggravate hot flashes.

Side effects generally include nausea, vomiting, headache, hot flashes, constipation, and abdominal pain.

tamoxifen citrate (Nolvadex). This antiestrogenic compound is similar to clomiphene. It competes with estradiol for receptor sites in tumors of the breast, uterus, and vagina and in other tumors with estrogen receptors. Its primary use is in the treatment of advanced breast cancer in postmenopausal women.

> **Dosage:**
> Adults: (Oral) 20 to 40 mg daily in two divided doses.

toremifene citrate (Fareston). Toremifene is indicated for the treatment of metastatic breast cancer in postmenopausal women. Side effects include hypercalcemia, leukopenia, and vaginal bleeding. It should not be used in patients with a history of thromboembolic disease.

> **Dosage:**
> Adults only: (Oral) 60 mg daily.

AROMATASE INHIBITORS

The aromatase inhibitors are used to treat advanced breast cancer in postmenopausal women. Many breast cancers contain aromatase, an enzyme that converts a naturally occurring adrenal hormone to additional estrone. This is a disadvantage when treating breast cancer. The aromatase inhibitors interfere with this process.

anastrozole (Arimidex).

> **Dosage:**
> Adults only: (Oral) 1 mg daily.

exemestane (Aromasin).

> **Dosage:**
> Adults only: (Oral) 25 mg once daily.

letrozole (Femara).

> **Dosage:**
> Adults only: (Oral) 2.5 mg daily.

INHIBITORS OF PITUITARY HORMONES

goserelin acetate (Zoladex). This synthetic analog of gonadotropin-releasing hormone is used as an antineoplastic agent, and is used in some cases for its endocrine effects. It is used for the treatment of prostate and breast cancer, as well as for endometriosis and dysfunctional uterine bleeding. Side effects include hot flashes, sexual dysfunction, headaches, blood pressure instability, rash, and dizziness.

Dosage:
Adults only: (Subcutaneous implant) 3.6 mg in implant every 4 weeks.

leuprolide acetate (Lupron). Another synthetic analog of gonadotropin-releasing hormone, leuprolide can be used for its antineoplastic and endocrine effects. Its uses and side effects are similar to those of goserelin acetate, but in addition it is used to treat precocious puberty.

Dosage:
Adults: (IM or subQ) 3.75 to 30 mg approximately every 4 weeks based on serum levels.
Children: (IM or subQ) 3.75 to 15 mg approximately every 4 weeks.

triptorelin pamoate (Trelstar). Also an analog of gonadotropin-releasing hormone, triptorelin pamoate has actions and uses similar to the other drugs in this category. It is used in the palliative treatment of prostate cancer.

Dosage:
Adults only: (IM) 3.75 to 11.25 mg monthly.

ANTITUMOR ANTIBIOTICS

dactinomycin, USP, BP (Actinomycin D, Cosmegen). Dactinomycin is an antibiotic that exerts its effect as an antineoplastic agent by interfering with RNA synthesis. It is used in the treatment of Wilms' tumor of the kidney and for control of the metastases of this tumor. It has been used in combination with other agents in the treatment of metastatic tumors of the testes, choriocarcinoma, and certain lymphomas. Toxic effects include bone marrow suppression and liver and kidney toxicity, as well as nausea, vomiting, oral stomatitis, anorexia, and various skin eruptions.

Dosage:
Adults and children: (IV) 15 mcg/kg daily for 5 days.

bleomycin sulfate, USP, BP (Blenoxane). The antibiotic action of this agent appears to occur by causing a splitting of the DNA chain. It is used in the treatment of Hodgkin's disease and squamous cell carcinomas of the skin, penis, vulva, head, neck, and larynx. Unlike most antineoplastic agents, this drug has a very low incidence of bone marrow toxicity. The most serious toxic effect is interstitial pneumonitis. Skin or mucocutaneous lesions, alopecia, fever, chills, and hypotension have been reported.

Dosage:
Adults: (IV, IM, subQ, Intraarterial, Intrapleural injection) 0.25 to 0.5 units/kg weekly.

mitoxantrone hydrochloride (Novantrone). This synthetic antineoplastic agent is used to treat acute nonlymphocytic leukemia and advanced prostate cancer. Side effects include bone marrow suppression, cardiac toxicity, nausea, vomiting, fatigue, and hemorrhage.

Dosage:
Adults only: (IV) 12 mg/m² daily.

doxorubicin hydrochloride, USP, BP (Adriamycin, Rubex, Doxil). Doxorubicin is an antibiotic produced by a strain of *Streptomyces*. As with the other antibiotics in this group, it has antiinfective properties but is generally considered to be too toxic to be utilized in this way. It is used in the treatment of solid tumors of the breast, ovaries, bladder, lung, thyroid gland, and bone. It is also of value in the treatment of neuroblastoma; Wilms' tumor; Hodgkin's disease; Ewing's sarcoma; squamous cell tumors of the head, neck, cervix, and vagina; and carcinomas of the testes, prostate, and uterus. The major side effects are found in bone marrow and the gastrointestinal tract. The patient should be monitored for cardiotoxicity, as manifested by electrocardiographic changes. Facial flushing, edema, alopecia, fever, chills, and skin rashes also occur.

Dosage:
Adults: (IV) 60 to 75 mg/m² body surface as a single dose at 21-day intervals.

valrubicin (Valstar). This agent is a semisynthetic analog of doxorubicin. It is used for instillation into the urinary bladder for carcinoma in situ of the bladder. Side effects include bladder spasm, hematuria, incontinence, pelvic pain, vomiting, diarrhea, and peripheral edema.

Dosage:
Adults only: (Intravesical) 800 mg once weekly for 6 weeks.

mithramycin, USP, BP (Mithracin). Also produced by a strain of *Streptomyces*, mithramycin is used primarily in the treatment of testicular tumors. It has been noted to lower serum calcium levels; thus it is also used in the treatment of hypercalcemia associated with a variety of neoplasms. The primary side effects are found in bone marrow and the intestinal tract. Facial flushing, malaise, depression, phlebitis, and skin rashes have also been noted.

Dosage:
Adults: (IV) 25 to 30 mg/kg daily for 8 to 10 days or until toxicity occurs.

mitomycin, USP, BP (Mutamycin). This antibiotic is used in the treatment of adenocarcinoma of the stomach, pancreas, colon, and rectum; squamous cell carcinomas of the lungs, cervix, head, and neck; and malignant melanoma. Bone marrow suppression, mouth ulcers, nausea, vomiting, and renal toxicity are among the side effects seen after administration.

Dosage:
Adults: (IV) 50 mcg/kg daily for 5 days.

daunorubicin hydrochloride (Cerubidine, Daunoxome). This antibiotic functions as an antineoplastic agent because of its effect as an inhibitor of DNA synthesis. It is used primarily to treat acute myelogenous leukemia. It has also been used in the treatment of lymphocytic leukemias and in disseminated neuroblastoma.
> **Dosage:**
> Adults and children: (IV infusion) 30 to 60 mg/m² daily for 3 to 5 days.

idarubicin hydrochloride (Idamycin). This agent is an analog of daunorubicin and also inhibits nucleic acid synthesis. It is used in combination with other antileukemic drugs for the treatment of acute myeloid leukemia in adults. Side effects include tissue necrosis at the site of injection, myocardial toxicity, nausea, vomiting, and peripheral neuropathy.
> **Dosage:**
> Adults only: (IV) 4 mg/m² every other week.

pentostatin (Nipent). Pentostatin is indicated for the treatment of hairy cell leukemia. Side effects include renal, liver, pulmonary, and central nervous system toxicities.
> **Dosage:**
> Adults only: (IV) 4 mg/m² every other week.

streptozocin (Zanosar). This antibiotic is produced by *Streptomyces achromogenes*. It is used to treat pancreatic islet cell carcinoma, carcinoid tumor, Hodgkin's disease, and colorectal cancer. The most serious side effect is its nephrotoxicity, which occurs in up to 75% of patients. Nausea, vomiting, bone marrow suppression, tissue necrosis, confusion, and depression have also been reported.
> **Dosage:**
> Adults only: (IV or Intraarterial) 500 mg/m² daily for 5 days.

epirubicin hydrochloride (Ellence). Related to doxorubicin, its uses include the treatment of breast cancer. Side effects are similar to those of its parent compound.
> **Dosage:**
> Adults only: (IV) 100 to 120 mg/m² monthly.

ENZYME INHIBITORS

asparaginase (Elspar). This enzyme, derived from *Escherichia coli*, is mainly used in combination chemotherapy for childhood acute lymphocytic leukemia, but is used in adults as well. Side effects include skin rashes and a variety of hepatic, renal, and hematologic effects.
> **Dosage:**
> Adults and children: (IM or IV) 6000 units on certain days of the protocol.

imatinib mesylate (Gleevec). This inhibitor of tyrosine kinase is used primarily in the treatment of chronic myel-

ogenous leukemia. Side effects include neutropenia, liver toxicity, and fluid retention.
> **Dosage:**
> Adults only: (Oral) 400 to 600 mg daily.

irinotecan hydrochloride (Camptosar). A DNA topoisomerase, irinotecan is used in the treatment of gastrointestinal, cervical, and lung cancer. Side effects include neutropenia, diarrhea, fever, and cardiovascular toxicity.
> **Dosage:**
> Adults only: (IV) 125 mg/m² weekly.

pegaspargase (Oncaspar). A conjugated asparaginase, this agent is used in the treatment of childhood acute lymphocytic leukemia. Side effects include hypotension, cough, epistaxis, malaise, nausea, and vomiting.
> **Dosage:**
> Children and young adults: (IM) 2500 units/m² at 14-day intervals.

IMMUNOMODULATING AGENTS IN CANCER

In the 1950s, when it was discovered that there was an interference phenomenon between viruses, subsequently labeled "virus-inhibitory factor," there was no recognition that the scientists had stumbled upon one of the arsenals of the body's own defense mechanism. This interference substance, then called interferon, was found to be produced by leukocytes (white blood cells), and it demonstrated antitumor effects in tissue cultures and animal experiments. A new form of cancer treatment has been introduced with the current development of interferons via **recombinant** DNA techniques—techniques in which a cell or organism receives genes from different parental strains.

interferon alfa (Roferon-A, Intron A, Alferon N, Rebetron). Interferon alfa is actually a family of proteins that possess complex antiviral, antineoplastic, and immunomodulating activities. Interferons for human use are of human origin, produced by means of cultured cells or recombinant techniques. Recombinant techniques use human genes that are grown in cultures of *Escherichia coli*. At least 23 structurally similar subtypes are known.

When used in cancer therapy, the interferons have a growth-inhibiting effect on normal and malignant cells. Interferon alfa-2a and -2b are used in the treatment of hairy cell leukemia; Kaposi's sarcoma in patients with acquired immunodeficiency syndrome; renal cell carcinoma; bladder, cervical, and ovarian cancer; and also melanoma and multiple myeloma.

Side effects include a flulike syndrome, myalgia, arthralgia, anorexia, mental disturbances, elevated liver enzymes, and skin rashes.
> **Dosage:**
> Adults only: (subQ or IM) 3 million units daily for 16 to 24 weeks.

levamisole hydrochloride (Ergamisol). This immunomodulator can be administered orally for the treatment of advanced colon cancer. Side effects include encephalopathy, peripheral neuropathy, seizures, confusion, and coma.

Dosage:

Adults only: (Oral) 50 mg three times daily for 3 days.

aldesleukin (Proleukin). This human recombinant interleukin is used for the treatment of adults with metastatic renal cell carcinoma and metastatic melanoma. Side effects include ventricular tachycardia, cardiac tamponade, renal failure, toxic psychosis, and gastrointestinal bleeding.

Dosage:

Adults only: (IV) 600,000 International Units/kg/dose every 8 hours for 14 days.

MOLECULAR MEDICINE AND GENE THERAPY

Continuing studies aimed at bringing treatment to the cellular level have produced many advances in cancer therapy. Treatment using agents developed through the techniques of molecular medicine and gene therapy is often more specific for a certain type of cancer than is the case with the other classes of antineoplastic agents. These agents are discussed in Chapter 31.

MISCELLANEOUS CANCER TREATMENT AGENTS

The following agents have many different modes of action, and do not fit into the previously mentioned classes. For information on other miscellaneous agents, see Table 29–1.

vincristine sulfate, USP, BP (Oncovin). Vincristine acts by interfering with normal cellular division. It must be administered intravenously and is used especially in the treatment of acute leukemias when the disease has become resistant to other orally administered drugs. Side effects include bone marrow suppression, neurologic symptoms, vomiting, diarrhea, and abdominal pain.

Dosage:

Adults: (IV) 1.4 mg/m^2 weekly.
Children: (IV) 1.5 to 2 mg/m^2 weekly.

vinblastine sulfate, USP, BP (Velban). Like vincristine, this drug acts primarily by interfering with cell division. It is also administered intravenously and has been used with limited success in the treatment of Hodgkin's disease, lymphosarcoma, and choriocarcinoma. It is of no practical value in the treatment of leukemias. Side effects are similar to those of vincristine.

Dosage:

Adults: (IV) 5.5 to 7.4 mg/m^2 weekly.
Children: (IV) 2.5 mg/m^2 as a single dose.

procarbazine hydrochloride, USP, BP (Matulane). This drug has been shown to be somewhat effective in the oral treatment of Hodgkin's disease but has no clinical effect in other types of malignancies. Side effects include leukopenia, nausea, vomiting, muscle and joint pain, and neurologic symptoms. This drug accentuates the central nervous system depressant action of sedatives, tranquilizers, narcotics, and antihistamines; thus, it should not be given simultaneously with these drugs. It should be used with caution in patients with kidney or liver damage.

Dosage:

Adults: (Oral) 100 to 300 mg daily.
Children: (Oral) 50 mg daily.

hydroxyurea, USP, BP (Hydrea). This derivative of urea is an antineoplastic drug believed to act by interfering in the formation of DNA. It is used orally in the treatment of malignant melanoma, ovarian carcinoma, and chronic granulocytic leukemia when the patient is resistant to other forms of therapy. Side effects are bone marrow suppression, nausea, vomiting, diarrhea, ulceration of the buccal mucosa and gastrointestinal epithelium, neurologic symptoms, alopecia, and dermatoses.

Dosage:

Adults: (Oral) 20 to 30 mg/kg daily.
Children: No standard dosage is established.

azathioprine, USP, BP (Imuran). Although the exact mechanism of action of this drug is not known, it is believed to inhibit RNA and DNA synthesis. At this time it is administered orally primarily to prevent the rejection of kidney transplants (see Chapter 30). Bone marrow suppression, nausea, vomiting, jaundice, mucous membrane ulcers, a

Table 29-1	*Other Miscellaneous Drugs for Treatment of Cancer*	
DRUG	**USES**	**ADULT-ONLY DOSAGE**
bexarotene (Targretin)	T-cell lymphoma	300 mg/m^2 orally once daily
docetaxel (Taxotere)	Breast and lung cancer	60–100 mg/m^2 IV, repeat in 3 wk
etoposide (VePesid)	Leukemias, lymphoma	50–100 mg/m^2 oral or IV daily
mitoxantrone HCl (Novantrone)	Acute myeloid leukemia	12 mg/m^2 IV daily
paclitaxel (Onxol)	Ovarian, breast, lung cancers	175 mg/m^2 IV every 3 wk
teniposide (Vumon)	Acute lymphocytic leukemia	165 mg/m^2 IV twice weekly
topotecan HCl (Hycamtin)	Ovarian and lung cancer	1.5 mg/m^2 IV daily
oxaliplatin (Eloxatin)	Colorectal cancer	85 mg/m^2 IV daily

persistent negative nitrogen balance, and muscle wasting have been observed after administration.

Dosage:
>Adults and children: (Oral) 3 to 5 mg/kg/day.

mitotane, USP, BP (Lysodren). This agent is believed to suppress the adrenal cortex and alter the utilization of steroids. It is used in the treatment of adrenocortical carcinoma. Gastrointestinal disturbances, somnolence, dizziness, anorexia, nausea, vomiting, and diarrhea have occurred following administration.

Dosage:
>Adults only: (Oral) 2 to 6 gm daily in three or four divided doses.

SUPPORTIVE AGENTS

epoetin alfa (Epogen, Procrit). Epoetin alfa is a biosynthetic form of the hormone erythropoietin. It is used for the treatment of chronic anemia. Patients who have anemia that is related to cancer or its treatment may benefit from administration of this drug. It is also used to treat anemia associated with chronic renal failure, hemodialysis, and other sources, such as human immunodeficiency virus infection. There is some potential for abuse by athletes to increase the oxygen-carrying ability of cells. Side effects include hypertension, seizures, nausea, and vomiting.

Dosage:
>Adults and children: (IV or subQ) 75 to 150 units/kg/week.

CLINICAL IMPLICATIONS

1. The patient receiving antineoplastic agents is often anxious and upset. Efforts should be made to provide emotional support to the patient and family.
2. The nurse should instruct the patient about the importance of good nutrition and his or her nutritional requirements. A diet high in protein but low in saturated fat is optimal (e.g., fish, lean poultry, eggs, nonfat dairy products, nuts, seeds, and legumes). Healthy choices include whole grains, legumes, fruits, and vegetables. Dietary supplements may be beneficial, but cannot replace a nutrient-rich diet.
3. Assess the patient's understanding of his or her illness and the possible side effects of medication.
4. Nursing procedures such as an ice cap placed on the scalp before the administration of intravenous antineoplastic agents may decrease hair loss. The patient should be advised that the hair will grow back in time, even if total alopecia results from the treatments.
5. Oral lesions and bleeding from the gums may result from treatment with antineoplastic agents. Good oral hygiene should be promoted, such as the use of lemon-glycerin swabs and the avoidance of irritating foods or acidic juices.
6. Common side effects of these agents are fever, sore throat, blood dyscrasias, and infections. The patient should be monitored for these effects.
7. The patient on antineoplastic medication is susceptible to untoward effects from minor illnesses. The patient and family should be counseled about avoiding contact with possibly infected persons.
8. Sedation or antiemetic medication before the administration of intravenous agents may minimize the nausea and vomiting produced as side effects. Administration in the evening may allow remission of the nausea before the next morning. The patient should be encouraged to eat small, frequent meals.
9. The site of injection should be observed carefully for signs of extravasation, because these agents may produce sloughing of tissues.
10. Observe the patient for therapeutic effects, such as reduction in tumor size and weight gain.
11. The patient may be depressed as a result of having cancer. Observation for depression and recommendation for treatment help in the overall management of the patient.

Online Resources

For updated drug information and Web activities, go to http://evolve.elsevier.com/Asperheim.

CRITICAL THINKING QUESTIONS

1. The child is undergoing treatment for acute lymphocytic leukemia and is receiving methotrexate presently. She has now noticed that her long hair is falling out rapidly and is very upset. What would you say to her?

2. The patient is receiving therapy with multiple antineoplastic agents for metastatic breast carcinoma. She has been resisting all attempts to brush her teeth because of extreme soreness in her mouth and throat. What nursing procedures may make her more comfortable?

3. The patient is undergoing treatment for Hodgkin's disease with uracil mustard. This morning when you made his bed you noticed a deep-purple rash on his back and thighs. Should you report this to the physician or merely assure the patient that this, like his recent hair loss and mouth ulcers, is a side effect to be expected and tolerated?

4. The patient is improving with the antineoplastic agents, but has become more and more quiet and listless. What may be the problem? What suggestions may be made?

REVIEW QUESTIONS

1. Neoplasms are caused by:
   a. carcinoma.
   b. uncontrolled cell division.
   c. cell growth of certain genes.
   d. rapidly dividing healthy tissues.

2. An antimetabolite, when used to treat cancer, works by:
   a. interfering with abnormal cell growth .
   b. alkylating the offending cells.
   c. interfering with some phase of normal cellular metabolism.
   d. interfering with abnormal metabolic processes.

3. An example of an antimetabolite is:
   a. carboplatin.
   b. thiotepa.
   c. methotrexate.
   d. nilutamide.

4. Methyltestosterone may be used to treat:
   a. breast cancer.
   b. leukemia.
   c. prostate cancer.
   d. testicular cancer.

5. An example of an antiandrogen is:
   a. testosterone.
   b. gemcitabine.
   c. nilutamide.
   d. nikethimide.

6. An example of an antitumor antibiotic is:
   a. goserelin.
   b. dactinomycin.
   c. angiotensin.
   d. amoxicillin.

7. Interferon alfa may be used in the treatment of:
   a. melanoma.
   b. colon cancer.
   c. acute leukemia.
   d. myalgia.

8. An enzyme that is used in cancer chemotherapy is:
   a. pancrelipase.
   b. ptyalin.
   c. pegaspargase.
   d. asparaginase.

9. Hydroxyurea is believed to function in cancer therapy by:
   a. interfering with cell wall formation.
   b. suppressing cell metabolism.
   c. functioning as an immunosuppressive.
   d. interfering with the formation of DNA.

10. An agent used to treat the anemia that often occurs after chemotherapy is:
    a. mitroxantrone.
    b. vitamin E.
    c. epinephrine.
    d. epoetin alfa.

Immunizing Agents and Immunosuppressives

Key Terms

Active immunity, p. 186
Immunity, p. 186
Immunizing agent, p. 186
Immunosuppressives, p. 191
Passive immunity, p. 186
Vaccine, p. 186

IMMUNIZING AGENTS

Immunity, the status of being protected against an infectious disease, may be brought about by actual contact with the disease or by the administration of a substance called a vaccine. A **vaccine,** or **immunizing agent,** is a preparation that uses an altered or killed microorganism to produce active immunity to a disease. Immunity may be gained by using a vaccine without the accompanying adverse effects of the disease itself.

Active immunity is achieved when the antigen, or altered microorganism, is injected into the body, and natural antibodies are produced against it.

Passive immunity is obtained when previously formed antibodies are injected into the body. This provides a faster immunity; however, it is short lived, lasting only a few weeks or months.

Because of the proven success of the vaccines against infectious diseases, childhood immunization is now required by law, generally before admission to school (Fig. 30–1). There are usually only minor complications from childhood vaccines. Rare serious effects do occur, but considering the

illness and death previously associated with these diseases in infants and children, there can be no doubt that the vaccines provide a safe and effective way to ensure the health of the population.

Considerations for Children

Immunizations

Encourage parents to immunize their children in a timely manner. Immunity to some diseases may not develop if booster doses of the immunizing agents are not given at the recommended intervals. Explain the importance of the immunization schedule during well-baby and well-child checkups.

Despite the effectiveness of immunization in adults, diphtheria/tetanus, influenza, hepatitis A and B, and pneumococcal vaccines continue to be underutilized. Health care workers should encourage the use of adult vaccines (Fig. 30-2).

Special Considerations

Immunizations

Immunizations are not just for children anymore. Everyone should receive tetanus toxoid every 10 years. Older adults should also receive pneumococcal vaccine. Health care workers, older adults, and anyone with an underlying respiratory illness should receive an annual influenza vaccine (flu shot). The hepatitis B vaccine series is required for most health care workers. Hepatitis A is recommended for endemic areas.

AGENTS THAT PROVIDE ACTIVE IMMUNITY

diphtheria and tetanus toxoids and acellular pertussis vaccine (DTaP) (Tripedia, Infanrix). This vaccine differs from earlier DPT vaccine in that the pertussis vaccine is prepared from inactivated acellular pertussis. It gives fewer adverse reactions than are produced by the whole-cell pertussis, while retaining the immunogenic properties. Side effects include local reactions of erythema and swelling at the injection site, mild fever, and malaise following injection. Immunocompromised individuals will have a diminished immunologic response.

Dosage:

Children to 6 years: (IM) 0.5 mL per schedule in Figure 30–1.

Recommended Childhood Immunization Schedule

United States, 2002

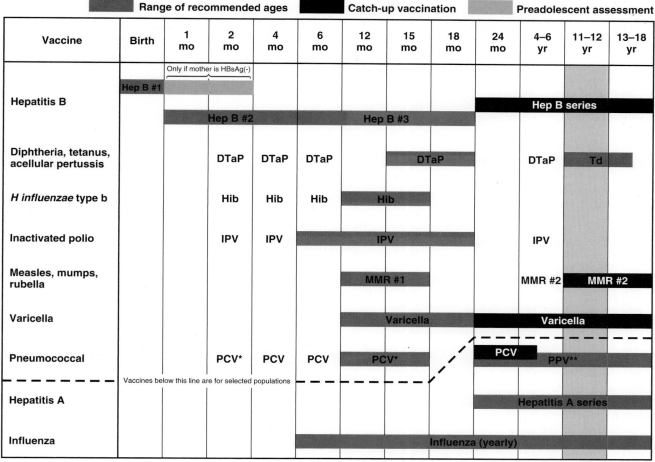

*Pneumococcal conjugate vaccine   **Pneumococcal polysaccharide vaccine

1. This schedule indicates the recommended ages for routine administration of currently licensed childhood vaccines, as of 11/1/00, for children through 18 years of age. Additional vaccines may be licensed and recommended during the year. Licensed combination vaccines may be used whenever any components of the combination are indicated and its other components are not contraindicated. Providers should consult the manufacturers' package inserts for detailed recommendations.

2. *Infants born to HBsAg-negative mothers* should receive the 1st dose of hepatitis B (Hep B) vaccine by age 2 months. The 2nd dose should be at least one month after the 1st dose. The 3rd dose should be administered at least 4 months after the 1st dose and at least 2 months after the 2nd dose, but not before 6 months of age for infants.
   Infants born to HBsAg-positive mothers should receive hepatitis B vaccine and 0.5 mL hepatitis B immune globulin (HBIG) within 12 hours of birth at separate sites. The 2nd dose is recommended at 1-2 months of age and the 3rd dose at 6 months of age.
   Infants born to mothers whose HBsAg status is unknown should receive hepatitis B vaccine within 12 hours of birth. Maternal blood should be drawn at the time of delivery to determine the mother's HBsAg status; if the HBsAg test is positive, the infant should receive HBIG as soon as possible (no later than 1 week of age).
   All children and adolescents who have not been immunized against hepatitis B should begin the series during any visit. Special efforts should be made to immunize children who were born in or whose parents were born in areas of the world with moderate or high endemicity of hepatitis B virus infection.

3. The 4th dose of DTaP (diphtheria and tetanus toxoids and acellular pertussis vaccine) may be administered as early as 12 months of age, provided 6 months have elapsed since the 3rd dose and the child is unlikely to return at age 15-18 months. Td (tetanus and diphtheria toxoids) is recommended at 11-12 years of age if at least 5 years have elapsed since the last dose of DTP, DTaP, or DT. Subsequent routine Td boosters are recommended every 10 years.

4. Three *Haemophilus influenzae* type b (Hib) conjugate vaccines are licensed for infant use. If PRP-OMP (PedvaxHIB® or ComVax® [Merck]) is administered at 2 and 4 months of age, a dose at 6 months is not required. Because clinical studies in infants have demonstrated that using some combination products may induce a lower immune response to the Hib vaccine component, DTaP/Hib combination products should not be used for primary immunization in infants at 2, 4, or 6 months of age, unless FDA-approved for these ages.

5. An all-IPV schedule is recommended for routine childhood polio vaccination in the United States. All children should receive four doses of IPV at 2 months, 4 months, 6-18 months, and 4-6 years of age. Oral polio vaccine (OPV) should be used only in selected circumstances. (See MMWR May 19, 2000/49(RR-5);1-22).

6. The heptavalent conjugate pneumococcal vaccine (PCV) is recommended for all children 2-23 months of age. It also is recommended for certain children 24-59 months of age. (See MMWR Oct. 6, 2000/49(RR-9);1-35)

7. The 2nd dose of measles, mumps, and rubella (MMR) vaccine is recommended routinely at 4-6 years of age but may be administered during any visit, provided at least 4 weeks have elapsed since receipt of the 1st dose and that both doses are administered beginning at or after 12 months of age. Those who have not previously received the second dose should complete the schedule by the 11-12 year old visit.

8. Varicella (Var) vaccine is recommended at any visit on or after the first birthday for susceptible children, i.e., those who lack a reliable history of chickenpox (as judged by a health care provider) and who have not been immunized. Susceptible persons 13 years of age or older should receive 2 doses, given at least 4 weeks apart.

9. Hepatitis A (Hep A) is shaded to indicate its recommended use in selected states and/or regions, and for certain high risk groups; consult your local public health authority. (See MMWR Oct. 1, 1999;48(RR-12); 1-37).

***For additional information about the vaccines listed above, please visit the National Immunization Program Home Page at http://www.cdc.gov/nip/
or call the National Immunization Hotline at 800-232-2522 (English) or 800-232-0233 (Spanish).***

FIGURE 30-1 Recommended schedule for childhood immunization.

Recommended Adult Immunization Schedule
United States, 2002–2003

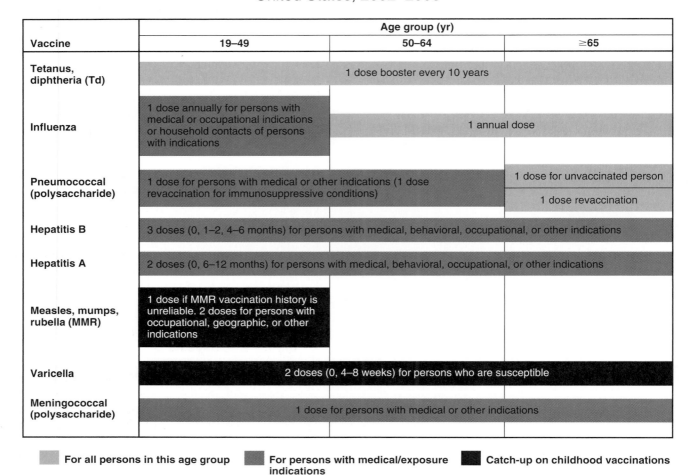

Vaccine	Age group (yr)		
	19–49	50–64	≥65
Tetanus, diphtheria (Td)	1 dose booster every 10 years		
Influenza	1 dose annually for persons with medical or occupational indications or household contacts of persons with indications	1 annual dose	
Pneumococcal (polysaccharide)	1 dose for persons with medical or other indications (1 dose revaccination for immunosuppressive conditions)		1 dose for unvaccinated person
			1 dose revaccination
Hepatitis B	3 doses (0, 1–2, 4–6 months) for persons with medical, behavioral, occupational, or other indications		
Hepatitis A	2 doses (0, 6–12 months) for persons with medical, behavioral, occupational, or other indications		
Measles, mumps, rubella (MMR)	1 dose if MMR vaccination history is unreliable. 2 doses for persons with occupational, geographic, or other indications		
Varicella	2 doses (0, 4–8 weeks) for persons who are susceptible		
Meningococcal (polysaccharide)	1 dose for persons with medical or other indications		

▓ **For all persons in this age group**   ▓ **For persons with medical/exposure indications**   ■ **Catch-up on childhood vaccinations**

FIGURE 30–2 Recommended adult immunization schedule.

diphtheria and tetanus toxoids, acellular pertussis, hepatitis B, and inactivated poliovirus vaccine (Pediarix). This is the first 5-in-l vaccine available and it has the ability to greatly reduce the number of vaccine injections necessary for infants and young children. Side effects include injection-site reactions such as pain, swelling, redness, and fever. This agent is associated with higher rates of reactions involving fever than are seen with the separately administered vaccines. It is contraindicated in infants with known sensitivity to any component of the vaccine, including yeast, neomycin, and polymyxin B. It should not be administered to any infant before 6 weeks of age, or to any child over 7 years old. It is a suspension and should be shaken vigorously before administration. It should not be used if all the material in the vial is not in the form of a suspension.

Dosage:
Children to 7 years: (IM) Three 0.5-mL injections at 6- to 8-week intervals.

poliovirus vaccine, inactivated (IPV, Salk vaccine) (Poliovax). Inactivated poliovirus vaccine is a noninfectious suspension

containing three strains of poliovirus. It may be administered IM or subQ.

The major disadvantage of the formerly used live oral polio vaccine was the risk of associated paralytic poliomyelitis in vaccine recipients and their contacts. It has been replaced by the injectable inactivated form.

The duration of immunity when using the inactivated virus has yet to be determined.

Dosage:
Children and adults: (IM or subQ) 0.5 mL per schedule in Figure 30–1.

Haemophilus b conjugate vaccine (Hib). This vaccine is a noninfectious bacteria-derived vaccine used to prevent *Haemophilus influenzae* infections in infants and young children. Several different types of conjugated vaccines (vaccines made by linking the inactivated bacteria to a carrier molecule) are available, differing in the protein carrier, the polysaccharide carrier, and the method of conjugation. Whatever type is chosen, it should be continued for the duration of the immunization schedule. The PedvaxHIB, ActHIB, and

HibTITER vaccines may all be used in infants and children up to 5 years of age. The ProHIBiT vaccine may be used in children 15 months to 5 years of age.

Dosage:

Children to 5 years: (IM) 0.5 mL per schedule in Figure 30–1.

Haemophilus **b and hepatitis B vaccine (Comvax).** This combination vaccine may be used in children under 5 years of age. It should not be administered to any infant under 6 weeks of age. If one dose of the hepatitis B vaccine was administered to the child as a newborn, this combination may still be used for the subsequent doses on the same schedule as follows.

Dosage:

(IM) 0.5 mL at 2, 4, and 12 to 15 months of age.

measles, mumps, and rubella virus vaccine, live, USP, BP (MMR) (M-M-R II). Although all these virus vaccines are available as single vaccines, it has been shown that immunity is conferred just as effectively with the triple live virus vaccine. Immunity is less than optimal if the vaccine is administered before 15 months of age, and if it is administered early because of a community epidemic, the dose must be repeated at a later time. Side effects are minimal with this vaccine; however, occasionally the patient may experience a low-grade fever and light pink rash 10 to 14 days after administration.

Dosage:

Children 15 months or older: (subQ) 0.5 mL per schedule in Figure 30–1.

varicella virus vaccine, live (Varivax). This vaccine stimulates immunity to varicella virus, or chickenpox. Long-term studies are necessary to determine the duration of protection after the use of this vaccine. Development of antibodies following vaccination does not occur in all cases, and breakthrough epidemics may still occur.

Dosage: Children: (IM) 0.5 mL.

diphtheria and tetanus toxoids, adsorbed (DT, Td). This agent is used for boosting immunity to diphtheria and tetanus when pertussis immunization is not necessary. It is used in late childhood and adulthood.

Dosage:

Adults and children: (IM) 0.5 mL.

tetanus toxoid, USP; tetanus vaccine, BP. Tetanus toxoid is a preparation of the formaldehyde-treated by-products of the tetanus bacillus *Clostridium tetani*. Although combined with other vaccines in the DPT and DT series given routinely in childhood, the tetanus toxoid alone is often chosen for periodic boosters after childhood. An effective serum level is sustained for 10 years after the booster dose; however, boosters can be given as often as every 5 years if there is concern that the patient may develop tetanus from an extremely dirty wound.

Dosage:

Adults: (IM) 0.5 mL.

influenza virus vaccine, USP, BP (Fluvirin, Fluzone). This vaccine contains virus material from several different strains of influenza A and B. It is prepared anew every year based on the influenza viruses seen at various places in the world, which presumably will be responsible for the following year's epidemic. It is given annually and is no longer restricted to the elderly and those with respiratory diseases. It is recommended annually even for children.

Dosage:

Adults and children: (IM) 0.5 mL in the autumn, annually.

influenza virus vaccine live, intranasal (Flumist). The intranasal form of influenza vaccine is recommended for persons 5 to 49 years of age. The effectiveness of the vaccine compares favorably with the injectable form. Immunized individuals should avoid contact with immunocompromised persons in the same household. Its safety in patients with asthma and reactive airway disease has not been established.

Dosage:

Adults and children: (Intranasal) 0.5 mL, followed by a repeat dose in 6 weeks.

hepatitis A virus vaccine, inactivated (Havrix, Vaqta). This vaccine is a noninfectious inactivated virus vaccine used for individuals at high risk for hepatitis A. It is routinely given to children who reside in areas where the incidence is high, generally in less developed regions in the western states. It is not believed to be necessary for the general population in the United States at this time. The two vaccines have different unit strengths, thus the dose is given here for each. A single dose only is given.

Dosage:

Havrix: Adults: (IM) 1440 units.
Children 2 to 18 years: (IM) 720 units.
Vaqta: Adults: (IM) 50 units.
Children 2 to 18 years: (IM) 25 units.

hepatitis B vaccine (Recombivax HB, Engerix-B). Hepatitis B vaccine (recombinant) is a noninfectious subunit viral vaccine containing hepatitis B surface antigen. It is prepared from a strain of *Saccharomyces cerevisiae* using recombinant DNA technology. The strain of *Saccharomyces* used has been genetically altered to contain the hepatitis B virus gene coding. Immunization is given to infants beginning at birth and should be given to all high-risk groups, particularly those in the health professions.

At least 90% of children and adults develop antibodies with this vaccine, but the duration of the immunity has not been established. Further booster doses may be necessary in the future. Recombivax HB and Engerix-B have different unit strengths, so their dosages are given separately here. Three doses are necessary, the first two given 1 month apart and the third given 6 months after the first dose, according to the schedule in Figure 30–1.

Dosage:
Recombivax: Infants to 19 years: (IM) 5 mcg.
Adults over 19 years: (IM) 10 mcg.
Predialysis patients: (IM) 40 mcg.
Engerix-B: Infants to 19 years: (IM) 10 mcg.
Adults over 19 years: (IM) 20 mcg.
Predialysis patients: (IM) 40 mcg.

pneumococcal vaccine, polyvalent (Pneumovax 23). Polyvalent pneumococcal vaccine is a sterile solution containing antigenic polysaccharides extracted from *Streptomyces pneumoniae*. It is used to stimulate immunity to 23 types of pneumonia that are represented in the vaccine. The polysaccharides in the vaccine promote production of antibody-specific immunity for each type. Antibody levels remain protective for at least 5 years after immunization. It is recommended for adults, particularly those over 50 years of age.

Dosage:
Adults and children over 2 years: (IM) 0.5 mL.

pneumococcal 7-valent conjugate vaccine (Prevnar). This agent is used for the active immunization of infants and toddlers against invasive disease caused by *Streptococcus pneumoniae*. It is recommended for administration at 2, 4, 6, and 12 to 15 months of age. This agent is NOT to be used for adult populations. It is NOT to be substituted for the pneumococcal polysaccharide vaccine in geriatric populations. It has been noted that not all individuals establish immunity after administration of this vaccine.

Dosage:
Children only: (IM) 0.5 mL per schedule in Figure 30–1.

AGENTS THAT PROVIDE PASSIVE IMMUNITY

Various preparations of antibodies are available to provide a short-lived but immediately effective protection or prophylaxis against disease.

diphtheria antitoxin, USP, BP
Dosage:
Adults: (IM) Prophylactic: 10,000 units. (IM, IV) Therapeutic: 10,000 to 200,000 units.

tetanus antitoxin, USP, BP (Equine Antitoxin)
Dosage:
Adults: (IM, subQ) Prophylactic: 3000 to 10,000 units. (IV) Therapeutic: 40,000 to 100,000 units.

tetanus immune human globulin, USP, BP
Dosage:
Adults: (IM) Prophylactic: 250 units. (IM) Therapeutic: 300 to 600 units.

botulism antitoxin, USP, BP
Dosage:
Adults: (IV) 1 mL (1000 units) in diluted solution 1:10 with 10% glucose solution injected slowly over 5 minutes. Subsequent dosage administration based on individual requirements.

pertussis immune human globulin, USP, BP
Dosage:
Adults: (IM) Prophylactic: 1.25 to 2.5 mL, repeated in 1 to 2 weeks. (IM) Therapeutic: 1.25 mL every 24 to 48 hours.

mumps immune human globulin, USP, BP
Dosage:
Adults: (IM) Prophylactic: 3 to 4.5 mL. (IM) Therapeutic: 15 to 20 mL.

immune human serum globulin, USP, BP
Dosage:
Adults: (IM) Prophylactic: 1.3 to 2 mL/kg every 6 to 8 weeks. (IM) Therapeutic: For dysgammaglobulinemia therapy, 20 to 50 mL monthly.

hepatitis B immune globulin
Dosage:
Adults: (IM) 0.06 mL/kg within 7 days of exposure.

Rh$_o$(D) immune human globulin, USP (RhoGAM). This antibody preparation is used to desensitize Rh-negative mothers after delivery of an Rh-positive infant. The sensitization of the mother occurs when infant blood cells enter the mother's bloodstream, thus causing antibody formation, which then causes erythroblastosis fetalis in subsequent Rh-positive infants that she may carry.

When administered within 72 hours of delivery, the immune globulin diminishes antibody formation in the mother.

Slight temperature elevations and mild local reactions at the site of injection may occur after administration.

Dosage:
Adults: (IM) 2 mL.

IMMUNOSUPPRESSIVE AGENTS

The immune system has its origins in the fetal thymus gland. A process occurs during intrauterine life whereby the infant recognizes certain substances and tissues as its own and develops two types of lymphoid cells, the T cells and the B cells, which are activated to recognize and destroy foreign substances and tissues.

With the development of technology for organ transplants, the body's attempts to reject foreign tissue had to be prevented. A great deal of improvement has occurred in the matching of tissue samples to provide the person receiving a transplant with an organ that matches his or her own tissues as closely as possible. This process, similar to but much more complex than typing blood, has improved the outcome of organ transplants, but **immunosuppressives,** agents that interfere with the development of antibody response to a foreign substance, are also needed to prevent organ rejection.

General complications of the immunosuppressives include increased susceptibility to infections and potentially fatal adverse effects when otherwise minor illnesses such as chickenpox are contracted. Central nervous system toxicity may be observed, and symptoms include dizziness, headache, confusion, slurred speech, and paresthesias. Jaundice from liver damage and symptoms of bone marrow suppression, such as sore throat, oral mucosal lesions, and excessive bruising, may also occur. Immunosuppressed patients may contract poliomyelitis from the live virus shed by infants after oral administration of live poliovirus vaccine. Family members of immunocompromised patients are generally administered the inactivated or Salk vaccine for this reason.

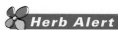 **Herb Alert**

Echinacea

Echinacea is taken to prevent or reduce the severity of colds. Echinacea reduces the effects of immunosuppressants, cyclosporine, and azathioprine. It should be avoided in patients with autoimmune disorders and multiple sclerosis. See Chapter 35 for more information on echinacea.

THE CORTICOSTEROIDS

The synthetic corticosteroids prednisone, prednisolone, and dexamethasone are used most often for immunosuppression. Side effects specific to this group include salt and water retention, with the characteristic moon facies and fat distribution noted as the administration is prolonged.

Prednisone and prednisolone
  Dosage:
    Adults: (Oral) 10 to 100 mg daily in divided doses.

Dexamethasone
  Dosage:
    Adults: (Oral) 0.75 to 9 mg daily in divided doses.
    Children: (Oral) 0.3 mg/kg daily in divided doses.

OTHER IMMUNOSUPPRESSIVE AGENTS

azathioprine, USP, BP (Imuran). Because of its similarity to the naturally occurring purines, this agent acts as an antagonist to RNA and DNA synthesis, thus interfering with cell metabolism.

This agent is primarily used in the treatment of renal transplant patients to prevent rejection. It is occasionally used in the treatment of other autoimmune disorders such as systemic lupus erythematosus, hemolytic anemias, and idiopathic thrombocytopenia.

Liver damage, increased susceptibility to infection, and bone marrow suppression are the most common side effects of this agent.

  Dosage:
    Adults and children: (Oral) 3 to 5 mg/kg daily initially, then 1 to 2 mg/kg daily as a maintenance dosage.

lymphocytic immune globulin, antithymocyte globulin (ATG, Atgam). This agent exhibits immunosuppressive activity and is used for the prevention or treatment of kidney transplant rejections. In addition it is used for the treatment of aplastic anemia and for the prevention of graft-versus-host disease following bone marrow transplant. Many adverse effects have been reported during therapy with this agent. They include fever, chills, leukopenia, thrombocytopenia, serum sickness, anaphylaxis, and infectious complications due to the immunosuppression.

  Dosage:
    Adults: (IV) 10 to 30 mg/kg/day.
    Children: (IV) 5 to 25 mg/kg/day.

tacrolimus (Prograf). This agent can be used orally or IV for its immunosuppressive effect. It is used to prevent rejection of kidney transplants, generally in combination with other agents. Side effects include nephrotoxicity, neurotoxicity, insomnia, paresthesias, and psychological disorders.

  Dosage:
    Adults only: (Oral or IV) 0.03 to 0.05 mg/kg/day.

cyclophosphamide, USP, BP (Cytoxan). By interfering with DNA and RNA activities, this agent disrupts cellular function and destroys multiplying lymph cells. It is used to treat autoimmune disorders, such as systemic lupus erythematosus, rheumatoid arthritis, and the nephrotic syndrome and to prevent organ transplant rejection. Cyclophosphamide is also covered in Chapter 29 in its role as an antineoplastic agent.

  Dosage:
    Adults and children: (Oral and IV) 1 to 5 mg/kg daily.

cyclosporine. This agent acts primarily against the T lymphocytes and inhibits the factors that stimulate T-lymphocyte growth. For this reason it is used to prevent rejection of organ and bone marrow transplants. Other uses include the treatment of rheumatoid arthritis, psoriasis, and other conditions that have an immunologic basis. Administration of this drug with grapefruit juice apparently causes decreased serum clearance of cyclosporine, thus raising the serum levels of the drug. Bioavailability has been increased by as much as 20% to 200% in various studies of this effect.

  Dosage:
    Adults and children: (Oral) 10 to 25 mg/kg daily.
    The dosage varies widely based on its use.

interferon beta (Betaseron). Interferons are species-specific proteins that possess complex antiviral, antineoplastic, and immunomodulating activities. This agent is used to treat multiple sclerosis and is believed to act principally by inhibiting the production of interferon gamma, thought to be involved in the increase in severity of the disease. Current evidence suggests that the frequency and severity of relapses is statistically lower in the treated patients than in controls.

Dosage:

Adults: (subQ) 0.25 mg every other day, with rotation of injection sites.

CLINICAL IMPLICATIONS

1. The nurse should be familiar with the childhood and adult diseases now prevented by the routine immunizations. All health care workers should be familiar with both childhood and adult immunization schedules.
2. The nurse has an effective role in promoting adherence to routine infant immunization.
3. When administering immunizations, the nurse should shake the vial carefully before withdrawing the required dose.
4. All biologic agents have an expiration date; this should be checked before administration of the vaccine.
5. Immunizations are often withheld when the patient is receiving corticosteroids or antineoplastic agents. In some cases immunization is deferred when close family members are immunologically compromised.
6. Before administration of a biologic vaccine from an animal source, the patient should be closely questioned for allergic reactions.
7. The patient should be counseled about expected side effects of the vaccines (i.e., pain, erythema, and swelling at the site of injection and a fever that may last for 24 to 48 hours).
8. When patients are receiving immunosuppressive medications, they should be observed for side effects such as fever, sore throat, bone marrow suppression, and bleeding disorders.
9. Oral hygiene should be maintained when a patient is receiving immunosuppressives. Lemon-glycerin swabs may be used in lieu of vigorous tooth brushing to prevent gingival bleeding.
10. Signs of renal toxicity in a patient receiving immunosuppressives should be observed; these include dark urine, decreased urine output, and peripheral edema.
11. Liver damage as a side effect of the immunosuppressives is manifested by jaundice, dark urine, clay-colored stools, and abdominal pain or swelling.
12. The patient should be observed for signs of skin rashes or petechiae when receiving immunosuppressives.
13. Foods such as grapefruit juice enhance the activity of certain drugs.

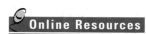 **Online Resources**

For updated drug information and Web activities, go to http://evolve.elsevier.com/Asperheim.

CRITICAL THINKING QUESTIONS

1. Your neighbor, who is the proud parent of a 1-month-old daughter, is confused by what she hears of the dangerous effects of the "baby shots." She wants your honest opinion as to whether these are really necessary. How would you respond?

2. The patient is alarmed and dismayed at the fat face she now has after her kidney transplant. She is being treated with Imuran and prednisolone. How would you discuss this problem with her?

3. The patient has never had a tetanus injection or any other childhood immunizations. He has just sustained deep lacerations after a fall off his tractor. How do you think tetanus immunity would be best attained?

4. The patient will be traveling extensively in the Middle East and will be doing missionary work in small villages in India. He wants to know where to check for required immunizations. Where would he go in your community? Which of the vaccines discussed in this chapter would be beneficial, even if not required?

REVIEW QUESTIONS

1. Active immunity is produced when:
   a. the previously formed antibodies are injected into the body.
   b. the antigen is injected into the body and natural antibodies are formed.
   c. the person is exposed to a disease.
   d. an antiserum is injected.

2. Passive immunity is produced when:
   a. a live virus vaccine is injected.
   b. a killed virus vaccine is injected.
   c. an antitoxin is injected.
   d. a toxin is injected.

REVIEW QUESTIONS—cont'd

3. Which vaccine must be administered every year?

   a. tetanus toxoid
   b. diphtheria and tetanus toxoids and acellular pertussis
   c. influenza vaccine
   d. pneumonia vaccine

4. Which gland is responsible for the infant's immune system?

   a. thyroid
   b. thymus
   c. parathyroid
   d. adrenal glands

5. An example of an immunosuppressive agent is:

   a. hepatitis B immune globulin.
   b. tetanus antitoxin.
   c. diphtheria antitoxin.
   d. prednisone.

6. An agent that may be used to prevent rejection of kidney transplants is:

   a. RhoGAM.
   b. Energix-B.
   c. tacrolimus.
   d. lymphocytic live vaccine.

7. Adults should get periodic injections of all except:

   a. influenza vaccine.
   b. pneumococcal vaccine.
   c. polio vaccine.
   d. tetanus toxoid.

8. An agent that may be used to treat multiple sclerosis is:

   a. cyclophosphamide.
   b. interferon beta.
   c. tacrolimus.
   d. azathioprine.

9. Varicella is another word for:

   a. chickenpox.
   b. smallpox.
   c. rubella.
   d. rubeola.

10. A serious side effect of the immunosuppressives is:

    a. an increased susceptibility to infections.
    b. increased blood coagulation.
    c. rejection of foreign tissues.
    d. increased antibody formation.

After completing this chapter, you should be able to do the following:

1. Begin to understand the genetic basis of many diseases.
2. Obtain an overview of the methods used in gene therapy.
3. Become familiar with the terms used in gene therapy.
4. Have an understanding of the various mechanisms of action of the genetically engineered drugs.
5. Understand the role of the health care worker in recognizing the serious side effects of these very potent agents.

Key Terms

Double helix, p. 194
Deoxyribonucleic acid (DNA), p. 194
Gene therapy, p. 194
Genome (JĒ-nōm), p. 194
Monoclonal (MŎN-ē-KLŌ-něl) **antibody,** p. 195
Oncogene (ŎNG-kō-jēn), p. 196
Stem cells, p. 194
Vector, p. 194

In 1953, Watson and Crick discovered a component of genes called **deoxyribonucleic acid (DNA)** and changed biology forever. Only four bases—adenine, guanine, cytosine and thymine—make up DNA in a twin-coil structure, or **double helix** (Fig. 31–1). Since this discovery, tremendous advancements have been made in our understanding of heredity (the genetic transfer of traits from parents to offspring), and at last the composition of the entire human **genome** (the complete set of chromosomes) has been determined. We now have a very limited understanding of the workings of inheritance (the acquisition of traits or conditions through heredity), both good and bad. The challenge of transferring these novel discoveries to the bedside is just beginning. Medicine undoubtedly will undergo an enormous change in the coming years, with the goal of individualizing treatment based on the human genome.

THE GENETIC BASIS OF DISEASE

By understanding the genetic basis of disease, researchers can hope to develop predictive tests for the disease. If a diagnosis is made before the disease becomes apparent, treatment may be started early and the disease prevented or at least treated more effectively.

The development of breast cancer in women with the *BRCA1* I and *BRCA2* II genes, and the existence of the Philadelphia chromosome as a marker for chronic myelogenous leukemia are now well known, and there are various steps that can be taken to avoid development of these diseases or at least treat them with early intervention. Other diseases with a confirmed genetic cause include cystic fibrosis, Huntington's disease, Alzheimer's disease, diabetes, hypertension, asthma, obesity, and certain heart disorders.

GENE THERAPY

The term **gene therapy** can be defined as the application of genetic principles to the treatment of human disease. The earliest predecessor to gene therapy was the development and use of vaccines. A vaccine works at the cellular level and produces a long-term change in the body's recognition of and response to infection.

Certain diseases occur because the body does not make a necessary substance, such as insulin or blood-clotting factors. If we can place the faulty or missing gene that manufactures these substances within a cell, the body then could manufacture its own missing protein. Gene therapy in this instance would have as its goal the permanent placement of the missing gene within the body's cells.

Viruses are known to invade the body's cells and transfer their genetic material for further manufacture by the cell, so one approach to this gene transfer is the use of viral **vectors,** or carriers. The use of nonviral vectors is also under study.

STEM CELLS

Stem cells are primitive cells that have the potential to develop into any of the tissues of the body. They can be harvested from human embryos, from umbilical cords, from shed baby teeth, and in small numbers from peripheral blood. When implanted, they would manufacture a missing substance or create new tissue cells to replace damaged tissue. Research on the implantation of stem cells in the brains of patients with Parkinson's disease is now in its early stages. Stem cells are also used in bone marrow transplants to treat

DNA

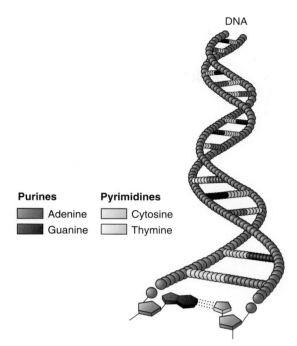

Purines
■ Adenine
■ Guanine

Pyrimidines
□ Cytosine
□ Thymine

FIGURE 31-1 The double helix structure of DNA.

various disorders. Continuing research will provide many developments in this field.

MONOCLONAL ANTIBODIES

Humans and animals have the ability to make antibodies that recognize and bind to virtually any antigen. Antibodies have been discussed previously in this text in their application as immunizing agents to protect against diseases (see Chapter 29). Human antibodies made in response to vaccines or in response to a disease or other antigen are often polyclonal, that is, they attach to many different receptors on the antigen.

A **monoclonal antibody** will attach only to one specific site or receptor; thus it may have more use in the treatment of specific disorders. In order to manufacture a monoclonal antibody, mice are immunized with the desired antigen, and then spleen cells from the mice are used in a complicated procedure to produce the specific desired monoclonal antibodies from human myeloma cells.

One problem with this technique has been that the mouse antibodies are seen as foreign and often the human patients mount an immune response against them, producing human antimouse antibody (HAMA). Not only does this cause the therapeutic antibodies to be quickly eliminated, but the immune complexes that form can cause damage to the kidneys.

Two approaches have been used in an attempt to reduce the problem of the HAMA response:

1. *Chimeric antibodies*—using genetic engineering, the antigen-binding part of the mouse antibody is fused to the part of a human antibody that controls its function. Infliximab and abciximab are examples.
2. *Humanized antibodies*—the mouse amino acids responsible for making the antigen binding site are inserted into a human antibody molecule. Daclizumab, rituximab, Vitaxin, gemtuzumab, trastuzumab, and omalizumab are examples.

Monoclonal antibodies are used therapeutically in several ways:

1. To suppress the immune system.
2. To treat various types of cancer.
3. As angiogenesis inhibitors to prevent tumors from getting an adequate blood supply.
4. As agents with variable modes of action against disease processes.

AGENTS USED TO SUPPRESS THE IMMUNE SYSTEM

daclizumab (Zenapax). This antibody binds specifically to a site on the surface of lymphocytes. It is used to prevent acute rejection of transplanted kidneys. It is often used as part of an immunosuppressive regimen that includes cyclosporine and corticosteroids. Adverse reactions are generally mild, occurring in less than 5% of the patients, and include gastritis, renal insufficiency, nausea, diarrhea, and headache. There is a precaution with this agent, because it is not known if this drug will have a long-term effect on the ability of the body to react normally to an antigen first encountered after the patient has begun receiving daclizumab therapy.

Dosage:
Adults: (IV) 1.0 mg/kg, diluted. The standard therapy is 5 doses, the first given no more than 24 hours before transplantation, the others at 14-day intervals.

infliximab (Remicade). Infliximab binds specifically to human tumor necrosis factor-alpha (TNFa). Elevated levels of TNFa have been found in the joints of rheumatoid arthritis patients and the stools of Crohn's disease patients. In rheumatoid arthritis, treatment with infliximab reduced passage of the inflammatory cells into joints. In Crohn's disease there is a reduction in passage of inflammatory cells in the intestine. After treatment these patients had decreased levels of C-reactive protein and other inflammatory proteins. Adverse reactions include infusion-related reactions of dyspnea, flushing, headache, and rash. Anaphylactic reactions have occurred, including laryngeal edema, severe bronchospasm, and seizures.

Dosage:
Adults: (IV) 3 to 5 mg/kg as an infusion, repeated in 2 to 6 weeks.

etanercept (Enbrel). By binding to tumor necrosis factor, this agent has shown promise in the treatment of rheumatoid arthritis. It is used to reduce signs and symptoms and inhibit progression of structural damage in patients with severe rheumatoid arthritis, psoriatic arthritis, and juvenile rheumatoid arthritis. It can be used in combination with methotrexate in patients who did not adequately respond to methotrexate alone. Glucocorticoids, nonsteroidal antiinflammatory drugs, or analgesics may be continued during treatment. Adverse reactions include sepsis, allergic reactions, aplastic anemia, and neurologic disorders such as transverse myelitis, demyelinating diseases, and seizures.

> **Dosage:**
> Adults: (subQ) 25 mg given twice weekly 72 to 96 hours apart.
> Children 4 to 17 years: (subQ) 0.4 mg/kg (up to 25 mg) twice weekly 72 to 96 hours apart.

adalimumab (Humira). Also used in the treatment of rheumatoid arthritis, this agent is similar to etanercept in actions and adverse reactions.

> **Dosage:**
> Adults: (subQ) 40 mg every other week.
> Children: No standard dosage is established.

omalizumab (Xolair). This agent is used in moderate to severe asthma to control symptoms in patients who do not respond to corticosteroids. It binds to immunoglobulin E (IgE), thus preventing the IgE from binding to mast cells. Adverse reactions include headache, sinusitis, anaphylaxis, and a possibility of malignant neoplasms.

> **Dosage:**
> Adults and children over 12 years: (subQ) 150 to 375 mg every 2 to 4 weeks.

AGENT IN DEVELOPMENT

Another immunosuppressive agent is in development, but full prescribing information is not available yet.

natalizumab (Antegren). Natalizumab has shown promise in the treatment of multiple sclerosis as well as Crohn's disease.

AGENTS USED TO TREAT CANCER

Viruses have been associated with cancers in animals for many years. Epstein-Barr virus has been accepted as a cause of lymphomas and certain carcinomas. It can be confusing to realize that many people are infected with a virus, but few develop the associated cancers. This pattern of individual immunity to infections as well as malignant diseases is well known but poorly understood. Eliminating or successfully treating cancers caused by viruses with antiviral therapies is a goal that has not yet been achieved.

It is now abundantly clear that genetic mutations, whether they are inherited or, as is more common, they appear in cells of various tissues later in life, can cause cancer. These mutations abnormally enhance the function of genes that may promote malignant processes when activated (the **oncogenes**) or cause other genes that may interfere with the growth of malignant cells (the tumor-suppressor genes) to lose function. There is continuing evidence of abnormal

silencing of genes in cancer cells, and much research is aimed at understanding and working with this process. The aim is to bring the treatment of cancer to a cellular level, rather than just blindly targeting cancer cells, which are known to be the "fast-growing" cells, while trying to spare "normal" cells, which has been the purpose of many of the earlier cancer drugs.

Treatment using these newer agents is generally more specific to a certain type of cancer than is the case with the other classes of antineoplastic agents.

aldesleukin (Proleukin). A biosynthetic agent of recombinant DNA origin, this agent can be used in the treatment of several types of cancer, including renal cell cancer and melanoma. It possesses complex antineoplastic and immunomodulating properties. Adverse effects include renal and hepatic toxicity and cardiovascular effects.

> **Dosage:**
> Adults only: (IV) 600,000 units/kg every 8 hours for 14 days.

alemtuzumab (Campath). A DNA-derived monoclonal antibody, this drug is used in the treatment of chronic lymphocytic leukemia. It binds to CD22, a molecule found on white blood cells. Adverse effects include immunosuppressive complications, including lymphopenia and infection.

> **Dosage:**
> Adults only: (IV) 3 mg daily.

rituximab (Rituxan). Rituximab binds to the CD20 molecule found on most beta cells and is used to treat beta cell non-Hodgkin's lymphomas. Adverse reactions include infusion reactions that in some cases have resulted in death within 24 hours. Infusion reactions can include hypoxia, myocardial infarction, cardiogenic shock, and acute respiratory distress syndrome. Approximately 80% of the infusion reactions occur with the first infusion.

> **Dosage:**
> Adults: (IV) 375 mg/m^2 as an infusion once weekly for 4 weeks.

trastuzumab (Herceptin). Trastuzumab is the first monoclonal antibody that is effective against solid tumors. It binds to HER2, a receptor for epidermal growth factor (EGF) that is found on some tumor cells (some breast cancers and some lymphomas). Adverse effects include the development of left ventricular dysfunction and congestive heart failure. Left ventricular function should be evaluated prior to treatment.

> **Dosage:**
> Adults: (IV) 4 mg/kg as a 90-minute infusion, repeated weekly as 2 mg/kg per infusion.

gemtuzumab ozogamicin (Mylotarg). This monoclonal antibody binds CD33, a cell-surface molecule found on the cancerous cells in acute myelogenous leukemia. CD33 is not found on stem cells or nonhematopoietic cells. It should be used alone, not combined with other agents. Adverse effects include hypersensitivity reactions of chills, fever, nausea, hepatotoxicity, and respiratory distress syndrome. In most cases the hypersensitivity reactions occur during the transfusion or within 24 hours after the transfusion.

> **Dosage:**
> Adults: (IV) 9 mg/m^2 administered as a 2-hour infusion. A second dose may be given in 14 days.

denileukin diftitox (Ontak). This agent is a recombinant DNA–derived cytotoxic protein related to diphtheria toxin. It is used to treat T-cell lymphoma. Adverse effects include hypersensitivity reactions, hypotension due to vascular leak syndrome, and a predisposition to infections.

> **Dosage:**
> Adults: (IV) 9 to 18 mcg/kg/day.

ibritumomab tiuxetan (Zevalin). This agent is used in combination with rituximab to treat refractory non-Hodgkin's lymphoma. It is supplied as a kit with instructions for use. Adverse effects include infusion reactions, thrombocytopenia, hemorrhage, and infections.

> **Dosage:**
> Adults: (IV) 250 mg as an infusion, repeated in 7 days.

AGENTS IN DEVELOPMENT

The following antineoplastic agents are in development, and full prescribing information is not available at this time.

LymphoCide—binds to CD22, a molecule found on some B-cell leukemia cells.

Lym-1 (Oncolym)—binds to an HLA-DR–encoded histocompatibility antigen that can be expressed on lymphoma cells.

cetuximab (Erbitux)—blocks HER1, another EGF receptor. It is used in the treatment of breast cancers and certain lymphomas.

ANGIOGENESIS INHIBITORS

These agents act to prevent the tumor from getting an adequate blood supply, thus starving it of essential nutrients for further growth. These agents are in development; full prescribing information is not available at this time.

Vitaxin—binds to a vascular integrin found on the blood vessels of tumors but not on the blood vessels supplying normal tissues. It has shown some promise in shrinking solid tumors without harmful effects.

bevacizumab (Avastin)—blocks the vascular endothelial growth factor receptor.

MISCELLANEOUS AGENTS

abciximab (ReoPro). This agent binds to the glycoprotein receptor of human platelets and prevents clumping of the platelets. It is helpful in preventing the recurrent obstruction of coronary arteries in patients after angioplasty. The risk of bleeding is increased with the use of this drug, particularly in the presence of anticoagulants.

> **Dosage:**
> Adults: (IV) 0.25-mg/kg bolus followed by an infusion of 125 mcg/kg/min over 12 hours.

CLINICAL IMPLICATIONS

1. When the immune system is suppressed, the patient is susceptible to many common infections. The patient should be cautioned against exposure to infected individuals.
2. Live virus vaccines administered in childhood, such as the measles, mumps, and rubella vaccine and the varicella vaccine, are potential sources of infection for an immunosuppressed patient, because live virus may be shed by the child for some time after administration of the vaccine.
3. There should be general recommendations by the health care worker to encourage the patient to continue good lifestyle habits, with regular exercise, good nutrition, and a positive outlook on life.
4. Serious adverse effects occur during and after administration of many of these agents. The health care worker should become familiar with the adverse effects and prepare to report them as soon as possible.
5. There are many other drugs and herbal products that react adversely with these drugs. A careful prescription drug and over-the-counter drug history should be taken. The patient should be advised against taking any drug or herb without knowledge of the practitioner.
6. Expiration dates should be carefully checked on these agents, as well as recommendations for storage (i.e., in a refrigerator, in a freezer, or at room temperature).
7. Patients should be observed frequently for skin rashes, signs of bleeding, or other untoward effects. They should be discreetly questioned about their own observations of side effects.
8. The use of lemon-glycerin swabs is helpful in maintaining oral hygiene.
9. Many drug programs are sponsored by the pharmaceutical manufacturers for the administration of these agents to indigent or uninsured patients. The patient may need assistance in obtaining this information.
10. The older patient may be more susceptible to the adverse effects of these agents than the younger individual.

Online Resources

For updated drug information and Web activities, go to
http://evolve.elsevier.com/Asperheim.

CRITICAL THINKING QUESTIONS

1. The patient presents for his monthly infusion of infliximab (Remicade). In the general conversation he reports that he has been to his dermatologist twice in the past month for his persistent skin rash, which he attributes to eating a lot of seafood lately. What advice may be given to him?

2. The patient has been on ibuprofen for over a year for the self-treatment of his rheumatoid arthritis. He is now going to begin treatment with etanercept (Enbrel). He wants to know if he has to stop his ibuprofen. How would you respond? He then admits he takes Darvocet-N from another doctor, and is a great believer in herbal therapies. Should he stop these?

3. The patient is receiving daclizumab (Zenapax). He had a mild headache after the last treatment, as well as some nausea. He wants to know if this means he can't take this drug any more. How would you respond?

REVIEW QUESTIONS

1. The human gene is composed of:
   a. DNA strands.
   b. a genome.
   c. an oncogene.
   d. transfer RNA.

2. A monoclonal antibody is:
   a. the cause of genetic diseases.
   b. a curative agent for genetic diseases.
   c. a specific antibody that binds to one receptor only.
   d. more heterogeneous than a polyclonal antibody.

3. An agent that is used to treat rheumatoid arthritis is:
   a. aldesleukin.
   b. omalizumab.
   c. infliximab.
   d. Vitaxin.

4. An angiogenesis inhibitor works by:
   a. increasing blood flow to any body part.
   b. reducing the size of the aorta.
   c. stopping antibody reproduction.
   d. preventing the tumor from getting an adequate blood supply.

5. Gene therapy means:
   a. using genetic knowledge to treat human diseases.
   b. giving genes by transplant.
   c. increasing the DNA in cells.
   d. suppressing all genomes.

6. Gene transfer into humans or animals can be made by:
   a. oral agents.
   b. viral vectors.
   c. insect vectors.
   d. combining cell nuclei.

7. An adverse reaction to daclizumab may be:
   a. hypertension.
   b. hypotension.
   c. gastritis.
   d. increased urine output.

8. Aldesleukin is used in the treatment of:
   a. melanoma.
   b. leukemia.
   c. lymphoma.
   d. brain neoplasms.

9. Vitaxin is an example of a(an):
   a. viral vector.
   b. monoclonal antibody.
   c. angiogenesis inhibitor.
   d. antiplatelet agent.

10. Stem cells are:
   a. cells found in the stems of plants.
   b. cells found in the nucleus.
   c. specialized cells in the brain.
   d. cells that are can develop into any tissue.

CHAPTER

32 Drug Therapy in Older Adults

Objectives

After completing this chapter, you should be able to do the following:

1. Define specific health problems seen in older adults.
2. Become aware of the differences in drug metabolism in older adults.
3. Become aware of nutritional problems in older adults and their solutions.
4. Recognize health problems in older adults, such as hypothyroidism, that may be confused with senility.
5. Recognize structural changes in the aging body, particularly those of the bone and connective tissue.
6. Recognize and assist in the solution of social problems when older adults are cared for in the home or a nursing facility.
7. Be aware that standard adult doses of many drugs may produce symptoms of a toxic overdose in the older adult.
8. Be aware that many drug interactions and toxic effects are caused by the addition of drugs and herbal remedies that the older patient buys at the drugstore.
9. Recognize that complicated drug schedules are often the reason for noncompliance in older adult patients.

Key Terms

Dementia (dĭ-MĔN-shě), p. 204
Geriatric (JĔR-ē-ĂT-rĭk), p. 199
Metabolism (mě-TĂB-ē-LĬZ-ěm), p. 200

About 6% of the world's population is 65 years of age or older. In the United States, about 35 million people, or 13% of the total population, are in this age group. By the year 2030, an estimated 70 million persons, or about 20% of the population, will be 65 or older. As a result, **geriatric** medicine, or therapy for the aged, has emerged as a vital and necessary health care discipline. The American Geriatrics Society has been formed to increase the number of health professionals trained in geriatrics and to expand and implement geriatric education and training for physicians, nurses, allied health personnel, and the general public.

Adults 65 years and older consume one third of all medications, and most take multiple prescribed and over-the-counter (OTC) drugs. Age-related physiologic changes and the presence of underlying disease, coupled with inappropriate prescribing and polypharmacy (the use of a number of different drugs), may predispose older patients to adverse drug reactions and drug-drug, drug-disease, or drug-food interactions (Box 32–1). To further confuse the problem, many older adults have several physicians for their many health problems, and this also accounts for many drug reactions.

One of the most important advances in the last few years has been the greater attention paid to what distinguishes the effects of aging from other influences on the health of older adults that may be modified or helped in some way. For example, disease conditions that some people acquire and some do not, environmental changes, and lifestyle factors such as diet, use of alcohol or drugs, smoking, and exercise all have an impact on a person's health status.

A great deal of interest is focused in the areas of health promotion, disease prevention, and maintenance of good health and maximum independence as long as possible throughout the life span. Interactions of the older adult with society should be productive, satisfying, and rewarding for all involved.

This chapter is designed to promote thinking about the treatment of the older adult and to address some specific problems seen in this group of patients.

DRUG THERAPY IN OLDER ADULTS

Appropriate and effective drug therapy for older adult patients presents many challenges. Five points should be kept in mind when prescribing drugs for the older adult:

1. *Obtain an accurate history.* Each patient should carry a list of current medications, or even better, should bring all medicine bottles to each visit. This should include any OTC drugs the patient uses. Similar or interacting drugs may be prescribed by different doctors, or the patient may still be continuing to take a drug that is no longer necessary.
2. *Dosages may need to be adjusted.* The usual adult dosage is based on the amount of drug needed for a healthy 150-pound man. Age-related disorders may require a dosage that is 25% to 50% of the usual adult dosage. The gastrointestinal tract may not have the "average" pH due to deficient acid production, the gastric emptying time may be slowed, and the gastric blood flow may be

Box 32-1 *Examples of Common Drug Interactions in Older Adults*

DRUG-DRUG INTERACTIONS

digoxin and thiazide diuretics (hypokalemia causes digoxin toxicity)

cimetidine and warfarin (warfarin is potentiated)

cimetidine and phenytoin (phenytoin blood level is increased)

quinolone antibiotics and warfarin (warfarin is potentiated)

NSAIDs and diuretics (decreased effectiveness of diuretics)

NSAIDs and aspirin (increased erosion of stomach lining)

ACE inhibitors and potassium-sparing diuretics (hyperkalemia)

warfarin and aspirin or NSAIDs (increased action of warfarin)

Increased use of fiber or bulk laxatives (inhibits absorption of any drug)

Antacid use (may inhibit absorption of many medications)

phenytoin and magnesium-based antacids (decreased absorption of phenytoin)

DRUG-FOOD INTERACTIONS

carbidopa/levodopa and food protein (decreased absorption of drug)

cyclosporine and grapefruit juice (increased serum level of cyclosporine)

tetracycline and dairy products (decreased absorption of tetracycline)

quinolone antibiotics and dairy products (decreased absorption of drugs)

monoamine oxidase inhibitors and wine or cheese (causes severe hypertension)

Sedatives and alcohol (increased sedation)

warfarin and psyllium (decreased absorption and decreased effectiveness of warfarin)

warfarin and vitamin E (increased effectiveness of warfarin)

iron tablets and tea, bran, or eggs (decreased absorption of iron)

DRUG-DISEASE INTERACTIONS

Anticholinergic agents (urinary retention)

Beta-blockers (worsen asthma)

ACE, Angiotensin-converting enzyme; *NSAIDs,* nonsteroidal antiinflammatory drugs.

deficient. The distribution of a drug depends on body composition (amounts of lipid, water, and lean body mass), and these obviously change with age. Decreased levels of albumin resulting from suboptimal nutrition affect the binding and distribution of drugs. Drug **metabolism** (that is, the sum of chemical changes that occur as a drug is processed) in the liver depends on blood flow and the enzyme system; both may be altered.

Age-related declines in renal function affect drug elimination from the body.

3. *Be vigilant about drug interactions.* It is not possible to remember every drug interaction, and new interactions are discovered frequently. Drug interactions should be checked for every drug combination. Drugs that have frequent interactions and are commonly used in older adults include coumadin, sedatives, antibiotics, and nonsteroidal antiinflammatory drugs (NSAIDs) (see Box 32–1 for more interactions).

4. *Consider drug costs.* On average, older adults take 4.5 prescription drugs and 2.1 nonprescription medications. Generic medications and less expensive alternatives should be used whenever possible.

5. *Discontinue drugs whenever possible.* Older people tend to hoard drugs and resist change in their medications, but an effort should be made to make the drug therapy as efficient as possible, reducing the number of medications taken.

Medication compliance is also a factor that must be considered. If the patient has several different drugs that must be taken on different schedules—for example, one taken before meals, one that must be taken 2 hours after meals, one taken four times a day, one taken three times a day, and so on—there are bound to be mistakes or forgotten doses. The regimen should be simplified whenever possible with once-a-day drugs. Alternate-day therapy should be avoided if possible. Most importantly, the regimen must be reviewed at each visit and revised as needed. Medications that can be taken together should be reviewed and explained. The daily or weekly pillbox should be recommended and explained.

The patient must be counseled about illness and medications. Should they take certain medications if they are nauseated and not eating? Insulin dosage needs to be adjusted as illnesses occur.

The patient's overall situation should be periodically assessed. Older adults often have many and chronic illnesses. Diminished liver or kidney function dramatically changes the effects of drug therapy. Changes in the patient's mental function, hearing, and vision must be evaluated periodically. The health care worker should not be hasty in attributing a new disability to "normal aging," when it may in fact be a drug-induced effect (Box 32–2). All prescription bottles should be easy to open. The patient must be able to read the labels on the bottles. A cursory examination should also be made to make sure the patient is actually able to read.

Box 32–3 lists several factors that contribute to noncompliance in older adults.

NUTRITION IN OLDER ADULTS

The older adult who is still in his or her home often becomes malnourished because of inattention or inability to obtain a sufficient supply of fresh food for a balanced diet. Depression and isolation are common problems that seem to increase as the patient ages, and they are accompanied by

Box 32-2 *Medications That Contribute to Cognitive Impairment in Older Adults*

ANALGESICS

codeine
meperidine
morphine
NSAIDs
pentazocine
propoxyphene

ANTIHISTAMINES

diphenhydramine
hydroxyzine

ANTIHYPERTENSIVE AGENTS

clonidine
diuretics
hydralazine
methyldopa
propranolol

ANTIMICROBIALS

gentamicin
isoniazid

ANTIPARKINSON AGENTS

amantadine
bromocriptine
carbidopa/levodopa

CARDIOVASCULAR DRUGS

atropine
digoxin
lidocaine
quinidine

HYPOGLYCEMICS

sulfonylureas

PSYCHOTROPICS

barbiturates
benzodiazepines
chlorpromazine
haloperidol
lithium
risperidone
SSRI antidepressants
tricyclic antidepressants

MISCELLANEOUS

cimetidine
corticosteroids
phenytoin

NSAIDs, Nonsteroidal antiinflammatory drugs; *SSRI,* selective serotonin reuptake inhibitor.

a decreased ability for and interest in self-care and nutrition. Social programs, such as Meals-on-Wheels, have improved the lives of these patients because they address both their isolation and their nutrition inadequacies.

Box 32-3 *Contributors to Noncompliance in Older Adults*

Complex treatment and dosing regimens
High cost of drugs
Inadequate understanding of therapy
Physical disability (e.g., dysphagia)
Medication side effects
Cognitive impairment
Inability to read drug label due to visual problems
Poor communication

Poorly fitting dentures or missing teeth create mechanical problems in chewing food. Dental needs may have to be addressed before nutrition deficits can be improved.

Many patients are on modified diets (e.g., a bland diet for ulcers, a low-fat or low-sodium diet, or a low-purine diet for the prevention of gout). Often older adults do not comprehend the instructions or simply do not know what they *can* eat. Patients then often restrict their diets so much that they lose weight and become malnourished. Vitamin and mineral supplements are very beneficial, but they do not provide additional calories. Dietary supplements are available that can enhance vitamin and mineral nutrition, as well as provide additional calories.

Enrich is a liquid nutritional supplement with fiber. Eight ounces contain 260 calories and 3.4 gm of dietary fiber. It is low in sodium and cholesterol and contains a complement of vitamins and minerals.

Ensure provides nutritional and caloric enrichment. There are 250 calories per 8-ounce serving. Like Enrich, it is low in sodium and cholesterol. *Ensure Plus* is similar to Ensure but has 355 calories per 8-ounce serving.

PREVENTIVE NUTRITION IN THE PATIENT WITH A CHRONIC DISEASE

Many factors have been recognized as affecting the course of many diseases of aging, such as coronary heart disease, hypertension, cancer, glucose intolerance, and osteoporosis.

Coronary Artery Disease

A diet including reduced fats, increased soluble fiber, vitamins with the trace elements copper and chromium, and a supplement of fish oil capsules has been found helpful. Fish oil capsules reduce serum lipids and appear to decrease prostaglandin synthesis, which reduces inflammation. The patient can increase fish consumption to three to four times a week instead of taking supplement capsules.

Hypertension

Hypertensive patients should decrease sodium intake and, particularly if diuretic medications are prescribed, should increase potassium intake. Potassium supplements can be given, or intake of foods high in potassium, such as oranges, bananas, and raisins, should be increased. Calcium and magnesium supplements or increases in dairy products and beans, brown rice, broccoli, and fish may be in order.

Cancer

A diet high in fiber appears to be protective against colon and breast cancers. Fiber is provided naturally in fruits, vegetables, beans, and whole grains, or it can be given as a supplement using wheat bran or commercial fiber supplements. The antioxidant vitamins A, C, and E and the trace mineral selenium are being studied as protective against cancer. Antioxidants probably function as scavengers of "free radicals," products of tissue oxidation that cause cellular damage. Oranges and dark green vegetables also provide beta-carotene, as do many dietary supplements.

Diabetes

A diet with complex carbohydrates and 25 to 30 grams of dietary fiber daily has been shown to increase control of diabetes. A diet deficient in chromium has been shown to increase the incidence of type 2 diabetes; thus chromium supplements should be given. Food sources of chromium include brewer's yeast and nuts.

Vision Problems

Macular degeneration and cataracts may be slowed by administration of zinc supplements. Food sources of zinc include wheat germ, wheat bran, and oysters. Vitamin E and C supplements have been found to be beneficial in lowering the incidence of cataracts.

Osteoporosis

Calcium, vitamin D supplements, and trace minerals such as magnesium and manganese have been used in the treatment of osteoporosis.

ARTHRITIS IN OLDER ADULTS

Many improvements have been made in the treatment of osteoarthritis, which is no longer looked on as a simple "wear and tear" disease. The articular cartilage has been found to be an active tissue that can undergo changes, rather than the unresponsive substance it was once thought to be.

Articular cartilage serves a number of important functions. It minimizes friction between joint surfaces, thereby minimizing wear; it increases the contact area between bones within the joint, thus decreasing contact stress; and it helps dissipate energy and absorb shock.

One of the earliest changes seen in osteoarthritis is an increase in the water content of cartilage. This is clinically important because this change increases the porosity (the number of openings through which fluids can pass) of the cartilage and thus decreases its strength and load-carrying capacity.

The NSAIDs have been shown to interrupt this inflammatory process and the subsequent thinning and breakdown of cartilage. Some NSAIDs have more effect on cartilage metabolism than others. Aspirin, ibuprofen (Motrin), and fenoprofen (Nalfon) have been shown to be the most beneficial in treating osteoarthritis. These agents are discussed in Chapter 24 (see Prostaglandin Inhibitors).

OSTEOPOROSIS IN OLDER ADULTS

As the life span increases, so do the long-term problems seen with osteoporosis in the older woman. The rates of illness and early death resulting from vertebral compression and fractures of various bones are very significant.

The most rapid bone loss in women occurs in the first 5 years after menopause, or the stopping of menstrual periods. It has been demonstrated that calcium supplements and exercise will slow this process somewhat, but research has proved that the only true "treatment" is prevention in the form of supplemental hormone therapy. The vasomotor symptoms, or "hot flashes," are also reduced or eliminated with hormone therapy. The continued use of hormones in menopausal women is controversial at present. Annual physical examinations are necessary when hormone therapy is given to detect the early presence of hormone-dependent cancers such as breast or gynecologic cancer.

Many of the commercially available estrogens can be given to prevent osteoporosis (see their discussion in Chapter 27). Conjugated estrogen (Premarin) is most commonly prescribed. Calcium supplements should be recommended in the dosage range of 1000 to 1500 mg/day.

MEDICATIONS USED IN THE PREVENTION OR TREATMENT OF OSTEOPOROSIS

alendronate (Fosamax). Alendronate is an agent that inhibits bone resorption. It has been shown to increase the mineral density of bone.

> **Dosage:**
> Adults only: (Oral) 10 mg in the morning 30 minutes before the first food is eaten.

calcitonin (Miacalcin, Calcimar). Calcitonin may be administered by nasal spray or by injection for the treatment of osteoporosis. It inhibits bone resorption.

> **Dosage:**
> Adults only: (subQ or IM) 100 International units daily. (Nasal spray) One spray (200 International Units) daily, alternating nostrils.

raloxifene hydrochloride (Evista). This agent is a selective estrogen receptor modulator. Its actions, like those of estrogen, are mediated through binding with estrogen receptors. In postmenopausal women, it preserves bone mass and increases bone mineral density. Compared with estrogen therapy, raloxifene appears to be associated with a lower risk of breast cancer in the postmenopausal woman.

> **Dosage:**
> Adults only: (Oral) 60 mg daily.

risedronate sodium (Actonel). Risedronate inhibits bone resorption and modulates bone metabolism. It is used for the treatment of Paget's disease of bone and for osteoporosis.

Dosage:

Adults only: (Oral) 30 mg daily.

PAIN AND AGING

Continuous or recurrent pain due to malignancies, degenerative conditions, and other diseases is extremely common in older adults. Chronic pain causes both physical and mental distress and has profound effects on the quality of life. Current estimates are that as many as 80% of older adults have some illness or degenerative condition that predisposes them to chronic pain.

The painful manifestations of arthritis and osteoporosis have been discussed. Other causes of pain include atherosclerotic disease, angina, cancer, diabetic neuropathy, herpes zoster, and temporal arteritis. There is much evidence that pain in older adults continues to be underassessed and underreported, and therefore undermanaged. The consequences of poorly controlled pain include impaired ambulation, reduced socialization, decreased independence in activities of daily living, and overall reduced quality of life. Pain and depression are strongly associated with each other, and each may exacerbate the other.

The potential for drug interactions and side effects is high when analgesic medications are administered, and careful dosage adjustment should be made. The concern about addiction is not as great in older adults as in younger adults. Older patients take the analgesics until they get pain relief. Pain relief is their only concern; they normally have no separate underlying need for the drugs. It would be very rare for them to increase their use of opioids and exhibit the drug-seeking behaviors typical of a drug addict. These concerns should be put to rest when considering pain therapy. Long-acting and transdermal dosage forms may give the best results.

THE AGING THYROID AND HOW IT AFFECTS OLDER ADULTS

Changes in thyroid function occur as a natural consequence of aging. These are associated with a lowered rate of thyroid hormone secretion and clearance from the body or, less commonly, hyperthyroidism or carcinoma of the thyroid.

Hypothyroidism occurs commonly in the older adult. It has been found that the pituitary secretion of thyroid-stimulating hormone (TSH) does not change with aging. When elevated levels of TSH are found in the blood, even if there are no recognizable signs of hypothyroidism, it is believed that the patient has subclinical hypothyroidism and should be given replacement therapy.

When hypothyroidism occurs in older adults, it may differ greatly from the disorder in a younger person. The fol-lowing clinical signs should increase the suspicion of hypothyroidism in an older adult:

- Unexplained elevations in plasma cholesterol or triglycerides
- Congestive heart failure
- Fecal impaction
- Macrocytic anemia
- Vague arthritic complaints
- Mild psychiatric disturbances
- The presence of a thyroidectomy scar
- A history of treatment with thyroid hormone
- Previous treatment with radioactive iodine
- Goiter

The treatment of hypothyroidism is replacement therapy with thyroid hormone. This can be given in the form of the natural gland (Armour Thyroid Tablets) or in the form of synthetic thyroxine (Synthroid). In most cases the need for thyroid hormone replacement is permanent. The dosage is individualized according to the patient's needs and responses. These agents are discussed in Chapter 27.

When hyperthyroidism, or Graves' disease, occurs in older adults, the signs may be muted or masked. Congestive heart failure is the most common presenting symptom of hyperthyroidism. Weight loss, muscle weakness, palpitations, eyelid tremor, eyelid lag, exophthalmos (protruding eyeballs), and nervousness are also seen.

The principal treatment for hyperthyroidism in older adults is radioactive iodine. The antithyroid drugs propylthiouracil and methimazole are used in younger patients, but they are less satisfactory in the older adult.

Thyroid cancer, or papillary carcinoma, is a more aggressive malignancy in older adults. The aggressiveness includes a more rapid rate of growth, metastases to distant sites, and recurrence after surgery. Surgery remains the treatment of choice, followed by antineoplastic drug therapy.

HYPERTENSION IN OLDER ADULTS

Hypertension in older adults must be treated more carefully than in the younger patient. Older adults have slower sympathetic nervous system responsiveness and impaired autoregulation; thus therapy should be slow and gradual, avoiding drugs such as prazosin that cause postural hypotension or aggravate other medical problems that patients may have.

In the past it was thought that older adults needed to maintain a slightly higher systolic blood pressure in order to maintain adequate passage of blood in the brain. This is no longer thought to be true. The blood pressure goal in older adults is to maintain a blood pressure under 140/90 mm Hg. The diastolic pressure should not be allowed to drop below 70 mm Hg.

Many home monitoring kits are available, and patients should be encouraged to use them. Weight loss, exercise, limiting alcohol consumption, and a diet low in fat, salt, and sugar should be recommended, as well as drug therapy when necessary.

The patient's OTC medications should be monitored. NSAIDs, pseudoephedrine, caffeine preparations, and asthma inhalers all may increase blood pressure.

Diuretics may be used, even though they are no longer the drugs of choice for the older patient. Beta-blockers should be used with caution; calcium channel blockers are a good choice, as are angiotensin-converting enzyme inhibitors in certain patients. Long-acting dosage forms should be chosen whenever possible to keep the number of medication doses at a minimum.

ANTIINFECTIVE THERAPY IN OLDER ADULTS

Older adults experience a higher incidence of vascular, metabolic, degenerative, and neoplastic disorders. They are also very susceptible to infectious complications of all their disorders. Antibiotic therapy can be challenging because the infection is often well advanced before the older adult seeks treatment, and, when treatment is begun, drug penetration into infected tissues is inadequate because arteriosclerosis has narrowed the arteries, limiting the drug's access to the tissues.

In addition, physiologic changes associated with aging result in alteration of drug metabolism. Renal plasma flow declines with age; thus drugs dependent on "average" renal function for excretion may build up in the body to toxic levels. Congestive heart failure may slow circulation further.

Several categories of antiinfective drugs must be monitored in the older adult patient.

AMINOGLYCOSIDE ANTIBIOTICS

Kanamycin, gentamicin, tobramycin, amikacin, and netilmicin are used in older adults for infections caused by *Enterobacter* and *Pseudomonas* strains. Excretion of these agents is often delayed, however. Thus blood levels must be monitored carefully. Nephrotoxicity and ototoxicity are common toxic effects.

PENICILLINS

Patients with impaired renal function may develop acute renal failure or hemolytic anemia when large doses of penicillin are given parenterally. Neurotoxic symptoms of muscle twitching, myoclonic jerking, and seizures have been reported as well. Large parenteral doses may be necessary for life-threatening, severe infections; thus choices may be limited.

CEPHALOSPORINS

Life-threatening hemorrhage may occur from wound sites or the gastrointestinal tract when the cephalosporins are used to treat infection. The risk of hemorrhage is greatest in the poorly nourished patient who has cancer and who has undergone a surgical procedure. It has been theorized that the cephalosporins interfere with intestinal production of vitamin K.

NITROFURANTOIN

Elderly patients who have been administered this agent for urinary tract infections have been reported to have increased risk of agranulocytosis, hepatitis, and chronic pulmonary fibrosis. It is believed that this agent should be used with caution in older adults if at all.

THE QUINOLONES

This class of antimicrobial agents has been shown to be highly favorable for use in older adults. These agents (norfloxacin, ciprofloxacin, and ofloxacin) have a broad spectrum of activity, are active orally in twice-daily dosages, and can be prescribed for penicillin-sensitive patients. They are contraindicated in patients with seizure disorders and are inactivated by the concurrent use of liquid antacids containing aluminum or magnesium. The drug interaction between quinolones and coumarin should be particularly noted. The effect of coumarin is enhanced when used with quinolones; thus careful monitoring and possible dosage adjustment may be necessary.

ANXIETY IN OLDER ADULTS

Anxiety is a prominent problem in older adults. The older patient is likely to suffer from a wide array of medical illnesses that can produce symptoms that either mimic or trigger anxiety. These illnesses include cardiovascular disease; drug-related problems; endocrine, hematologic, immunologic, neurologic, or pulmonary problems; and some forms of cancer. In addition, older adults are often engaged in fewer productive activities and, therefore, have more time to worry than do younger people.

Buspirone (BuSpar) has been shown to be the drug of choice in many studies for the treatment of anxiety in older adults. It is discussed in Chapter 23. Drugs such as the benzodiazepines (e.g., alprazolam, diazepam, and triazolam) are better avoided in older adults because these patients have a decreased ability to detoxify these agents, and impaired mental and motor function symptoms are intensified.

DRUGS USED TO TREAT ALZHEIMER'S DISEASE

Alzheimer's disease (AD) is the primary cause of **dementia**, or the loss of cognitive and intellectual functions, in older adults. It is often underrecognized and undertreated. The prevalence of AD doubles every 5 years after age 65 years, and an estimated 30% of people 85 years of age or older have some form of the disease. Impairment is cognitive, functional, and behavioral.

The diagnosis can be made by using the Mini-Mental State Examination (MMSE). This test provides an easy-to-administer mental examination for preliminary and serial

Table 32-1	*Drugs Used to Treat Alzheimer's Disease*	
GENERIC NAME	**TRADE NAME**	**DOSAGE**
donepezil hydrochloride	Aricept	5–10 mg/day
rivastigmine	Exelon	6 mg twice daily
tacrine hydrochloride	Cognex	10 mg 4 times daily

assessment of cognition (the ability to be aware, think, reason, and remember). A perfect score is 30; a score of 20 or less is found in patients with dementia. More information on this examination can be found at *www.minimental.com.*

Another test is the Alzheimer's Disease Assessment Scale–Cognitive Subscale (ADAS-Cog). Healthy nondemented patients score 0 to 1 on this test, and the scores of demented patients usually increase by 6 to 12 points per year.

Neuroimaging using computed tomography, positron emission tomography, or magnetic resonance imaging can also establish the diagnosis.

Drugs used to treat Alzheimer's disease (Table 32–1) are reversible inhibitors of the enzyme acetylcholinesterase, allowing an increase in the level of acetylcholine in the brain. The cholinergic system, which uses acetylcholine to transmit nerve impulses, is involved with memory and attention. Results of treatment are often subjective and difficult to quantify, but they appear to demonstrate improvement when compared with administration of placebos. Side effects include bradycardia, increased gastric secretion and ulcers, and liver impairment.

FAMILY CARE OF OLDER ADULTS AND CAREGIVER STRESS

When the older patient is living at home, a caregiver is usually required. Meeting the needs of the older adult causes increased stress in the caregiver. There is often a sense of ambivalence because the son, daughter, or spouse who is the caregiver would otherwise be at a stage of life when most responsibilities are fulfilled, and this is the long-awaited free time for travel or other interests.

Parental care is different from child care. Child care is naturally expected to lessen as time goes on. The reverse is true with elder care. Adult children begin with grocery shopping and transportation, then add housecleaning and meal preparation, bathing and dressing, and, finally, feeding and coping with incontinence.

Concerns about the seemingly increasing incidence of elder abuse reflect emotional problems in the caregiver as normal coping mechanisms fail to relieve the stress of caring for an older adult. Health care personnel can play an important role in screening for elder abuse and offering appropriate support, education, advice, and intervention for the older adult and his or her caregiver.

Caregiver stress can present as vague symptoms of fatigue, anxiety, depression, back strain, anger, guilt, frustra-

tion, social isolation, and a perception of poor health. Elements to screen for when interviewing the caregiver include a history of drug or alcohol abuse in the older adult or the caregiver, a family history of violence, a mention of "punishment" of the older adult by the caregiver, or a recent life stress for the caregiver.

Caregivers need specific advice. They must be encouraged to set realistic limitations on the amount of care they can give. Other family members should be encouraged to become involved and give relief to the primary caregiver. The use of adult day centers for the older adult and temporary nursing home placement for time off should be encouraged.

Self-help or support groups for caregivers are available in many communities. In addition, there are support groups for those dealing with Alzheimer's disease in older adults. The health care worker should become familiar with support groups and services for the older adult in his or her community so that support and intervention can be given whenever necessary.

CLINICAL IMPLICATIONS

1. The metabolism of the older adult differs significantly from that of the younger adult. The patient should be observed for signs of drug overdose.
2. Aging patients should not be considered as merely senile when behavior and abilities begin to change. A look at the possibility of underlying diseases or drug reactions is always in order.
3. The older adult patient should be counseled thoroughly on the choices in his or her special diet. Careful attention should be given to nutrition, with the recommendation of supplemental vitamins and minerals and dietary supplements.
4. Drug compliance is a problem in older adults. They should be counseled regarding the importance of taking the medications as prescribed. Long-acting medications and simplified drug dosage schedules should be used as much as possible.
5. Falling, confusion, and decreased cognitive abilities may be signs of overdosage of a sedative medication.
6. The use of over-the-counter medications such as aspirin and ibuprofen can alleviate many of the symptoms of osteoarthritis.
7. Congestive heart failure may point to thyroid abnormalities as well as specific problems with the myocardium of the heart.
8. The health care worker should be aware of problems with the older adult's caregiver. Skilled counseling is possible only if the social problems are recognized.
9. Anxiety is a common problem of older adults. The use of anxiolytic agents can significantly relieve many of these symptoms.
10. Chronologic aging does not in itself mean a loss of function or a poor quality of life. Good medical care and the proper use of community services can provide many improvements for older adults.
11. Preventive nutrition may prevent or minimize some chronic illnesses in older adults.

12. Hypertension must be treated carefully to avoid conditions such as postural hypotension.
13. When infections become more numerous and severe, the tolerance to many antibiotics is decreased.
14. Drug interactions must be checked whenever a patient is on more than one medication.
15. Dementia should be assessed. If it is progressive, medications are available to alleviate the condition.

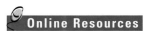

For updated drug information and Web activities, go to http://evolve.elsevier.com/Asperheim.

CRITICAL THINKING QUESTIONS

1. The patient came to the heart clinic today for her 6-month checkup. The chart shows a slow but steady weight loss for the past year. Minnie says that she is so tired that it is hard to get to the grocery store, and mostly she just has toast and coffee for lunch and a sandwich for dinner. What may be some of her additional problems? How may they be improved?

2. The patient is admitted to the hospital for a broken hip. The physician ordered blood studies because of the large bruises over his shoulder and upper back. The blood studies are normal. His daughter says he "just falls a lot." Should further investigation and studies be made?

3. The patient has become more and more confused when she is seen in follow-up for her hypertension. Her medications include digoxin, Lasix, Slow-K, Valium, and Dalmane. Should any of the medications be considered part of her problem?

4. The patient came to her physician for "burnout." She works full time and has two teenage children, an elderly father with Alzheimer's disease, and a married daughter with a new baby. With no time for herself, her marriage is suffering, and she complains of sleep problems and anxiety. What suggestions may be made to improve her situation?

REVIEW QUESTIONS

1. A careful medication history should be taken from older adults because:
   a. they take very few medications.
   b. they often combine herbal products with their medicines.
   c. they are careful generally to see only one doctor.
   d. they have few underlying diseases.

2. When treating older adults, a great effort should be made to:
   a. get all medications on an every-4-hours schedule.
   b. make sure the patient has a medication for each illness.
   c. simplify the drug regimen as much as possible.
   d. get a specialist for each illness.

3. A symptom of osteoporosis may be:
   a. a swollen knee joint.
   b. painful hands in the morning.
   c. back pain and shortening of stature.
   d. weight gain.

4. Hypothyroidism in the older adult may have all the following symptoms except:
   a. goiter.
   b. fecal impaction.
   c. intolerance to heat.
   d. congestive heart failure.

5. A drug of choice for the treatment of anxiety in the elderly is:
   a. buspirone.
   b. phenobarbital.
   c. alprazolam.
   d. triazolam.

6. A side effect of donepezil may be:
   a. tachycardia.
   b. hypertension.
   c. bradycardia.
   d. increased renal output.

7. When giving medication to an elderly person, the usual dose of a medication may need to be:
   a. increased.
   b. decreased.
   c. not changed.
   d. divided into two doses.

8. When prescribing various medications to an elderly person, compliance with the drug schedule may be affected by:
   a. confusion.
   b. too many caregivers.
   c. osteoporosis.
   d. drug addiction.

9. Nitrofurantoin is one of the medications not recommended for the elderly because of the risk of:

a. agranulocytosis.

b. pleocytosis.

c. elevated white blood cell count.

d. anemia.

10. The most common presenting sign of hyperthyroidism in the elderly is:

a. hypotension.

b. intolerance to heat.

c. slowed heart rate.

d. congestive heart failure.

33 Home Health and End-of-Life Care

Home health care is professional health care in the home, offering many services formerly available only in a hospital setting. Home health care has grown rapidly, and with it have grown the opportunities for nurses and allied health care workers.

Home care offers an acceptable, effective alternative to extended hospitalization. Cost-containment efforts by payers, newer techniques, and the increasing availability of sophisticated home health care providers have made all sectors in the health care field believe that this trend will only increase in the future.

The home health care professional is a part of a collaborative team of nurse, physician, and other health care providers. Usually the home health worker is the only one seeing the patient on a regular basis; thus he or she must be responsible for the assessment of the patient and must keep sufficiently detailed records so that changes in the patient's condition, mental state, blood pressure, and so on may be noted and reported in a timely fashion.

The health care worker must be acutely aware of the medications that each patient is taking and be knowledgeable of the effects, side effects, and potential toxic effect of each medication so that untoward events may be avoided. Appropriate corrective actions may be taken by other members of the team only if problems are reported.

A reassessment of nursing theories and responsibilities must be made. The new role of providing home care places more emphasis on responsibility and decision-making skills for the nurse or health professional.

Some aspects of home health care are covered in this chapter, but it cannot be all-inclusive.

HOME INFUSION THERAPY

Infusion is the introduction of a fluid other than blood into a vein. Home infusion can shorten or prevent hospitalization for selected patients needing intravenous antibiotics, chemotherapy, hydration, pain management, immunoglobulins, transfusions, and parenteral nutrition.

The main advantage of home infusion is that it offers the patient a more normal lifestyle with reduced medical costs. Home infusion is generally safe and effective. The following list includes many of the home infusion therapies now considered standard:

- Short- and long-term antibiotics
- Antifungal and antiviral therapy
- Blood transfusions
- Total parenteral nutrition
- Pain management
- Chemotherapy
- Anticoagulation with heparin

Patients who are referred for home infusion often have no previous experience in this type of therapy. They must be screened for intellectual, psychological, social, and environmental factors that could negatively affect therapy before home infusion is offered.

The patient should be medically stable after discharge, with the exception of the need for intravenous therapy. Patients with hypotension, unexplained fevers, respiratory distress, active bleeding, recent emboli, or other conditions that render them medically unstable are poor risks for home health care. Medications that may cause allergic or severe adverse reactions should not be started in the home but should simply be continued by home therapy after initial doses are administered in a hospital setting.

Long-term central catheters are commonly used for home infusions. Blocked catheters may sometimes be reopened by infusing small amounts of acid or base solution, and clotted catheters may be opened by the infusion of urokinase. Pumps that can be programmed offer new alternatives for the administration of various medications at different times.

HOME INFUSION FOR CHILDREN

Home infusion therapy for children presents another set of obstacles and opportunities.

Hospitalization is a stressful and expensive event for a child and the family. The trend toward moving even high-technology care into the home is very beneficial. Particular problems occur with the young patient, however. Fear and its associated lack of cooperation and the limited intellectual ability and maturity of the child will cause problems. Maturity and cooperation of the parent or caregiver cannot be ensured either. Parents may be of limited intelligence and may be visually or physically handicapped as well, and they may not be dependable as allies in the care of the child.

Hematology and oncology patients are often candidates for home care. Blood and blood product administration, intravenous medication administration, and total parenteral nutrition are often done in the home.

Families should be encouraged to discuss the procedures with the home health caregiver, and the child's questions should be answered truthfully; the child should be given as much explanation as the situation warrants. Much of the anxiety and fear experienced by the child and the family are associated with a lack of comfort in their roles with regard to the infusion. Effective communication here is essential.

HOME THERAPY FOR THE BONE MARROW TRANSPLANT PATIENT

With the new ability to treat malignant and nonmalignant diseases by means of bone marrow transplants come the attendant problems of long-term therapy for these patients, often in a home setting.

The patient first has the bone marrow destroyed by myelosuppressive therapy of one sort or another and then receives a compatible marrow by infusion. After the bone marrow transplantation, immunosuppressive drugs are given to prevent rejection.

Prophylactic therapy, that is, treatment that may prevent an illness or disorder, is aimed at preventing infections in the immunocompromised state that follows transplantation. Antibiotics and antifungal and antiviral agents are used. Anemia is treated with whole blood transfusions or with packed cells after these blood products are irradiated.

There is often general loss of the epithelium of the mouth and even the entire gastrointestinal tract. Pain control, oral hygiene, adequate nutrition, and fluid intake must be managed. Hepatic, renal, and pulmonary dysfunction occur and must be managed appropriately. Pain associated with all the attendant problems must be managed within the guidelines of chronic pain management.

DIABETICS IN THE HOME CARE SETTING

The severe diabetic with secondary problems resulting from the disease often becomes a candidate for home health services.

Diabetic retinopathy often leaves the patient severely visually compromised or even totally blind. The patient then cannot self-administer insulin injections or attend to personal hygiene, foot care, or skin care properly.

Syringes prefilled by a home health worker may facilitate continued partial self-sufficiency for the visually impaired patient. Continual observation of the patient for skin breakdown or infections and monitoring of blood glucose levels are necessary. Detailed inquiries about any diet management issues and assessment of the patient's level of skill in taking any other medications must be made.

PSYCHIATRIC HOME CARE

The move to decentralize health care and provide more services in the home has extended to psychiatric patients as well. Some patients may believe that discharge from the hospital means that "there is no more hope for me" rather than seeing it as a sign of improvement. At the other extreme, the "I'm cured" way of thinking may prompt the patient to stop taking medications altogether.

The home health care worker must be skilled in the assessment of the pyschiatric patient's medication needs and compliance in taking them. An understanding of adverse side effects of the psychotropic drugs and recognition that the dose may be too small or too large are important factors in providing home care.

Home health care workers who care for clients being treated for mental illness must be trained to collaborate with psychiatrists to provide adequate care. Assessing psychiatric issues requires that the nurse be trained to listen; most assessment involves interviews and observation.

When assessing a patient whose behavior indicates mental illness, the nurse must ask her- or himself four questions:
1. Does the aberrant behavior reflect a new primary disorder, or is it secondary to another disease, or is it a medication side effect?
2. Is the behavior precipitated by stress, or is it a sign that medication effects are different than predicted?
3. What is the level of aberrant behavior, and does it constitute a threat to the patient or to others?
4. How does the behavior relate to the culture and environment?

Imbalances of activity and rest, an inability to make appropriate food choices, poor self-care, and a deteriorating environment may be early signs that the mental status is declining.

END-OF-LIFE CARE

About the middle of the 20th century, care for the dying began to move out of the home and into the hospital. With the advent of modern medicine, and the techniques and procedures available in the hospital, more and more attempts to prolong life at any cost were made. As a result, death was often endured essentially alone, away from friends and family, in an intensive care unit, in the midst of painful and invasive procedures.

How do we know when a medical procedure is making the dying process unnatural and burdensome, or when it offers promise of cure or freedom from pain? How can we prepare for the death of a loved one and make the experience as meaningful and pain-free as possible? The hospice movement has led the way in answering these questions. A **hospice** is an institution that provides a centralized program of palliative and supportive care to dying persons and their families. This movement has taught us that to let someone die naturally does not mean we stop treating or caring for the patient with **terminal illness** (that is, a disease expected to cause death within a short period).

Health care professionals' inadequate knowledge of pain management, symptom control, and other dimensions of terminal care have been cited as the major barrier to good end-of-life care. The issues and methods of pain management are covered later in this chapter and in more depth in Chapter 21.

Although pain has been identified as the predominant symptom in a terminal illness, other critical symptoms and needs in the dying patient are being recognized through the practice of palliative care. For many people, fear of the unknown is at least as great as fear of death itself. Fear of uncontrollable pain, nausea, vomiting, embarrassment, and especially abandonment are very prominent in the patient's list of concerns. Presenting hospice as an option for treating a terminal illness can help with many of these unknowns. Good care of a dying person means making the body as comfortable as possible so that the patient can prepare for death mentally and spiritually. It means allowing the patient to live as fully as possible until the time she or he dies.

The needs of the dying have been described as follows:
- The need to be treated as a living human being.
- The need to maintain a sense of hopefulness.
- The need to be cared for by those who will help him or her maintain hopefulness.
- The need to express feelings and emotions about death in one's own way.
- The need to participate in decisions concerning one's care.

- The need to be cared for by compassionate, sensitive, and knowledgeable people.
- The need to expect continuing medical care, even though the goals may change.
- The need to have all questions answered honestly and fully.
- The need to seek spirituality.
- The need to be free of physical pain.
- The need to express feelings and emotions about pain in one's own way.
- The need of children to participate in death.
- The need to understand the process of death.
- The need to die in peace and dignity.
- The need not to die alone.
- The need to expect that the sanctity of the body will be respected after death.

There are many ways the health care professional can assist the dying patient, by dealing with the subject of death in a forthright manner in accordance with the patient's needs and wishes.

ISSUES TO RESOLVE IN END-OF-LIFE CARE

Delivering good palliative care requires a particular set of skills. These include knowledge of pain management and the ability to communicate about end-of-life issues such as advanced care planning, the use of cardiopulmonary resuscitation, and artificial life support. Other elective options include intubation, mechanical ventilation, surgery, dialysis, blood transfusions, artificial nutrition and hydration, antibiotics, and other medications and treatments, as well as future admissions to the hospital or the intensive care unit. The treatment choices and the complexities increase as a patient's condition worsens. Many patients who initially choose a do-not-resuscitate (DNR) order make changes as time goes on. It is much better for all concerned to make these decisions well ahead of time.

The first step in palliative care is to establish goals. What is important to the patient and the family? This may be a continuing process because the goals may need to be adjusted as time passes. Preferences and understanding about death and the dying process vary widely, so they must be addressed.

Specific issues that should be discussed with the patient and the family include the following:
1. What do they know about the illness and the treatment options?
2. How much information do they want to have?
3. What decisions should be made by the patient, by the family, and by the health professional?
4. What defines an acceptable quality of life for the patient?
5. What roles will the physician and nurse play?
6. Which family member will be the liaison between the patient and the health care team?
7. Where would the patient like to die?
8. Does the family have issues or preferences about being with the patient when he or she dies?

PAIN CONTROL

Pain control is a critical subject for discussion with the patient. Patients need to know that most pain can be controlled with relatively simple therapies. The pain relief can be increased as the disease progresses. One question that patients should be asked is whether they are willing to trade full consciousness for pain relief, since adequate control of pain may in some cases require sedation. In the final hours of life the patient often experiences transient distress caused by dyspnea, agitation, and restlessness. Treatment for those symptoms also may require sedating medications.

Patients who cannot verbalize pain may still be experiencing it and are at risk for undertreatment. This is especially true for patients with dementia. In one study of patients who had been hospitalized for treatment of hip fracture, it was noted that patients with dementia received less than one half the analgesic relief provided to patients with the same hip fracture but normal cognitive function. The health care worker should recognize that signs of restlessness, anxiety, or fearfulness in the patient who is unable to communicate may be a reaction to pain. An appropriate analgesic may be given to see whether the symptoms abate.

Drug Selection

It is obvious that there are many different choices for the various levels of pain that the patient may have. A general rule is that, as the pain progresses, a sustained-release form of the narcotic may be administered by mouth, and a short-acting "rescue" drug may be given for breakthrough pain between doses. Frequent use of the rescue drug (more than three to four times daily) may signal the need for an increase in the baseline long-acting drug. The usual dosage of the short-acting drug should be equivalent to 5% to 15% of the 24-hour baseline dosage of the long-acting drug.

Pain control is discussed in more detail in Chapter 22, which also contains a list of oral and transdermal analgesic agents that are considered equivalent in potency to the effect of 10 mg of morphine intramuscularly (see Table 21–1).

Tolerance to Opioids

The use of opioids often raises fear of addiction in patient and health professional alike. Such fear is almost always unwarranted. The risk of addiction is extremely small in patients with pain and no history of substance abuse.

Severe pain allows patients to tolerate the sedative effects of opioids. Whether tolerance develops to the pain-relieving effects of opioids is a matter of controversy. Most of the data on opioid tolerance and physical dependence in humans come from studies involving subjects who were not in pain. Studies of patients with chronic pain who have taken opioids for a long time indicate that, once the dose required for pain relief is established, it generally remains stable unless the underlying disease progresses.

With long-term use of opioids, sudden withdrawal of the opioids or a significant reduction in dosage will give withdrawal symptoms such as sweating, nausea, diarrhea, and irritability. This type of physical dependence, of course, can occur with other drugs also, such as antihypertensives and sedatives. Slowly tapering the dose will avoid the withdrawal symptoms.

When treating chronic pain, it is important to remember that there is no ceiling or maximal opioid dose. Extremely large doses of morphine, such as several hundred milligrams every 4 hours, may be needed to relieve severe pain.

NUTRITION AND HYDRATION

Nutrition and hydration deserve special attention. There is perhaps no issue more common than concerns over the feeding of the dying patient. Very often the struggle over eating is really about fear of dying and losing a loved one. It is often easier for the patient than it is for the family to accept that the patient just cannot eat as much as she or he previously did.

Food is the way we energize our body. It is the means by which we keep our body moving and alive. In other words, we obviously eat to live. When a patient is preparing to die, it is perfectly natural that eating should stop. This is one of the hardest concepts for the family to accept. There is a gradual decrease in eating habits, with meats generally being refused first, then vegetables, followed by a preference for softer foods, and then liquids only. It must be remembered that it is okay not to eat. A different kind of energy is needed now, the spiritual energy to complete the task at hand.

Feeding tubes are often placed as a quick and easy solution to the time-consuming process of feeding a reluctant patient. Families may fear that the patient will "starve to death" rather than die of the disease. There is some evidence that artificial feeding may not lengthen the life of a patient, but instead may just add to his or her problems by overloading a poorly functioning gastrointestinal tract.

Removing the guilt and anxiety about this issue does everyone a service. The patient may be offered food and liquids and encouraged to take as much as desired without placing undue burdens or responsibilities on anyone.

HOSPICE CARE
Goals

1. Patients can live at home. After all, this is where they are most comfortable. They have the opportunity to see friends and relatives and enjoy time with cherished pets and belongings.
2. They can stay as active as possible. Some limited trips with skilled assistance may be possible, or patients may help with daily living tasks as long as they are able.
3. Patients should be encouraged to express their feelings. The discussion of death and dying produces great anxiety in many family members, obviously in relation to their own fear of death. It is very important to patients that this be discussed, however. They may need to resolve old issues with family members, or merely say goodbye, or they may wish to dispose of their possessions without relatives "shushing" them about talk of death.
4. Pain and other symptoms will be relieved as much as is possible.

5. Hospice care should help people feel at peace. As the end of life approaches, it creates a loving environment where family members can say goodbye.

Palliative Performance Scale

The Palliative Performance Scale (PPS) is often used to evaluate the status of the patient. It gives a shortcut method of describing the patient's status (Table 33–1).

Drugs Used for Hospice Patients

While effective pain management is paramount to the effective treatment of the hospice patient, other conditions may need attention and treatment as well. Many of these agents are discussed elsewhere in this text; therefore, only a list is provided in Table 33–2, with some typical dosages given to hospice patients. Dosages of all of these agents may vary greatly, of course, depending on the patient and the circumstances of the illness.

Table 33-1 | *Palliative Performance Scale*

%	AMBULATION	ACTIVITY AND EVIDENCE OF DISEASE	SELF-CARE	INTAKE	CONSCIOUS LEVEL
100	Full	Normal activity, no sign of disease	Full	Normal	Full
90	Full	Normal activity, some sign of disease	Full	Normal	Full
80	Full	Normal activity with effort, some evidence of disease	Full	Normal/less	Full
70	Reduced	Unable to work normal job, some evidence of disease	Full	Normal/less	Full
60	Reduced	Unable to do hobby/housework, significant disease	Occasional help	Normal/less	Full/confusion
50	Mainly sit/lie	Unable to do any work, extensive disease	Considerable help	Normal/less	Full/confusion
40	Mainly in bed	As above	Considerable help	Normal/less	Full/drowsy or confusion
30	Bed bound	As above	Total care	Reduced	As above
20	As above	As above	Total care	Minimal sips	Drowsy/coma
10	As above	As above	Total care	Mouth care only	Drowsy/coma
0	Death				

Table 33-2 | *Drugs Used for Hospice Patients*

DRUG	DOSAGE
DRUGS FOR ANXIETY	
lorazepam (Ativan)	0.5–1 mg 3 times daily
alprazolam (Xanax)	0.25–0.5 mg 3 times daily
haloperidol (Haldol)	1–5 mg up to 4 times daily
diazepam (Valium)	10 mg 4 times daily
hydroxyzine (Atarax, Vistaril)	25 mg 3 times daily
chlorpromazine (Thorazine)	25–50 mg 4 times daily
DRUGS FOR SLEEPLESSNESS	
flurazepam (Dalmane)	15–30 mg at bedtime
temazepam (Restoril)	15–30 mg at bedtime
triazolam (Halcion)	0.25–0.5 mg at bedtime
DRUGS FOR DEPRESSION	
sertraline hydrochloride (Zoloft)	50–200 mg in the morning
paroxetine hydrochloride (Paxil)	20–50 mg in the morning
amitriptyline hydrochloride (Elavil)	50–150 mg at bedtime
desipramine hydrochloride (Norpramin)	10–150 mg at bedtime
DRUGS FOR NEUROPATHIC PAIN	
valproate sodium (Depakene)	250 mg 3 times daily
carbamazepine (Tegretol)	200 mg twice daily
gabapentin (Neurontin)	100 mg twice daily
divalproex (Depakote)	125 mg twice daily
phenytoin (Dilantin)	100 mg 3 times daily

Table 33-2 | *Drugs Used for Hospice Patients—cont'd*

DRUG	DOSAGE
DRUGS FOR NAUSEA OR VOMITING	
prochlorperazine (Compazine)	5–10 mg 4 times daily
promethazine hydrochloride (Phenergan)	25 mg 3 times daily
DRUGS FOR DIARRHEA	
diphenoxylate hydrochloride (Lomotil)	5 mg 4 times daily
DRUGS FOR CONSTIPATION	
Stool softeners such as Colace, Peri-Colace	
Other laxatives such as Senokot, Dulcolax tablets, or suppositories	
DRUGS FOR ABDOMINAL CRAMPING	
hyoscyamine (Levsin)	0.125 mg 3 times daily
scopolamine (Transderm Scōp)	1–2 patches every 3 days
DRUGS FOR ORAL *CANDIDA*	
nystatin suspension (Mycostatin)	4 mL 4 times daily
clotrimazole (Mycelex)	10-mg troches 5 times daily
ketoconazole (Nizoral)	200 mg twice a day
DRUGS FOR VIRAL INFECTIONS	
acyclovir (Zovirax)	400 mg 5 times daily
DRUGS FOR REFLUX ESOPHAGITIS OR PEPTIC ULCERS	
cimetidine (Tagamet)	300 mg 4 times daily
ranitidine (Zantac)	150 mg twice daily
DRUGS FOR MUSCLE SPASMS	
baclofen (Lioresal)	5 mg 3 times daily
diazepam (Valium)	5 mg 3 times daily
DRUGS FOR DYSPNEA	
Mild	
hydrocodone bitartrate (Hycodan or Lortab)	5 mg every 4 hr
Tylenol with codeine	30 mg 4 times a day
Severe	
morphine sulfate syrup	3–10 mg every 4 hr
hydromorphone hydrochloride (Dilaudid)	0.5–2 mg every 4 hr
The dosages for severe dyspnea can be increased by 50% every 4–12 hr until relief is obtained.	
Terminal	
midazolam hydrochloride (Versed)	0.25 mg/hr subQ, increased as necessary
DRUGS FOR PAIN CONTROL	
Mild Pain	
acetaminophen (Tylenol)	Up to 3–4 gm/day
aspirin	Up to 3–4 gm/day
ibuprofen (Motrin)	600–800 mg 4 times daily
indomethacin (Indocin)	25 mg 3 times daily
ketorolac tromethamine (Toradol)	10 mg 4 times daily
naproxen sodium (Naprosyn, Anaprox)	500 mg twice daily
Moderate Pain	
codeine sulfate (with aspirin or Tylenol)	130–200 mg every 3–4 hr
hydrocodone bitartrate (Dilaudid)	30 mg every 3–4 hr
oxycodone hydrochloride (Percodan, Percocet)	30 mg every 3–4 hr
tramadol hydrochloride (Ultram)	50–100 mg every 4–6 hr (to 400 mg/day)

Continued

| Table 33-2 | *Drugs Used for Hospice Patients—cont'd* |

DRUG	DOSAGE
Severe Pain	
morphine sulfate	30–60 mg every 3–4 hr
morphine sulfate controlled release (Oramorph SR, MS Contin)	90–120 mg every 12 hr
fentanyl citrate (Duragesic patch)	25–100 mcg/hr; parenteral, 0.1 mg/hr
hydromorphone hydrochloride (Dilaudid)	7.5 mg every 3–4 hr; parenteral, 1.5 mg every 3 hr
levorphanol tartrate (Levo-Dromoran)	3 mg 4 times daily; parenteral, 2 mg every 6 hr
meperidine hydrochloride (Demerol)	100–150 mg every 3–4 hr; parenteral, 100 mg every 3 hr
methadone hydrochloride (Dolophine)	20 mg every 6–8 hr; parenteral, 10 mg every 6 hr
oxymorphone hydrochloride (Numorphan)	parenteral, 1 mg every 3–4 hr

CLINICAL IMPLICATIONS

1. The role of the home health care provider places new responsibilities on the nurse or other health care provider.
2. Often the nurse is the only professional who sees the patient on a regular basis. It is important to remain alert for any changes in the patient's status.
3. Detailed records must be kept with regard to the patient's mental condition and personal hygiene, as well as the medical signs of blood pressure, pulse, and so on.
4. If there are signs that the patient is not medically stable, the medical provider should be notified immediately.
5. Children may have excessive fears that interfere with therapy.
6. The abilities of the patient's home caregiver also should be assessed.
7. Effective communication skills with the patient, family, and others on the health team are essential.
8. New skills may need to be learned for infusions at the home site.
9. Pain management for the terminally ill patient has different goals than those for the acutely ill patient.
10. Concerns regarding narcotic tolerance and habituation are not applicable when treating a terminally ill patient.
11. Skills in assessing patient compliance with medication are particularly important when visiting the psychiatric patient at home.
12. Clues from the home environment are often helpful when assessing the patient.
13. The dying process is natural, and death at home in a hospice environment has many advantages over death in a hospital, where frantic procedures may be done to prolong life at any cost.
14. Palliative care differs from therapeutic care in that a cure is no longer expected, but the patient is made as comfortable as possible.
15. A good quality of life may be experienced by the dying patient.
16. It is essential to be able to speak of death and dying with a terminal patient.
17. Much of the suffering of terminally ill patients has occurred because no one would let them speak of death or prepare themselves to die.
18. It is possible to relieve almost any level of pain with the medications available.
19. Patients who are not communicating well may be suffering significant pain.
20. Anxiety and depression in the terminally ill patient may be masked as anger at those around him or her.
21. Long-acting pain medication should be given routinely. The patient should not have to experience pain before each dose.
22. The dose and frequency of the rescue drug will signify when an increase in the long-acting analgesic is necessary.

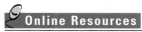

Online Resources

For updated drug information and Web activities, go to http://evolve.elsevier.com/Asperheim.

CRITICAL THINKING QUESTIONS

1. The patient, age 67 years, has been diagnosed with terminal colon cancer. He has had many surgical and radiation procedures and is now admitted to hospice care. The very anxious daughter who will be the primary caregiver states that she wants "everything possible" done for her father. How would you respond?

2. An 80-year-old patient, who has cancer and also Alzheimer's disease, has refused to eat more than a spoonful at each meal for the last 3 days. Her husband is afraid she will starve to death and wants a feeding tube put in. How should this request be handled?

3. The patient, 57 years old, has terminal metastatic breast cancer. She has just been admitted to hospice

care. You are meeting with her husband and daughter and the patient for the first time. What will you say?

4. Every time the patient, 74 years old and a terminal cancer patient, wants to talk about death, his children quickly change the subject, telling him that he is going to get well and "not to talk like that." How could you help?

5. The patient has been an insulin-dependent diabetic for many years. Her blood sugar levels have been unstable lately, with several high or low readings. After visiting with her, she asks you to set her oven because she is having trouble with the numbers. Would you have any recommendations for her care?

6. The patient, previously diagnosed as a schizophrenic, was sent home stable on his psychiatric medication. On your recent visit, you notice he is eating only bread, his appearance is becoming more disheveled, and he is obviously delusional. What would be your course of action?

7. A patient who is on intravenous medication for his colon cancer reports more sores in his mouth today. What would you advise?

REVIEW QUESTIONS

1. Home infusion therapy may be used for all except which of the following?
   a. Antibiotic infusion
   b. Antiviral therapy
   c. Pain management
   d. Suspected pulmonary emboli

2. Which of the following would be appropriate when working with a child undergoing home infusion?
   a. Tell the child everything will be all right, don't worry.
   b. Discuss the procedures truthfully with the child, while reassuring him or her.
   c. Don't talk at all to the child, explain everything to the parent.
   d. Don't explain anything, just do your work.

3. Which would not be expected to be a problem with a diabetic home health patient?
   a. Visual problems limiting the ability to adust the insulin dosage accurately
   b. Skin breakdown
   c. Confusion
   d. Strict adherence to an American Diabetes Association diet

4. A deficiency of good end-of-life care would be:
   a. not using the newest experimental drug.
   b. talking about death with the patient if she or he wishes.
   c. inadequate pain control.
   d. maintaining hopefulness even with a terminal illness.

5. With a Palliative Performance Scale score of 50, the patient may be able to:
   a. continue to do light housework.
   b. mainly sit or lie quietly.
   c. do all personal hygiene tasks.
   d. enjoy reading novels.

6. A drug that may be used for anxiety is:
   a. morphine.
   b. promethazine.
   c. nystatin.
   d. lorazepam.

7. An agent useful for oral monilia is:
   a. hyoscyamine.
   b. nystatin.
   c. sertraline.
   d. desipramine.

8. The dose of codeine that would be equivalent to 40 mg of hydrocodone would be:
   a. 30 mg.
   b. 100 mg.
   c. 200 mg.
   d. 400 mg.

9. A terminally ill patient has been on morphine for about 4 months. Over this time, would you expect his dose of morphine to have been:
   a. significantly increased.
   b. not changed.
   d. significantly decreased.
   c. discontinued.

10. The need to increase the dose of an opioid to get the desired analgesia over time is called:
    a. addiction.
    b. habituation.
    c. tolerance.
    d. depression.

34 Substance Abuse

After completing this chapter, you should be able to do the following:

1. Identify the risk factors that predispose patient's to substance abuse.
2. Identify particular risk factors in the teenager.
3. Have an understanding of drug addiction and its symptoms.
4. Recognize withdrawal symptoms in drug dependence.
5. Recognize the symptoms shown by a patient under the influence of drugs.
6. Become familiar with the short- and long-term effects of alcohol abuse.
7. Recognize drugs that are potentiated in their effects when taken with alcohol.
8. Identify the physical symptoms and dangerous sequelae of a drug overdose.

Key Terms

Habit formation, p. 217
Psychoactive (SĪ-kō-ĀK-tīv) **drug,** p. 216
Substance abuse, p. 216

Substance abuse is the use or overuse of a chemical or substance in a way that leads to dependence and has adverse effects on the health and well-being of the user and others. It has become a national and international problem of gigantic proportions and affects all of us in some way. The use of **psychoactive drugs** (drugs possessing the ability to alter mood, behavior, or cognitive processes) by children and adolescents is a fact no longer questioned. The most reasonable preventive effort is now focused on education. Rehabilitation programs have limited success but are increasing in numbers as the national problem persists.

According to a publication of the U.S. Department of Health and Human Services, more than 90% of adolescents in the United States will have used alcohol before graduating from high school, 50% will have used marijuana, 17% will have used cocaine, and 12% will have used hallucinogens. Of the 25,000 accidental deaths among youths annually, approximately 40% are alcohol related.

Studies have been done of the risk factors that predispose to substance abuse. The studies have shown that vulnerability to drug use is increased in children who have low self-esteem, a feeling of not belonging, a high need for social approval, inadequate bonding to family and society, inadequate communication and coping skills, an inability to defer gratification, and an inability to accept the consequences of their actions. A family history of alcoholism or substance abuse greatly increases the risk.

The substance-abusing teenager may first come to medical attention as a result of trauma related to intoxication or secondary to an acute drug overdose. The health care team should be responsible not only for treating the trauma but also for recognizing and assessing the substance abuse problem and, it is hoped, initiating some sort of remedial program. Most adolescents have three spheres of interaction: school, family, and peers. Adolescents who are having difficulty in any one of these spheres probably need referral for drug treatment. Convincing a patient and family members that a referral is needed may not be easy because there may be denial, a minimizing of the problem as a one-time occurrence, or a rejection of the values of society altogether.

During acute crises or overdoses in substance abusers, the health care worker has the responsibility of assessing the type of drug taken, the method of administration, the time the drug was taken, and the previous pattern of substance abuse. This information can be obtained from the abuser, if responsive, or the family or friends.

In the treatment and rehabilitation of the substance abuser, the health care worker is involved at many levels, assisting the patient through the withdrawal period, observing the patient for other problems, and observing the effects of therapy and the patient's level of cooperation.

SEVEN SIGNS OF POSSIBLE DRUG INVOLVEMENT

1. Change in school or work attendance or performance (e.g., the student whose grades begin to fall or the employee whose absentee rate is a matter of concern)
2. Alteration of personal appearance (e.g., the person who was once neat now appears disheveled and disorderly)
3. Mood swings or attitude changes
4. Withdrawal from family contacts

5. Association with drug-using friends
6. Unusual patterns of behavior or mannerisms
7. Defensive attitude concerning drugs

DEPENDENCE ON NARCOTICS

Heroin is the narcotic of choice for most addicts in the United States. Although this drug is outlawed in this country, illegal drug channels keep the addicts supplied. Paregoric, morphine, oxycodone (OxyContin), and hydromorphone (Dilaudid) are often abused also.

The desired sensation is a euphoria (an exaggerated sense of physical and emotional well-being) after administration of the drug, usually intravenously. With continued use, a tolerance to the drug occurs and higher doses are required for the euphoria. After a period of time, the addiction is so intense that the drug is taken for homeostasis and to prevent withdrawal symptoms. Accidental overdoses and death may occur inadvertently or in an attempt to obtain euphoria again.

The withdrawal symptoms from narcotics are severe and may be life-threatening. The first abstinence symptoms are malaise and weakness about 6 to 12 hours after the last dose. After 12 hours, yawning and perspiration occur, and the patient becomes anxious. After 24 hours, muscular contractions and pain, chills, increased rate and depth of respiration, blood pressure elevation, pupil dilation, and extreme agitation occur. The withdrawal symptoms peak in 48 hours and begin to subside in 72 hours. General symptoms of weakness and malaise may be present for several weeks.

Methadone maintenance programs have been developed to sustain narcotic addicts after withdrawal. Although methadone (Dolophine) is in itself an addicting narcotic, it produces little euphoria and allows the patient to function normally in society. Even with methadone, the percentage of addicts who are able to stop using narcotics is small.

SEDATIVE-HYPNOTIC ABUSE

Although these agents can be obtained through illegal channels, they are often abused by obtaining prescriptions for them, often from many physicians simultaneously. These drugs become dangerous with overuse, particularly when combined with alcohol or other depressive drugs.

Withdrawal is not as severe as with the narcotic agents and is primarily characterized by insomnia, irritability, and anxiety-related symptoms.

MARIJUANA ABUSE

Marijuana is an intoxicant derived from the leaves and flowering tops of the *Cannabis* plant. It is generally smoked in cigarette form and produces a feeling of euphoria and a dreamy state. The length of the effect lasts 3 to 12 hours.

Physical dependence most certainly occurs, although the question of true addiction is not settled. When a user demonstrates a preference for the use of a chemical or substance, but is not necessarily physiologically dependent, **habit formation** is said to have occurred. The term is generally used to mean a less severe state than addiction.

Various disorders have been attributed to long-term or chronic use of marijuana. These include chromosome breaks, personality and mental changes, cognitive problems, anxiety, and irritation when the drug is not available. Gynecomastia has been noted in males.

One of its more notable disadvantages is that it leads the dependent person to try other more addicting substances for a greater euphoric effect.

MEDICINAL USES OF MARIJUANA

Few ideas are so firmly held by the public and so doubted by the medical profession as the healing powers of marijuana. Believers speak of relief from premenstrual syndrome, the nausea and vomiting of chemotherapy, the physical wasting of acquired immunodeficiency syndrome and cancer, glaucoma, itching, insomnia, arthritis, depression, pain of childbirth, attention deficit disorder, peripheral neuropathy, and multiple sclerosis. Researchers are belatedly addressing this controversy to establish with scientific certainty whether such claims as pain relief, antinauseant effects, and muscle relaxant effects have any medical validity.

Research is also needed to compare smoked marijuana and orally administered delta-9-tetrahydrocannabinol (THC), the most active ingredient. THC has been available for some time in a synthetic tablet form called dronabinol (Marinol). Theoretically, the smoked and oral forms should do the same thing, but most participants prefer the smoked form, for control of both the dosage and the onset of action. Marinol when taken orally needs a couple of hours to take effect, and then the dose may be too high. When smoked, marijuana's chemicals reach the bloodstream in seconds and reach the brain soon thereafter. Users can regulate the effect puff by puff.

It is believed by some that marijuana has too many effects on the body to be readily controlled as a therapeutic drug. Some of its actions are readily apparent to those who have tried it: it produces a sense of well-being, a ravenous appetite, altered time and distance perception, and talkativeness, but users also experience a disruption of short-term memory and suppressed immune defenses. Research will undoubtedly shed light on this matter in the coming years.

COCAINE ABUSE

Although cocaine was once thought to be a relatively "safe" recreational drug, it is now considered one of the most potent of all the addictive drugs. In 1984 the highly potent, highly addictive "crack" form of cocaine was introduced, and its availability, along with its relatively inexpensive price, has greatly increased the number of addicts. It is believed that even one use of crack cocaine makes the user an addict because the urge for another "high" is so intense after even the first experience with this drug.

When applied locally, cocaine is a very effective anesthetic. When given systemically, cocaine is a central nervous system stimulant with effects that are similar to those of amphetamine. It produces a strong stimulant and euphoric effect and increases pulse rate, blood pressure, and respiratory rate. Many reports have documented cocaine-related myocardial ischemic events following systemic administration of cocaine. The risk of an acute myocardial infarction is increased by a factor of 24 during the 60 minutes after the use of cocaine. Cigarette smoking after taking cocaine induces vasoconstriction of the coronary arteries and increases the risk of myocardial events. The increase in systemic arterial pressure induced by cocaine has been implicated as a cause of aortic dissection or rupture.

The user feels a heightened sense of self-confidence, clarity of thought, and alertness as well as increased energy and well-being. Reductions in the need for sleep and food are common. The intoxicated individual has tremulousness, dysphoria, delirium, delusional thinking, and assaultive behavior.

Withdrawal symptoms include deep depression and profound exhaustion. Suicidal behavior is common during withdrawal. Medications are now used to treat the cocaine addict and to assist in the withdrawal with replacement drugs. These include antidepressants such as desipramine, imipramine, protriptyline, and trazodone. Lithium, usually prescribed for manic-depressive disorder, has been effective, especially if combined with an antidepressant. Amino acid supplements containing tyrosine and tryptophan, when combined with an antidepressant, seem to block the cocaine high.

ALCOHOL ABUSE

The most common "street drug" today, alcohol, is losing much of its social acceptability as the effects of its abuse become recognized.

Unlike the other abused agents, alcohol does have some beneficial effects in moderation. It has been shown to raise the level of high-density lipoproteins (the "good" type of cholesterol) and thus reduce the risk of coronary disease. Its effect on behavior is well known, from a sense of relaxation in small doses to abnormal behavior, a loss of sensorimotor control, and coma in overdose.

As intake progresses, the abuser loses the ability to perform fine motor movements, memory and discrimination become dulled, and nausea and vomiting result. It is believed that the cumulative effects on the central nervous system and liver progress with each dose.

Infants born to alcohol abusers have a cluster of birth defects known as the fetal alcohol syndrome. This is typified by a characteristic elfin facies and mental retardation. Some researchers believe that even small doses of alcohol during pregnancy may harm the fetus.

Many prescription drugs are potentiated by even small amounts of alcohol (Table 34–1). These generally are agents that have sedation as a side effect. They include antihistamines, tranquilizers, some antidepressants, sleeping medications, and many muscle relaxants. As a general rule, alcohol should be avoided when taking any prescription medication.

Table 34-1 | *Prescription Drugs Affected by Alcohol*

ALCOHOL COMBINED WITH	MAY CAUSE
Sleeping medication	Rapid intoxication with small amounts of alcohol
Tranquilizers	
Antidepressants	Excessive drowsiness
Motion sickness medication	Mental confusion
Pain relievers	
Muscle relaxants	
Antihistamines	
Allergy medicine	
Antiangina medication	Dizziness, fainting
Antihypertensives	Lack of muscle coordination, falling
Aspirin	Increase in gastric irritation and bleeding
Nonsteroidal antiinflammatory drugs	
Potassium tablets	
Anticoagulants	
Metronidazole (Flagyl)	Severe reaction, similar to that of disulfiram (Antabuse); nausea, tachycardia, dyspnea
Oral hypoglycemic agents	
Certain antibiotics	
Anticoagulants	Changes in the effectiveness of the drug controlling the condition
Oral hypoglycemic agents	
Seizure medications	

Table 34-2	*Comparative Symptoms of Drug Use*		
DRUG	**PHYSICAL SYMPTOMS**	**SIGNS TO LOOK FOR**	**DANGEROUS EFFECTS**
Inhalants (gas, aerosols)	Nausea, dizziness, headaches, lack of coordination	Odor of the substance on breath, intoxication symptoms	Unconsciousness, brain damage, sudden death
Heroin, narcotics	Euphoria, drowsiness, nausea, vomiting	Pinpoint pupils, needle tracks on arms	Death from overdose, AIDS, hepatitis from needles
Cocaine, amphetamine	Talkativeness, hyperalert state, increased blood pressure	History of weight loss, hyperactivity, ulcers in nasal mucosa	Sudden death, hallucinations, paranoia
Barbiturates, alcohol, tranquilizers	Intoxication, slowed heart and respiratory rate	Capsules and pills, history of seeing more than one physician, slurred speech	Death from overdose, especially in combinations with alcohol
Hallucinogens, LSD, PCP	Altered mood, panic, focus on detail	Capsules, blotter squares	Unpredictable and violent behavior
Marijuana	Altered perceptions, euphoria, laughing, red eyes, dry mouth	Cigarette papers, odor of burnt rope	Panic reaction, impaired memory

AIDS, Acquired immunodeficiency syndrome; *LSD,* lysergic acid diethylamide; *PCP,* phencyclidine hydrochloride.

SYMPTOMS OF DRUG ABUSE

Table 34–2 presents a general method to determine the agent that was most likely taken when a patient presents with abnormal drug-induced behavior. It should always be remembered that substance abusers may not have taken only a single substance. Drugs are often taken in combination, and they are often combined with alcohol.

CLINICAL IMPLICATIONS

1. Drug abuse among adolescents is very common. An assessment of the patient should include some questions about substance and alcohol abuse.
2. A vigorous denial of drug use should not be accepted at face value if the adolescent has risk factors for substance abuse.
3. The withdrawal symptoms from drug usage are unpleasant and may be severe and life-threatening. Many nursing interventions can be used to ease some of the discomfort and to prevent adverse outcomes.
4. After acute drug withdrawal, the addiction problem remains. Subsequent follow-up is vitally important, and abstinence must be reinforced and encouraged.

5. Substance abuse can occur using only prescription medications. Questioning the patient about drug compliance and about the use of several physicians as prescription drug sources can uncover this problem.
6. There is no "safe" recreational drug.
7. The most commonly abused substance is alcohol. Society provides many situations in which alcohol abuse is approved or tolerated. Societal norms are now found to be detrimental when attempting to control alcohol abuse.
8. Cocaine is a dangerous and extremely addicting drug, particularly in the "crack" form.
9. Many drugs are useful in the treatment of cocaine and heroin addiction. These agents both reduce the craving for the drug and prevent recurrence of the addictive pattern.
10. The symptoms of drug abuse, although not explicit in many cases, can enable the nurse to identify patients who may be under the influence of drugs.

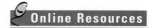 **Online Resources**

For updated drug information and Web activities, go to http://evolve.elsevier.com/Asperheim.

CRITICAL THINKING QUESTIONS

1. The patient has been brought to the emergency room after a car accident. She has a broken wrist and multiple bruises. Although it is expected that she would be worried and in pain, she is bright, cheerful, talkative, and alert. What other assessment may be made on this patient?

2. The patient is brought in for psychological testing by his parents. In grade school, he was an excellent student. He seems to have adjustment problems in high school, however. His grades are barely passing, he seems to have no friends, and his clothes seem disheveled and dirty. What line of questioning may be appropriate here?

3. The patient calls the clinic to say she needs a new prescription for Valium. Her entire bottle of tablets somehow was thrown out with the trash. You notice on her chart that her purse was stolen just 2 weeks ago, necessitating a new prescription. She also has headaches that require numerous pain medications, and requests are often called in just before the office closes. The doctors sharing night call report numerous requests for prescription refills. What additional problems may need to be pursued?

REVIEW QUESTIONS

1. A symptom of heroin withdrawal may be:
   a. sedation.
   b. tolerance.
   c. hypertension.
   d. pupil constriction.

2. A drug used frequently in maintenance programs for narcotic addicts is:
   a. heroin.
   b. morphine.
   c. hydrocodone.
   d. methadone.

3. A narcotic that is a central nervous system stimulant is:
   a. cocaine.
   b. procaine.
   c. marcaine.
   d. heroin.

4. For an opioid addict, the desired sensation after taking a drug is:
   a. sedation.
   b. euphoria.
   c. hypotension.
   d. enhanced school/work performance.

5. The dreamy state after smoking marijuana may last:
   a. 30 minutes.
   b. 2 hours.
   c. 3 to 12 hours.
   d. 2 weeks.

6. A beneficial effect of alcohol, consumed in moderation is:
   a. raised blood count.
   b. lowered blood count.
   c. lowered low-density lipoproteins.
   d. raised high-density lipoproteins.

7. The most commonly abused substance is:
   a. crack cocaine.
   b. heroin.
   c. prescription drugs.
   d. alcohol.

8. Which symptom may occur in a person secretly abusing drugs?
   a. A calm, reflective demeanor
   b. Withdrawal from family contacts
   c. A very neat appearance
   d. Improved school performance

9. When an addict does not take the drug of abuse, she or he is likely to experience:
   a. tolerance.
   b. increased level of addiction.
   c. lessening of tolerance.
   d. withdrawal symptoms.

10. Alcohol can potentiate the effects of all except which of the following prescription drugs?
    a. Tranquilizers
    b. Sleeping pills
    c. Muscle relaxants
    d. Oral contraceptives

Herbal Therapies and Drug-Herb Interactions

Objectives

After completing this chapter, you should be able to do the following:

1. Identify the common herbal medicines and their therapeutic actions.
2. Recognize prescription drugs that commonly interact with herbal products.
3. Recognize symptoms that may mean a patient is taking herbal medicines.
4. Understand the different ways herbs react with other drugs.
5. Assist the patient in choosing appropriate herbal remedies.

Key Terms

Health food products, p. 221
Herb, p. 221
Interaction, p. 221
Natural remedy, p. 221
Pharmacodynamic (FĂR-mĕ-kō-kī-NĔT-ĭk), p. 225
Pharmacokinetic (FĂR-mĕ-kō-dī-NĂM-ĭk), p. 225

It takes only a look around any drugstore or health food store to determine that herbal remedies are here to stay. Indeed, **health food products,** nutritional supplements or products that may or may not have the advertised effect, seem to proliferate daily.

In a historical context, of course, many of our drugs come from plants. The word "drug" comes from the French word *drogue,* meaning herb. Plant sources have provided aspirin, morphine, quinine, and digitalis, to mention a few of the currently used medications. As our skill in the laboratory has advanced, we have been able to extract only the active ingredients of plant sources, standardizing the dosage and reliably obtaining predictable results from each dose. In earlier forms of drugs, such as digitalis leaf, the entire leaf was pulverized and formed into a tablet. Early thyroid preparations were merely pulverized thyroid glands. There were obviously many more difficulties in determining the strength and potency of each preparation. Some of these difficulties persist with the use of nonstandardized herbal remedies.

One of the many problems with these self-healing products is that, at best, the money is wasted since there is no sci-entific basis for the sometimes outrageous claims made for these products; at worst, the product may be harmful to a person with certain medical conditions. Furthermore, to an increasingly alarming degree, they have been found to interfere with or alter the metabolism of many prescription drugs. The altered effect that occurs when two or more drugs and herbs are taken together is referred to as an **interaction,** and the results of such an interaction can be disastrous.

In the United States, at least five times as many people use medicinal herbs today as did at the start of the 1990s. The term **natural remedy** is used to refer to any treatment that can be used by nonprofessionals to alter a condition. The term **herb** is used to refer to any plant or plant part valued for its medicinal, savory, or aromatic qualities. Some surveys show that 35% to 48% of those surveyed had taken a natural remedy within the past year, and about one third took them every day. Many patients do not admit to using alternative therapies because of embarrassment or fear of censure. It is very important to assess the use of herbal remedies during any medical history (Box 35–1).

The difficulty in determining potency, pharmacologic activity, and standardization of doses in the products of the health food industry presents obvious problems. Furthermore, no regulatory agency such as the Food and Drug Administration oversees herbal products. When a manufacturer or health food store states that a natural remedy may be "good" for migraine headaches, for jittery nerves, for sleep, for memory enhancement, for colds, and so forth, it must be remembered that there is no guarantee that a product will do what the label says it does.

With these disclaimers in mind, this chapter attempts to sort out some of the literature and discuss the common herbal and natural remedies and their side effects, and then the interactions that may occur with prescription drugs when these are known. I have attempted to cover the common herbs and not include the ones that have no proven medicinal value, or those with less common usage. When a proved therapeutic dosage is available, this is given; in most cases there is merely a list of the forms that are commercially available.

HERBAL THERAPIES

aloe. Gel from the cactus-like leaves of the aloe plant has been used since prehistoric times. Rubbing aloe on skin to soothe minor burns, treat infections, and moisturize dry patches of skin is an accepted remedy. Its topical use to treat psoriasis is new and somewhat unproved, but it seems to work better than placebo. It has been taken internally as a cathartic, but this is not generally recommended due to side effects, which include heart arrhythmias, edema, and nephropathies when taken orally.

How supplied:
Capsule: 250 mg, 470 mg.
Gel: 72%, 99%.

angelica. The medicinal parts of this plant are the seeds, whole herb, and root. According to legend, angelica was revealed to a monk by an angel as a cure for the plague. Although its effect on the plague is not known, it has been shown to promote circulation to the extremities and produce a warming effect on the body. Women have found it useful in the treatment of menstrual cramps. Applied externally, it gives some relief to arthritic joints, and it is useful in the local treatment of lice. It has been used in folk remedies as a treatment for respiratory infections.

How supplied:
Comminuted root in a daily dose of 4.5 gm.
Tincture: 1:5 solution for internal or external use.

arnica. The medicinal parts of the arnica plant include the dried flowers, the leaves, and the dried rhizome and roots. Taken internally, it has been used to treat respiratory infections. Externally, it has been shown to be effective as an antiseptic and an analgesic. It relieves muscle spasms and joint pain when applied topically.

How supplied:
Whole herb.
Tincture: 1:10 using 70% ethanol.
Ointment: 15% arnica in a neutral base.

asafoetida. The oily gum-resin is the active ingredient of this plant. It has a mild intestinal disinfectant effect and has been used to treat dyspepsia and irritable bowel syndrome. Its effectiveness as a sedative is less certain. It has a putrid odor and a bitter taste, hence its nickname "devil's dung."

How supplied:
Tincture: 1:5 solution; recommended dose, 20 drops orally.

black cohosh. The roots and dark-colored rhizomes of this herb are used to treat the hot flashes of menopause, premenstrual tension, and dysmenorrhea. The old-time remedy "Lydia Pinkham's Vegetable Compound" contained many natural ingredients, including black cohosh. It appears that at least three fractions of the herb suppress luteinizing hormone and bind to estrogen receptors. It is contraindicated during pregnancy because it is associated with an increased risk of spontaneous abortion.

How supplied:
Capsule: Various strengths from 60 to 545 mg.

chamomile. Typically a cup of chamomile tea made from the flowers of the plant was used to relieve female anxiety. It is still a popular remedy for nervous stomach and is known for its calming effect on smooth muscle of the intestinal tract. Used externally, it relieves skin irritations and hemorrhoids, and used as a mouthwash it may relieve the pain of toothache.

How supplied:
Capsule: Various strengths from 125 to 354 mg.
Liquid: 1:4 dilution.
Tea: 3 gm of the herb in 1 cup of hot water; steep for 5 to 10 minutes, then strain.

cayenne (capsicum). Hot, spicy food may be good for your health. When taken orally, cayenne is a digestive aid. It stimulates the production of gastric juices and helps relieve gas. In addition, peppers contain vitamin C, as well as iron, calcium, phosphorus, and B-complex vitamins. Biting into a chili pepper triggers the release of endorphins in the brain, and this mechanism is known to relieve pain. Various antimicrobial effects have been shown after administration of cayenne pepper. Capsaicin, the active ingredient of the pepper, can be applied topically to relieve the pain of diabetic neuropathy, and for the topical treatment of muscle and joint disorders. It is a common ingredient of self-defense sprays. When sprayed into an attacker's eyes, it causes immediate blindness and irritation for up to 30 minutes, with no permanent effect.

How supplied:
Capsule: Various strengths from 400 to 500 mg.
Cream: 0.25% and 0.75% in a neutral base.

chaparral. The chaparrals are a group of related shrubs found in the southwestern United States and in Mexico. The leaflets and twigs are used medicinally to make tea. It has long been used by Native Americans to treat respiratory infections and painful conditions such as arthritis and abdominal pain. There have been reports of cancer patients benefiting from chaparral tea, and this effect is being studied. It has been shown to contain potent antioxidants.

How supplied:
Powdered leaflets

comfrey. The fresh root and leaves of comfrey are used medicinally. The healing effects of this plant are attributed to its active ingredient, allantoin, an agent that promotes cell proliferation. Poultices and ointments made from comfrey have been shown to have healing and antiinflammatory effects when applied topically. It has been taken internally for the treatment of gastritis and peptic ulcers, as well as for inflammatory conditions. It is hepatotoxic; thus long-term oral use is not advisable.

How supplied:

Comminuted herb.

Tea: 5 to 10 gm in 1 cup of boiling water; steep for 10 to 15 minutes.

echinacea. Extracts made from this root were all-time favorite cold remedies before antibiotics. It has been studied in Germany and some (of the many) types available have been shown in the laboratory to boost the immune system. Herbalists tend to prefer liquid tinctures made with alcohol because direct contact with the throat may enhance echinacea's effect. It may be taken prophylactically to prevent colds, or taken early in the infection.

How supplied:

Capsule: Various strengths from 100 to 500 mg.

Liquid: 120 mg/5 mL.

Tea: 1 teaspoon of the ground root in 1 cup of boiling water; steep for 10 minutes, then strain.

ephedra (ma-huang). The young canes and the dried rhizomes of this plant are the medicinal parts. It has been used for many centuries, particularly in Asia, to treat colds, asthma, and other respiratory symptoms. The use of the standardized ephedrine/pseudoephedrine has largely supplanted use of the crude drug for respiratory diseases. It has been used in the past in proprietary diet preparations. These have been removed from the market owing to the number of untoward side effects. When taken orally, there is a perceived increased energy, increased heart rate, and increased blood pressure, as well as nasal decongestion and bronchodilation. Toxic psychosis can be induced by this drug, as can life-threatening seizures, tachycardia, hypertension, and heart failure. Life-threatening poisonings are seen with very high dosages of the drug.

How supplied:

Powdered herb.

Tea: 1 to 4 gm in 1 cup of hot water.

Tincture: 1 part drug to 4 parts alcohol/water mixture; recommended dosage, 6 to 8 mL.

feverfew. Much interest has been focused on the activity of feverfew leaves in the prevention of migraine headaches, and some new studies appear to confirm its effectiveness for this purpose. Its effectiveness when used as a digestive aid, when used to treat intestinal parasites, arthritis, and menstrual cramps, or when used as a local anesthetic has not been confirmed. An increase in mouth ulcers has been reported with chronic use.

Recommended dosage for migraine prevention:

0.2 to 0.5 mg of parthenolide (the active ingredient) daily in fresh or dry powdered leaves.

How supplied:

Capsule: Various strengths from 80 to 1000 mg.

Tea: 2 teaspoonfuls of the herb in 1 cup of hot water; steep for 25 minutes.

garlic. Long a staple of both medicine and cuisine the world over, garlic was used in ancient times in poultices as an effective antibacterial. It has shown some effectiveness in the lowering of cholesterol and triglyceride levels while raising high-density lipoprotein levels. It interferes with platelet adhesiveness and reduces blood sugar levels, but studies have not shown a lowering of blood pressure, as claimed. Garlic's benefits appear to come from a compound called allicin, which breaks down into a number of other compounds. For the full benefit, it should be eaten raw.

How supplied:

Fresh garlic bulb, dried powder, oil, and aqueous extracts.

Capsule: Various strengths from 3 to 5000 mg.

ginger. The ginger root has been used for centuries for various ills. It is taken for heartburn, as an antiemetic, and as an antiinflammatory, and it increases the tone and peristalsis of the intestine. It has been compared favorably with scopolamine and dimenhydrinate when used to prevent motion sickness. It may be taken in moderation for the treatment of morning sickness in pregnant women. Some report that the cookie called a ginger snap works almost as well as the herb itself.

How supplied:

Powdered herb.

Capsule: Various strengths from 100 to 1000 mg.

Tea: 0.5 to 1 gm in 1 cup of boiling water; steep 5 minutes.

Ginkgo biloba. Studies have shown that seeds and leaves of the ginkgo tree can relieve the symptoms of intermittent claudication, increase walking performance, and somewhat diminish lower extremity pain. It has been studied in the treatment of Alzheimer's disease, and there are significant, if modest, benefits from the herb. It is known for its antioxidant effect as well. An increase in bleeding time and subdural hematomas have been observed after prolonged use. It should not be taken with warfarin because it enhances the anticoagulant effect.

How supplied:

Capsule: Various strengths from 30 to 500 mg.

Pulverized leaves: 3 to 6 gm as an infusion in 1 cup of hot water.

ginseng. In Chinese, *gin* means "man" and *seng* means "essence," a reflection of the root's human-like appearance and its supposed ability to cure just about everything. It has been used as a stimulant and as a tonic, and to treat menopausal hot flashes. It has been claimed to enhance cognitive function, but this has not been substantiated. It is currently used for the treatment of a subjective "lack of stamina." It should not be used with warfarin or nonsteroidal antiinflammatory drugs (NSAIDs) because it enhances the anticoagulant effect of these agents.

How supplied:
Comminuted root.
Capsule: Various strengths from 100 to 1250 mg.

goldenseal. The medicinal parts of goldenseal are the air-dried rhizome and root fibers, which contain the active alkaloids hydrastine, berberine, and canadine. It is poorly absorbed when given orally but has shown some effectiveness in the treatment of bacterial infections, notably with *Salmonella, Shigella,* and *Klebsiella* species, as well as in vitro activity against the intestinal parasites *Giardia lamblia, Trichomonas,* and *Entamoeba histolytica.* It has been used in the past for the treatment of eye infections, notably trachoma. It also has hypotensive, antisecretory, antitumor, and sedative properties. Prolonged use can cause digestive disorders and constipation, mucous membrane irritation, and occasionally hallucinations. It has an antagonistic effect on the anticoagulant activity of heparin.

How supplied:
Capsule: Various strengths from 500 to 1000 mg.
Extract: 5% hydrastine.

hops. This perennial plant has both male and female flowers. The female, conelike flowering parts are used medicinally. It has been used as an appetite stimulant, to treat neuropathies and headaches, and as a sedative. Its most common use, however, is in the commercial preparation of beer, to which it imparts the characteristic flavor.

How supplied:
Comminuted herb.
Liquid extract: 1:1 in 45% ethanol.
Tea: 1 teaspoonful in 1 cup of boiling water; steep for 10 to 15 minutes.

horse chestnut. The seeds and leaves of the horse chestnut are used medicinally. When taken internally, horse chestnut has been noted to reduce vascular permeability and exert a vascular tightening effect. It is used to treat lower extremity edema caused by venous insufficiency. Horse chestnut has a coumarin component; thus it enhances the effect of coumarin given therapeutically. Long-term use is not advisable due to the side effects of liver and kidney toxicity. It may be used topically for the treatment of hemorrhoids.

How supplied:
Capsule: Various strengths from 250 to 485 mg.
Tincture: 1:1 in 75% ethanol.

juniper. The berry cones of this plant, when administered orally, act as a diuretic. It also has an antihypertensive effect. The most common uses are as a flavoring for gin and as an ingredient in bath salts. Prolonged oral administration may result in nephrotoxicity.

How supplied:
Comminuted berries.

Capsule: 515 mg.
Tea: 0.5 gm in 1 cup of boiling water; steep for 10 to 15 minutes.

kava kava. South Pacific islanders have made a relaxing drink from the dried rhizome and roots of the kava plant for centuries. Ceremonial use has documented euphoria, muscle weakness, and, in higher doses, deep sleep. Several more recent, well-documented studies have shown that kava can relieve anxiety and stress. When chewed, it causes numbness in the mouth. Several cases of acute liver failure and cirrhosis have occurred following regular use. It should not be used by persons with underlying liver problems, or those who frequently imbibe alcoholic beverages.

How supplied:
Capsule: Various strengths from 100 to 500 mg.

milk thistle. The active ingredients of the milk thistle seed are silymarin and silybin. In vivo tests have shown that, after taking this agent, there is increased protein synthesis in the liver cells due to increased activity of ribosomal RNA. This reportedly activates the regenerative capacity of the liver through cell development. Hepatoprotection may also be attributed to its antioxidant properties and its alteration of the liver cell membrane, thus preventing the entrance of toxins into the cell. It is used as an adjunct in the treatment of alcoholic cirrhosis and hepatitis. It has been used in the treatment of *Amanita* mushroom poisoning. There is no evidence that it has a direct antiviral effect on the hepatitis virus; hepatitis B surface antigen levels remain unchanged. It is believed to aid in restoring hepatic function after viral or other damage.

Dosage:
140 mg of silymarin (active ingredient) three times daily.
How supplied:
Capsule: Various strengths from 70 to 1050 mg.

red clover. The dried flower heads of the clover may be taken internally to treat coughs and respiratory conditions. Externally it is used for the treatment of chronic skin conditions such as psoriasis and eczema. It has been used in combination with other herbs as the "Red Clover Combination" for the treatment of cancer. Its usefulness as an antineoplastic has not been proved. There is a coumarin-like anticoagulant effect; thus it is additive with warfarin and it enhances the antiplatelet effect of NSAIDs.

How supplied:
Comminuted herb.
Liquid extract: 1:1 prepared in 25% ethanol.
Tea: 4 gm in 1 cup of boiling water; steep for 10 to 15 minutes.

saw palmetto. The berries of the saw palmetto, a type of palm tree native to Florida, are the active parts of this plant. The mechanism of action for saw palmetto's effect in suppression of the symptoms of benign prostatic hypertrophy

(BPH) is poorly understood. It is believed to inhibit testosterone reductase, an enzyme that converts testosterone to 5-alpha-testosterone in the prostate. It does reduce the symptoms of BPH, including urinary hesitancy, nocturia, and frequent urination. It also has been shown to reduce blood levels of prostate-specific antigen. Concomitant prostate carcinoma should always be considered and ruled out when symptoms of prostate obstruction are present.

How supplied:
Capsule: Various strengths from 80 to 1000 mg.

slippery elm. The dried inner rind of the bark of this tree is used medicinally by many native peoples. The active ingredient is the mucilage that is derived from the inner bark when it is soaked in water. This may be used locally as a demulcent for the treatment of many topical conditions, including ulcers, wounds, abscesses, and toothaches. Taken internally, it is a soothing drink that relieves irritations of the mucous membrane.

How supplied:
Comminuted herb.
Capsule: 370 mg.

St. John's wort. The medicinal parts of St. John's wort include the fresh buds and flowers, but all above-ground parts of the plant may be used. It has been used effectively to treat mild to moderate depression in studies completed in Germany. It is now a component of various herbal remedies for the treatment of anxiety and depression. Its use in combination with selective serotonin reuptake inhibitors and tricyclic antidepressants is being studied.

How supplied:
Capsule: Various strengths from 125 to 1000 mg.
Tea: 2 to 3 gm of dried herb in 1 cup of hot water.
Liquid: 300 mg/5 mL.
Transdermal: 900 mg/24 hours.

tea tree oil. This oil comes from the leaves of the Australian tree *Melaleuca alternifolia.* It can be found as a pure oil and as an ingredient in skin creams and gels, toothpaste, dental floss, mouthwash, deodorant, shampoos, and even toothpicks. It is a topical antifungal and antibiotic for infections of the skin and mucous membranes. It is used as a topical treatment for acne, tinea pedis, head lice, cradle cap, gingivitis, canker sores, warts, and scabies, as well as in a douche for nonspecific vaginitis.

Dosage:
For toenail onychomycosis—100% oil applied to toenails twice daily. For acne or other topical conditions—5% to 15% oil preparations three or four times daily.

valerian. Hippocrates and Galen both used the root of the valerian plant for a sedative to treat insomnia, and it is used effectively for this purpose today. Its main disadvantage appears to be its disagreeable smell. It is often combined with hops or St. John's wort in commercial products.

Dosage:
For insomnia—300 to 600 mg 2 hours before bedtime.

How supplied:
Capsule: Various strengths from 100 to 1000 mg.
Tea: 1 teaspoonful (3 to 5 gm) of powdered root in 1 cup of hot water; steep for 10 to 15 minutes, then strain.

white willow. The bark of young (2- to 3-year-old) branches is harvested during early spring for medicinal use. The active ingredient is salicin, the precursor of salicylic acid, which is itself the precursor of acetylsalicylic acid, or aspirin. It has antirheumatic, antiinflammatory, and antipyretic effects. The tannin component of the bark has astringent properties on mucous membranes. White willow will also reduce platelet aggregation similar to aspirin. It should not be taken with warfarin or other NSAIDs.

How supplied:
Comminuted herb.
Tea: 2 to 3 gm in cold water; bring to a boil, then steep for 5 minutes.

DRUG-HERB INTERACTIONS

It is essential that health care professionals know what herbal preparations the patient is taking. Queries about the use of over-the-counter or proprietary drugs should be part of every medical history. If the patient senses that the health care worker is judgmental, a full and correct history may not be obtained.

Herbal medicines interact with drugs in two general ways: pharmacokinetically and pharmacodynamically. **Pharmacokinetic** effects include alterations in drug absorption, distribution, metabolism, or excretion. These biologic changes may act to either increase or decrease the amount of drug available to have the desired effect. **Pharmacodynamic** interactions change the way a drug affects a tissue or organ system. This may result in increased or decreased effect on the targeted end organ for the drug. Table 35–1 lists some known drug-herb interactions.

It is important to ask the right questions when interviewing a patient about the use of drugs and herbal remedies in order to avoid possible drug and/or herb interactions. Some additions to the interview may obtain the necessary information:

1. Remember to inquire about lifestyle, such as smoking. Smoking may alter the metabolism of certain drugs such as theophylline.
2. Ask about diet, specific types of food, and quantity. Diets with excessive amounts of green leafy vegetables may have sufficient amounts of vitamin K to interfere with the effects of warfarin (Coumadin). Diet is also important for patients taking monoamine oxidase inhibitors, because they must avoid foods with a high tyramine content, such as cheeses and wine.

Table 35-1 *Drug-Herb Interactions*

HERB	REDUCES EFFECT	ENHANCES EFFECT	AVOID USE WITH
aloe		Potassium loss of diuretics	
black cohosh		Antihypertensives, diuretics	Pregnancy
		Antiplatelet action of NSAIDs	
		Warfarin	
capsicum		Antihypertensives	
chamomile		Sedatives, warfarin	
		Antiplatelet action of NSAIDs	
comfrey			Preexisting liver disease
echinacea	Immunosuppressants, cyclosporine, azathioprine	Autoimmune disorders, multiple sclerosis	
ephedra	Antihypertensives, phenothiazines	Theophylline, epinephrine, caffeine, decongestants, stimulants	Hypertension, diabetes, psychiatric disorders, cardiac arrhythmias, MAO inhibitors
feverfew		Antiplatelet action of NSAIDs Warfarin	Pregnancy, lactation
garlic		Antiplatelet action of NSAIDs Warfarin	
Ginkgo biloba		Antiplatelet action of NSAIDs Warfarin	Tricyclic antidepressants
ginger		Antiplatelet action of NSAIDs Warfarin, digitalis	Gallstones, bleeding disorders
ginseng		Antiplatelet action of NSAIDs Warfarin, phenelzine	Diabetes, MAO inhibitors
goldenseal	Heparin	Antihypertensives, sedatives	G6PD deficiency
hawthorn		Digitalis, antihypertensives	
horse chestnut		Antiplatelet action of NSAIDs Warfarin	
juniper berries		Lithium, diuretics	Preexisting liver disease
kava kava	Levodopa and other antiparkinson drugs	Sedatives, hypnotics, antihistamines, alcohol, alprazolam	Depressive disorders; pregnancy, lactation
red clover		Antiplatelet action of NSAIDs Warfarin	
saw palmetto	Estrogens, androgens, adrenergic drugs, oral contraceptives		Pregnancy, lactation
St. John's wort	Theophylline, coumarin, digoxin, indinavir, cyclosporine, oral contraceptives	SSRIs, tricyclic antidepressants	MAO inhibitors
valerian		Sedatives, hypnotics, antihistamines, benzodiazepines	Pregnancy, lactation
white willow	probenecid	Antiplatelet action of NSAIDs Warfarin, phenytoin, methotrexate	Preexisting bleeding tendencies

G6PD, Glucose-6-phosphate dehydrogenase; *MAO*, monoamine oxidase; *NSAIDs*, nonsteroidal antiinflammatory drugs; *SSRIs*, selective serotonin reuptake inhibitors.

3. Ask to see all the prescription medications that a patient is taking. They can often remember only part of the list of medications.

4. Ask what the patient may take when he or she has a headache, indigestion, or pain or needs a laxative. Ask specifically about herbs or natural remedies.

5. Ask about alcohol consumption in a nonthreatening manner. The physician should be notified if the patient consumes more than four alcoholic drinks per day.

6. Medication compliance is an issue, particularly for the elderly. The spouse or caregiver should be questioned about the reliability of the patient managing her or his own medications.

CLINICAL IMPLICATIONS

1. Herbal remedies should not be disregarded as useless; many have significant pharmacologic actions.
2. A careful history should be taken to ascertain whether the patient is taking any herbal or other proprietary remedies. Patients may not answer questions truthfully if they feel the nurse is being judgmental about herbal remedies.
3. Plants have been the source of many of our commonly used pharmacologic agents, as well as herbal remedies.
4. The nurse should be particularly aware of the many herbal remedies that may cause bleeding problems when the patient is taking warfarin or NSAIDs.
5. Herbal remedies may have active ingredients that are similar to commonly used drugs.
6. Many herbs will alter the metabolism of another drug in the body. This alteration may be an increase or a decrease in the potency of the other drug.
7. Herbal remedies may affect many diseases such as hypertension or diabetes, as well as immune disorders. Particular care should be taken to advise patients with these diseases not to take herbal remedies without medical advice.
8. There is often an enhanced feeling of well-being when a person is taking proprietary medications. These should not necessarily be discouraged unless there is evidence that a combination may be harmful.
9. Many herbal remedies do not exert their advertised effect. There is no regulation to determine truth in advertising with regard to herbs.
10. The nurse should become familiar with common herbal formulations and advise the patient as to which may be helpful and which to avoid.

Online Resources

For updated drug information and Web activities, go to http://evolve.elsevier.com/Asperheim.

CRITICAL THINKING QUESTIONS

1. The patient arrives at the doctor's office to have his rash treated. You notice dark red patches on his forearms. He has a previous history of thromboembolic disorders and has been maintained for 9 months on a low dose of warfarin without any previous changes in his international normalized ratios, which have always been maintained in the optimal range of 2.5 to 3.5. What could be the cause of the rash? What questions would you ask the patient?

2. The patient arrives with some new herbal remedies he has begun taking. These are hawthorn, goldenseal, and angelica. You notice his regular medicines are verapamil (Calan SR), hydrochlorothiazide (HydroDIURIL), and Colace. Would there be any conflicts here? What do you advise?

3. The patient, a generally healthy elderly woman taking no medications except calcium and vitamins, is complaining of chronic insomnia. She doesn't want to take any prescription sedatives, fearing that they may be habit forming. What herbal remedies may be advised?

REVIEW QUESTIONS

1. The term *herb* may be applied to:
   a. any drug.
   b. any plant part used in medicine.
   c. any plant.
   d. a drug considered for prescription use.

2. A claim made about the intended use of an herbal product may be:
   a. not trusted at all.
   b. not proven by established medical standards.
   c. believed in its entirety.
   d. considered safe because it's a natural drug.

3. A drug used by some to relieve the symptoms of menopause is:
   a. asafetida.
   b. cayenne.
   c. black cohosh.
   d. angelica.

4. Garlic has been shown to:
   a. lower cholesterol levels.
   b. raise cholesterol levels.
   c. treat heartburn.
   d. help with weight loss.

5. An herb used as a cold remedy is:
   a. ginger.
   b. chaparral.
   c. echinacea.
   d. feverfew.

6. A sedative drink can be made from:
   a. Ginkgo biloba.
   b. kava kava.
   c. tea tree oil.
   d. saw palmetto.

7. Which herb is thought to relieve prostatic hypertrophy?
   a. Kava kava
   b. Slippery elm
   c. Red clover
   d. Saw palmetto

8. Which herb was a precursor of aspirin?
   a. White willow
   b. Valerian
   c. Asafetida
   d. Cayenne

9. Which herb should not be taken with warfarin?
   a. Valerian
   b. Aloe
   c. White willow
   d. Kava kava

10. When a patient is scheduled for surgery, all herbs should be discontinued:
    a. 1 day before surgery.
    b. 7 days before surgery.
    c. 3 weeks before surgery.
    d. No need to discontinue them.

Glossary

A

ACE inhibitor An agent that inhibits the angiotensin-converting enzyme (ACE).

acetylcholine (ăs-ē-tĭl-KŌ-lēn) A neurotransmitter agent widely distributed in body tissues, with a primary function of mediating synaptic activity of the nervous system and skeletal muscles.

achlorhydria (Ā-klŏr-HĪ-drē-ĕ) The absence of hydrochloric acid in the stomach.

acidosis (ĂS-ĭ-DŌ-sĭs) A decrease in the alkali reserve of the blood, notably in the bicarbonates, with lowering of the blood pH.

acne An inflammatory eruption of the skin.

active immunity Production of natural antibodies against an antigen, or attenuated microorganism, injected into the body.

addiction The state in which the use of drugs is compulsive; withdrawal symptoms occur if the drug is withdrawn.

Addison's disease Adrenal insufficiency, fatal if not treated with corticosteroid hormones. Symptoms include bronzing of the skin, emaciation, and anemia.

additive effect The combined effect of two drugs that is equal to the sum of the effects of each drug taken alone.

adjunct An additional drug or chemical substance used to increase the efficacy or safety of a primary drug or to facilitate its action.

adrenergic (ĂD-rĭ-NŪR-jĭk) An agent that produces stimulating effects on the sympathetic nervous system (adrenaline-like effects).

adrenergic blocking agent A drug that interferes with adrenergic, or sympathetic nervous system, actions.

adverse or untoward effect An action, usually negative, that is different from the planned effect.

aerosols Active pharmaceutical agents in a pressurized container.

agranulocytosis (ă-GRĂN-yū-lō-sī-TŌ-sĭs) A toxic condition often caused by reactions to drug therapy in which a certain type of white blood cells—those with very small granules in the cell body—is deficient or absent.

AIDS Acquired immunodeficiency syndrome.

alkaloid (ĂL-kĕ-loĭd) An organic substance, basic in reaction, often the active ingredient of plant medicinals.

alkalosis An increase in the bicarbonate content of the blood, with subsequent raising of the blood pH.

alkylating (ĂL-kĭ-LĀ-tĭng) **agents** Any substance that contains an alkyl radical and is capable of replacing a free hydrogen atom in an organic compound.

allergen A substance capable of producing an allergic reaction.

allergic reaction An untoward reaction that develops after the individual has taken a drug.

allergy A hypersensitivity reaction provoked by a sensitizing agent, or allergen.

amide A substance derived from ammonia.

amino acid An organic acid composed of carbon, hydrogen, and nitrogen. These are components of protein molecules.

analgesia (ăn-ăl-JĒ-zē-ă) The relief of pain.

analgesic A substance used to relieve pain.

analog A substance structurally or chemically similar to another related drug or chemical but that has different effects.

anaphylaxis (ĂN-ĕ-fĭ-LĂK-sĭs) A severe, life-threatening allergic reaction accompanied by vasodilation, lowered blood pressure, and shock.

androgen (ĂN-drĕ-jĭn) Any steroid hormone that increases male characteristics.

anemia A reduction in the hemoglobin content or number of red blood cells.

anesthesia (ăn-ĕs-THĒ-zē-ă) Loss of sensation resulting from pharmacologic depression of the central nervous system.

anesthetic (ăn-ĕs-THĒ-tĭk), **general** An agent that induces analgesia, then unconsciousness.

anesthetic, local An agent, usually injected, that interferes with local nerve transmission and produces deadening or anesthesia of a small area of the body.

angina pectoris (ăn-JĪ-nĕ PĔK-tĕr-ĭs) Severe chest pain resulting from ischemia of the cardiac muscle that may radiate to other locations, notably the left shoulder or arm.

anorexia (ĂN-ō-RĔK-sē-ă) A loss of appetite.

antacid An agent that destroys gastric acids either in whole or in part by neutralizing or adsorbing them, thus rendering them inactive.

antagonism The combined effect of two drugs that is less than the effect of either drug taken alone.

antagonist A drug that opposes a bodily system or expected effect.

antibiotic An agent that kills or inhibits microorganisms.

antibody A substance produced by the body as a reaction to the intrusion of a foreign compound, or antigen; the antibody is designed to counteract or neutralize the offending antigen.

anticoagulant (ăn-tĭ-kō-ĂG-ū-lănt) A substance used to delay blood clotting.

anticonvulsant (ăn-tĭ-kŏn-VŬL-sănt) A substance used to prevent or treat seizures.

antidepressant (ăn-tĭ-dĕ-PRĔS-ănt) A drug used to produce mood elevation or mild central nervous system stimulation.

antidote (ĂN-tĭ-dōt) An agent that neutralizes a substance or counteracts its effects.

antiemetic (ĂN-tĭ-ĭ-MĔT-ĭk) An agent that prevents vomiting.

antigen Any substance that stimulates the production of antibodies in the body or any substance that reacts with previously formed antibodies.

antihistamine (AN-tĭ-HIS-tă-mĭn) An agent that prevents or diminishes the pharmacologic effects of histamine, hence used in the treatment of allergy-type syndromes.

antihypertensive (ăn-tĭ-hī-pĕr-TĔN-sĭv) **drug** An agent used in the treatment of high blood pressure.

antilipidemic (ĂN-tĭ-LĬP-ĭ-DĒ-mĭk) **drug** A drug that reduces the amount of lipids in the serum.

antimetabolite (ăn-tĭ-mĕ-TĂB-ĕ-līt) A substance that competes with, replaces, or antagonizes a bodily function.

antineoplastic (ĂN-tĭ-NĒ-ō-PLĂS-tĭk) **drug** An agent used in the treatment of cancer.

antioxidant (ĂN-tĭ-ŎK-sĭ-dĕnt) An agent that inhibits oxidation and neutralizes the effects of free radicals.

antiplatelet (ăn-tĭ-PLĀT-lĭt) **agent** An agent that destroys platelets or inhibits their function.

antiprostaglandin (ăn-tĭ-PRŎS-tă-GLĂN-dĭn) An agent that counteracts the effect of a prostaglandin on a specific tissue.

antipyretic (ĂN-tĭ-pī-RĔT-ĭk) A substance used to lower body temperature.

antiseptic A substance that inhibits the growth of microorganisms.

antispasmodic An agent used to decrease peristaltic activity of the gastrointestinal tract.

anxiolytic (ĀNGK-sē-ō-LĬT-ĭk) **agent** An agent that is used to relieve anxiety.

aplastic anemia Dysfunction of the bone marrow, often occurring as a reaction to drug therapy, in which there is a severe decrease in the production of erythrocytes and white blood cells.

arachnoiditis Inflammation of the arachnoid membrane covering the brain.

arthritis Inflammation of joints.

ascites (ĕ-SĪ-tēz) The presence of large amounts of fluid in the abdominal cavity.

asphyxia (ăs-FĬK-sē-ĕ) Suffocation.

asthma (ĂS-mĕ) A condition in which there is constriction of the lung bronchioles in response to allergic or emotional phenomena, producing symptoms of dyspnea, constriction in the chest, coughing, and expiratory wheezing.

astringents (ĕ-STRĬN-jĕnts) Substances that cause tissues to contract, helping to reduce secretions.

ataxia (ĕ-TĂK-sē-ĕ) Muscular incoordination, with staggering gait.

atherosclerosis (ĂTH-ĕ-RŌ-sklĕ-RŌ-sĭs) The deposition of fatty material in the walls of the blood vessels.

athetosis (ĂTH-ĕ-TŌ-sĭs) Recurrent, slow, and continual body movements, usually the result of a brain lesion.

atrium (pl. atria) The upper chambers of the heart.

automatic stop policy An institutional policy that discontinues a drug order or prescription after a specified period of time.

autonomic (ăw-tō-NŎM-ĭk) **nervous system** The nervous system that controls many body organ systems automatically or involuntarily; composed of nerves leading from the central nervous system that innervate and control smooth muscle, cardiac muscle, and glands.

avitaminosis The condition that develops from a lack of vitamins.

B

bacteremia (BĂK-tĭ-RĒ-mē-ĕ) The presence of microorganisms in the bloodstream.

bactericide A substance that kills bacteria.

bacteriostatic A substance that inhibits the growth of bacteria.

barbiturates (băr-BĬCH-ū-rătĕs) Drugs derived from barbituric acid that act as sedatives or hypnotics.

beriberi A condition caused by a nutritional deficiency of thiamine (vitamin B$_1$), with symptoms and neurologic involvement such as weakness, paralysis, edema, and mental deterioration.

beta-lactam antibiotics The cephalosporin group, named by an element in their chemical structure.

biosynthesis Formation of a chemical compound by enzymes either within an organism (in vivo) or in the laboratory (in vitro) by fragmentation of cells.

biotechnology The field of pharmacology that involves using living cells, usually altered cultures of *Escherichia coli,* to manufacture drugs.

bladder The membranous sac that collects urine produced by the kidneys.

blood dyscrasia (dĭs-KRĀ-zhĕ) Any abnormal condition in the type or number of the formed elements (cells) of the blood.

Bowman's capsule The renal glomerular capsule.

bradycardia (BRĂD-ē-KĂR-dē-ĕ) Slowing of the heartbeat.

broad-spectrum antibiotic An antibiotic that is effective against a wide range of infectious microorganisms.

bronchiole (BRŎNG-kē-ōl) The tiny, thin-walled lung tubules near the alveoli.

bronchoconstrictor An agent that causes tightening or narrowing of the lung bronchioles.

bronchodilator An agent that causes relaxation and enlargement of the bronchi.

C

calibration Measurement of an intravenous solution delivered "per drop."

cancer A tumor or unnatural growth in the body.

Candida albicans (KĂN-dĭ-dĕ ĂL-bĕ-kănz) A yeastlike organism that produces cutaneous or mucus membrane infections.

candidiasis (KĂN-dĭ-DĪ-ĕ-sĭs) A superinfection with the fungus *Candida albicans.* May be in the form of diaper rash, oral mucous membrane involvement (thrush), vaginitis, or infection of the skin or nails. If superinfection occurs in the gastrointestinal tract, diarrhea commonly results.

capsules Powdered or liquid drugs placed in soft gelatin capsules (e.g., cod liver oil capsules, Benadryl capsules).

carcinogen An agent that produces cancer.

carcinoma (KĂR-sĭ-NŌ-mĕ) A malignant neoplasm caused by excessive cellular proliferation; also known as cancer.

carminative (kăr-MĬN-ĕ-tĭv) An agent used to expel gas from the gastrointestinal tract.

catalyst (KĂT-ĕ-lĭst) A substance that increases the speed of a chemical reaction but is not used up or permanently changed in any way by the reaction.

cathartic (kĕ-THĂR-tĭk) A strong laxative that produces frequent, watery stools.

CD4 cells A subpopulation of lymphocytes referred to as the helper T cells. The CD4 cell count corresponds to the severity of an AIDS infection.

cephalosporin (SĔF-ĕ-lō-SPŌ-ĭn) An antibiotic derived from the microorganism *Cephalosporium falciforme,* and similar to penicillin.

cerebral palsy A nonspecific term for motor, speech, and mental dysfunctions resulting from brain damage, usually at birth.

chancroid (SHĂNG-krŏĭd) Venereal infection, with lesions involving the genitalia, and enlarged, painful inguinal lymph nodes.

chemical substances Agents that may be made synthetically (e.g., sulfonamides, aspirin, sodium bicarbonate).

cholinergic (KŌ-lēn-ŬR-jĭk) An agent that produces the effects of stimulation of the parasympathetic nervous system (acetylcholine-like effects).

cholinergic blocking agent An agent that interferes with the cholinergic, or parasympathetic nervous system, functions.

coagulant (kō-ĂG-yĕ-lĕnt) An agent that causes a blood clot to form.

coanalgesic (KŌ-ăn-ăl-JĒ-sĭk) A drug that may be used to potentiate pain relief.

colitis Inflammation of the colon with accompanying diarrhea, often associated with mucus or blood.

congestive heart failure A condition in which the heart is unable to circulate blood satisfactorily.

constipation The condition whereby bowel movements are infrequent or incomplete.

contraceptive An agent that prevents conception.

Controlled Substances Act A law (effective May 1, 1971) that requires that every person who manufactures, dispenses, prescribes, or administers any controlled substance be registered annually with the Attorney General, under the direction of the Drug Enforcement Administration (DEA).

convulsion (seizure) Involuntary muscle contractions, either focal or generalized, usually occurring as a result of brain dysfunction.

corticosteroid (KŎR-tĭ-kō-STĬR-ŏyd) Any of the hormones produced by the adrenal cortex (other than sex hormones) that influence or control key processes of the body.

cortisone A glucocorticoid not normally secreted in significant amounts by the adrenal cortex. It exhibits no biological activity until converted to hydrocortisone.

coryza Engorgement of the nasal mucous membranes, accompanied by increased nasal discharge and often sneezing.

COX-2 inhibitor A class of NSAIDs that preferentially inhibit cyclooxygenase-2 over cyclooxygenase-1, to reduce side effects of the medication.

cretin (KRĒ-tĭn) Mentally retarded dwarf with congenital hypothyroidism.

crystalluria (KRĬS-tĕ-LŪR-ē-ē) Crystals in the urine.

Cushing's disease (or syndrome) A condition caused by overactivity of the adrenal gland, causing florid facies, edema, striae, demineralization of bone, and other effects.

cyanosis (SĪ-ĕ-NŌ-sĭs) Bluish tinge of the skin and mucous membranes, usually caused by excessive amounts of deoxygenated hemoglobin in the blood.

cyclooxygenase-2 (COX-2) An enzyme in the body that is involved in the inflammatory process.

cystitis (sĭs-TĪ-tĭs) Inflammation of the urinary bladder.

D

DEA Drug Enforcement Administration.

dementia (dĭ-MĔN-shē) The loss of cognitive and intellectual functions.

demulcent (dĭ-MŬL-sĕnt) A substance used to soothe or reduce irritation of a surface.

deoxyribonucleic acid *See* DNA.

dependence A severe attachment to a drug or agent; an addiction.

depressant An agent that causes reduction in activity of a bodily system.

depression (1) A decrease in activity of cells caused by the action of a drug. (2) An unnatural state of lethargy, inactivity, and sadness.

dermatitis An inflammatory condition of the skin.

diabetes insipidus A disease caused by a decrease in the hormone vasopressin, permitting large amounts of very dilute urine to be passed regardless of the body fluid status. The condition is accompanied by extreme thirst and dehydration.

diabetes mellitus A condition brought about by a deficiency of functional insulin from the pancreas, thus interfering with the body's ability to metabolize glucose. Hyperglycemia, glycosuria, atherosclerosis, decreased resistance to infection, retinal hemorrhages, and kidney damage are among the manifestations of the disease.

diagnostic Pertaining to the art or act of determining the nature of a patient's disease.

diarrhea Abnormally frequent bowel discharges.

digestant A drug that promotes the process of digestion in the gastrointestinal tract and constitutes a type of replacement therapy in deficiency states.

digestion The mechanical, chemical, and enzymatic process whereby food is converted to material suitable for use in the body.

disinfectant (germicide) A substance that destroys microorganisms on objects; usually too irritating to be used on human tissue.

diuresis (dĭ-ūr-RĒ-sĭs) The formation of urine.

diuretic A substance used to increase the output of urine.

DNA Deoxyribonucleic acid; the component of genes that carries information.

dosage The size amount, frequency, and number of doses of a therapeutic agent to be administered to a patient.

dosage forms The systems used to deliver drugs.

dose The amount of a drug or other substance to be administered at one time.

double helix The twin coil structure of DNA.

drug Any substance used as medicine (e.g., used to diagnose, cure, mitigate, treat, or prevent disease).

drug allergy An adverse reaction to a drug.

drug order Consists of the name of the drug, the dosage, when the drug is to be given, how it is to be given, how many times it is to be given, the date of the order, and the signature of the physician who wrote the order.

drug standards Published lists of the known value, strength, quality, and ingredients of various drugs.

dyscrasia (dĭs-KRĀ-zhĕ) An abnormal state.

dysmenorrhea (DĬS-mĕn-ĕ-RĒ-ĕ) Painful menstruation.

E

ED Erectile dysfunction.

edema (ĭ-DĒ-mĕ) The excessive accumulation of fluid in the tissue spaces.

elixirs Solutions containing alcohol, sugar, and water. They may or may not be aromatic and may or may not have active medicinals. Most frequently they are used as flavoring agents or solvents (e.g., terpin hydrate elixir, phenobarbital elixir).

embolus (pl. emboli) (ĔM-bĕ-lĕs) A blood clot, or portion of a clot, that has broken away from its site of formation and traveled via the bloodstream to another site within the body.

emesis (ĔM-ĕ-sĭs) Vomiting.

emetic (ĭ-MĔT-ĭk) A substance used to induce vomiting.

emollient (ĭ-MŎL-yĕnt) A substance that softens tissue, particularly skin and mucous membranes.

emulsions Suspensions of fat globules in water (or water globules in fat) with an emulsifying agent (e.g., Haley's MO, Petrogalar). (Homogenized milk is also an emulsion.)

endocrine gland A ductless gland that secretes internally.

enuresis (ĕn-ū-RĒ-sĭs) Involuntary discharge of urine.

enzyme A substance formed by living cells that promotes or enhances a particular chemical reaction in the body by functioning as a catalyst.

epilepsy A brain dysfunction in which abnormal electrical discharges occur at intervals, causing motor seizures or psychic phenomena.

epileptic equivalents Disorders that resemble epilepsy, but are caused by other conditions.

epinephrine (ĔP-ĕ-NĔF-rĭn) A natural adrenal medulla hormone.

erythema (ĔR-ĭ-THĒ-mĕ) Reddening of the skin.

erythrocyte (ĕ-RĬTH-rĕ-SĪT) Red blood cell; contains hemoglobin, which is responsible for carrying oxygen to body tissues.

essential fatty acids Molecules found within fats that are not produced by the body but are necessary for proper functioning.

estrogens (ĔS-trŏ-jĭns) One of a group of hormonal steroids that promote the development of female sex characteristics.

exocrine gland A gland with a duct, which secretes outwardly or onto a luminal surface.

F

fiber A food substance found only in plants that is not digested by gastrointestinal enzymes.

fibrillation Quivering of cardiac muscle fibers, rendering the heart unable to contract with sufficient force to circulate blood effectively.

fluid extract Alcoholic liquid extract of a drug made by percolation so that 1 mL of the fluid extract contains 1 gm of the drug. Only vegetable drugs are used (e.g., glycyrrhiza fluid extract).

follicle-stimulating hormone The hormone that stimulates the maturation of the graafian follicles in the ovary.

fungus A general term for a group of microorganisms that includes yeasts and molds.

G

ganglion (GĂNG-glē-ŏn) A group of nerve cell bodies.

gels Aqueous suspensions of insoluble drugs in hydrated form. Aluminum hydroxide gel, USP, is an example.

gene A functional unit of heredity that occupies a specific place on a chromosome.

gene therapy The application of genetic principles to the treatment of human disease.

genome (JĒ-nōm) A complete set of chromosomes.

geriatric (JĔR-ē-ĂT-rĭk) Pertaining to old age or the elderly.

gland An organized aggregation of cells that functions as a secretory or excretory organ.

glaucoma (glô-KŌ-mĕ) A serious eye disorder in which normal drainage of intraocular fluid is impaired, causing increased intraocular pressure. Blindness results if treatment is delayed.

glomerulus (glō-MĔR-yū-lĕs) The tuft of capillaries projecting into the glomerular capsule. The capillaries allow filtration of water, salt, and impurities from the blood and thus are responsible for the first stage in urine formation.

glycosuria (GLĪ-kō-SŎŎR-ē-ĕ) Sugar in the urine.

goiter (GŎY-tĕr) Enlargement of the thyroid gland; may occur with either hypothyroidism or hyperthyroidism.

gynecomastia Abnormal enlargement of one or both of the male breasts.

H

habit formation The condition in which drugs are routinely taken as a matter of course, not as a matter of necessity. Withdrawal symptoms are not seen on cessation of the habit.

health food products {AU: PLEASE SUPPLY DEFINITION}

hematinic (HĔM-ĕ-TĬN-ĭk) An agent that increases the number of erythrocytes or the hemoglobin concentration of the blood; examples are iron and B vitamins.

hemoglobin The red pigment in erythrocytes that reversibly combines with oxygen, thus transporting it to tissues.

hemosiderosis (HĒ-mō-SĪD-ĕ-RŌ-sĭs) A condition in which there is an excessive deposition of iron in the tissues, particularly in the liver, causing cirrhosis, and in the pancreas, causing diabetes mellitus.

hepatitis Inflammation of the liver.

herb Any plant or plant part valued for its medicinal, savory, or aromatic qualities.

herbal remedy A drug derived from a plant, generally available without a prescription.

hirsutism (HŬR-sū-TĬZ-ĕm) Excessive growth of facial or body hair.

histamine (HĬS-tă-mĭn) An amino acid that, when released in the body, produces the symptoms of allergic reactions; nasal secretions are increased, engorgement of capillary beds occurs, visceral muscles are stimulated, and lung bronchioles are constricted.

HIV Human immunodeficiency virus.

Hodgkin's disease A form of lymphoma characterized by enlargement and malignant degeneration of the lymph nodes, eventually spreading to involve the liver, spleen, and other internal organs.

home health care Professional health care, providing many services formerly available only in a hospital setting, in the home environment.

hormone An agent secreted by the endocrine glands into the bloodstream that produces or alters bodily functions.

hospice (HŌS-pĭs) An institution that provides a centralized program of palliative and supportive care to dying patients and their families.

hydrocortisone A glucocorticoid hormone secreted by the adrenal cortex.

hypertension Blood pressure persistently exceeding 140/90 mm Hg.

hypertensive An agent used to elevate blood pressure therapeutically.

hyperthyroidism (HĪ-pĕr-THĪ-rŏy-DĪZ-ĕm) A condition caused by excessive activity of the thyroid gland, with accompanying hypertension, nervousness, tachycardia, and exophthalmos.

hyperuricemia (HĪ-pĕr-ū-rĕ-SĒ-mē-ă) Increased uric acid levels in the blood, often associated with gout or gouty arthritis.

hypervitaminosis A condition that develops owing to an overdose of vitamins.

hypnotic An agent used to induce sleep.

hypochlorhydria (HĪ-pō-klŏ-RHĬD-rē-ē) A decrease in the amount of gastric hydrochloric acid.

hypotension Lowered blood pressure.

hypotensive An agent used to decrease blood pressure therapeutically.

hypothyroidism Decreased functioning of the thyroid gland, with subsequent slowing down of mental and motor functions.

I

idiosyncrasy (ĬD-ē-ō-SĬN-krĕ-sē) Abnormal sensitivity to a drug, or a reaction not intended.

immunity The state in which the individual is not susceptible to a certain disease.

immunizing agent A biologic preparation injected to produce immunity to disease.

immunosuppression (ĬM-yĕ-nō-sĕ-PRĔSH-ĕn) Interference with the development of antibody response to a disease.

immunosuppressive An agent that interferes with the body systems that resist infection and foreign materials.

immunotherapy (ĬM-yĕ-nō-THĔR-ĕ-pē) Treatment of conditions by enhancing or altering the immune system of the body.

incontinence (ĭn-KŎN-tĭ-nĕns) The inability to control the discharge of excretions, urine, or feces.

inflammation (ĬN-flĕ-MĀ-shŭn) A pathologic reaction by the body in response to an injury or abnormal stimulation by an agent.

infusion (ĭn-FYŪ-zhĕn) The introduction of fluid other than blood into a vein.

inotropic (ĬN-ō-TRŎP-ĭk) **drug** An agent that increases myocardial contractility.

INR International Normalized Ratio.

inscription The part of the prescription that states the name and quantities of the ingredients.

insulin The pancreatic hormone that aids in the utilization of glucose as energy, stores excess glucose as glycogen in the liver, and is responsible for the conversion of glucose to fat.

interaction The altered effect that occurs when two or more drugs/herbs are taken together.

International Normalized Ratio A standardized format for reporting thromboplastin values. It is used to adjust the dose of anticoagulant medications.

intraarterial injection Insertion of a needle into an artery to administer a drug or other substance.

intradermal injection Insertion of a needle into the dermis of the skin to administer a drug or other substance.

intramuscular (IM) injection Insertion of a needle into a muscle to administer a drug or other substance.

intravenous (IV) injection Insertion of a needle into a vein to administer a drug or other substance.

intrinsic factor A substance in the gastric wall that is necessary for vitamin B_{12} absorption.

J

jaundice Yellow pigmentation noticeable in the skin and mucous membranes that is caused by an increase in the amount of serum bilirubin, usually as a result of a liver disorder.

L

laxative A cathartic agent that evacuates the bowel by a mild action.

leukemia A condition characterized by uncontrolled proliferation of the leukocytes, or white cells, of the blood.

leukocyte (LŪ-kĕ-sīt) A white blood cell; responsible for antibody production and defense against infectious agents in the body.

leukopenia (LŪ-kō-PĒ-nē-ē) A decrease in the number of white cells in the blood.

liniment A mixture of drugs with oil, soap, water, or alcohol intended for external application with rubbing (e.g., camphor liniment, chloroform liniment).

local effects Effects limited to the site of application.

long-acting or sustained-release dosage forms Active pharmaceutical agents that are either layered in tablet form for release over several hours or placed in pellets within a capsule. The pellets are of varying size and disintegrate over a period of 8 to 24 hours. These dosage forms must not be broken or crushed because their efficacy depends on release of the various layers over time.

lotions Aqueous preparations containing suspended materials intended for soothing, local application. Most are patted on rather than rubbed (e.g., calamine lotion, Caladryl lotion).

luteinizing hormone The hormone that stimulates development of the corpus luteum.

lymphocyte (LĬM-fĕ-sīt) A white blood cell, formed in the lymph tissues of the body, such as the spleen, lymph nodes, and tonsils. Cells are active in antibody formation to counteract infection.

lymphoma (līm-FŌ-mĕ) Any of a group of malignant conditions involving lymphoid tissue.

lymphosarcoma (līm-FŌ-sär-KŌ-mĕ) A tumor of the lymph nodes in which the nodes contain masses of rounded malignant cells that resemble lymphocytes.

M

macrolide (MĂ-krō-līd) antibiotics The erythromycin family of antibiotics.

malaise (mă-LĀZ) Generalized, nonspecific discomfort or unease.

meningitis (MĬN-ĭn-JĬ-tīs) Infection of the meninges, the lining of the brain and the spinal cord.

menopause (MĔN-ĕ-pŏz) The time at which female fertility and menstruation cease.

menorrhagia (MĔN-ĕ-RĂ-jĕ-ĕ) Excessive menstrual flow.

metabolism (mĕ-TĂB-ĕ-LĬZ-ĕm) The chemical changes in living organisms by which energy is produced and tissue repairs are effected.

migraine Paroxysmal, intensely painful headache caused by vasomotor disturbances in a scalp artery, often accompanied by psychic phenomena, nausea, and vomiting.

mineral A naturally occurring, inorganic substance necessary to body function.

miosis (mī-Ō-sīs) Pupil constriction.

moniliasis (MŌ-nĕ-LĬ-ĕ-sīs) Superinfection with the fungus *Candida albicans* (*See* Candidiasis).

monoamine oxidase inhibitors (MAOIs) Agents that inhibit monoamine oxidase, a naturally occurring hormone that is involved in the breakdown of several neurotransmitters in the brain, including epinephrine, dopamine, and serotonin.

monoclonal (MŎN-ĕ-KLŌ-nĕl) **antibody** Very specific antibody that binds to one receptor only.

multiple myeloma A malignant disease of the bone marrow characterized by bone destruction, often with pathologic fractures, anemia, hyperglobulinemia, hypercalcemia, and increased numbers of immature cells in the bone marrow.

mycosis fungoides (mī-KŌ-sīs fŭng-GŎY-dēz) A form of lymphoma that has numerous cutaneous manifestations, such as eczema, nodules, tumors, infiltrations, and ulcerations.

mydriasis (mī-DRĬ-ĕ-sīs) Dilation of the pupil.

myxedema (MĬK-sĕ-DĒ-mĕ) Hypothyroidism, with onset usually in late childhood or adulthood, characterized by puffiness of the skin and a slowing of mental and motor functions.

N

narcotic (năr-KŎT-ĭk) Any drug derived from opium, or its synthetic equivalents.

narrow-spectrum antibiotic An antibiotic effective against only a few microorganisms.

natural remedy Any treatment that can be used by nonprofessionals to alter a condition.

neoplasm (NĒ-ō-PLĂZ-ĕm) An unnatural growth or tumor in the body; a cancer.

nephritis (nĕ-FRĬ-tīs) Inflammation of the kidney.

nephron (NĔF-rŏn) The functional unit of the kidney, consisting of the glomerulus, the glomerular capsule, and the collecting tubules.

neuron (NŪR-ŏn) One cell of the nervous system, the functional unit.

neurosis (nū-RŌ-sīs) An emotional disorder characterized by anxiety or depressive reaction, but in which the patient has not lost contact with reality.

neutropenia (NŪ-trō-PĔ-nĕ-ĕ) A decrease in the number of neutrophils (a type of white cell) in the blood.

nocardiosis (nō-KĂR-dĕ-Ō-sīs) A systemic fungus infection, often with granuloma formation in various organs.

nocturia (nŏk-TŪR-ĕ-ĕ) Purposeful urination during the night.

norepinephrine A hormone secreted by the adrenal medulla, released with epinephrine in response to stress.

NSAID Nonsteroidal anti-inflammatory drug; a drug that prevents the synthesis of prostaglandins at the site of inflammation.

O

ointments Mixtures of drugs with a fatty base for external application, usually by rubbing (e.g., zinc oxide ointment, Ben-Gay ointment).

oncogene (ŎNG-kō-jĕn) A gene that may foster malignant processes if activated.

opiates Drugs derived from opium.

opioid (Ō-pē-ŏĭd) An agent, natural or synthetic, that is similar in structure and effect to opium derivatives.

opisthotonos (Ō-pīs-THŌT-ĕ-nĕs) A tetanic muscle spasm characterized by arching of the back, inability to speak, and loss of muscle control; the patient is usually conscious. Occurs as a rare drug hypersensitivity reaction.

oral administration Introduction of a substance to the body via the mouth.

osmosis The process in which water travels through a semipermeable membrane to equalize concentrations of fluid on either side of the membrane.

osteoarthritis A condition caused by erosion of articular cartilage.

osteomalacia (ŎS-tē-Ō-mĕ-LĀ-shĕ) Softening of the bones, resulting from interference with calcium deposits in bony tissue.

osteoporosis Thinning and increased porosity of the bone, with resultant deformities or fractures; common in postmenopausal women.

oxytocic (ŎK-sī-TŌ-sĭk) A drug used to produce effects similar to those of oxytocin, especially stimulation of uterine contractions.

P

palliation Treatment that improves the comfort or well-being of the patient but does not cure him or her.

palliative An agent or measure that relieves symptoms.

pancytopenia (PĂN-sī-tĕ-PĒ-nĕ-ĕ) A condition in which there are decreased numbers of all blood cells.

Para-aminobenzoic acid (PABA) A substance needed to synthesize folic acid, an essential enzyme.

paralysis An inability to move an affected body part.

parasympatholytic An agent that counteracts the effects of the parasympathetic nervous system.

parasympathomimetic (PĔR-ĕ-SĬM-pĕ-THŌ-mĭ-MĔT-ĭk) An agent that produces stimulating effects on the parasympathetic nervous system.

parenteral administration Introduction of a drug or other substance to the body via injection.

paresis (pĕ-RĔ-sĭs) Weakness of an affected body part.

paresthesia (PĔR-ĕs-THĔ-zhĕ) The abnormal skin sensation of crawling, burning, or tingling, not caused by surface stimuli.

Parkinson's disease A progressive condition resulting primarily from deterioration of certain brain nuclei; characterized by rigidity, tremors, akinesia, and loss of spontaneous or automatic movement.

parkinsonism A syndrome, resembling Parkinson's disease but occurring instead as a side effect of certain drugs, notably the tranquilizers, and reversible following withdrawal of the drug.

passive immunity Injection of previously formed antibodies into the body.

penicillin Any of the group of antibiotics derived from cultures of species of the fungus *Penicillium*.

peptic Relates to the stomach, to gastric digestion, or to pepsin.

peptide A group of two or more amino acids.

peristalsis (PĔR-ĕ-STĂL-sĭs) Automatic contractions of the gastrointestinal tract.

pharmacodynamics (FĂR-mĕ-kō-kĭ-NĔT-ĭks) The study of how a drug acts on a living organism.

pharmacokinetics (FĂR-mĕ-kō-dĭ-NĂM-ĭks) The study of the body's actions on a drug, including the mechanisms of absorption, distribution, metabolism, and excretion.

pharmacology A broad term that includes the study of drugs and their actions in the body.

pharmacy The art of preparing, compounding, and dispensing drugs for medicinal use.

pheochromocytoma (FĔ-ō-KRŌ-mō-sī-TŌ-mĕ) A tumor of the sympathetic nervous system, usually located in the adrenal medulla, that may cause severe, intermittent, or persistent hypertension.

photosensitizer (FŌ-tō-SĔN-sĭ-TĪZ-ĕr) An agent that makes the skin more susceptible to burning and sun damage.

physical dependence A condition in which continuous use of a drug is required for proper functioning, and the user would experience withdrawal symptoms if the drug is discontinued.

pills Single-dose units made by mixing a powdered form of a drug with a liquid such as syrup and rolling it into a round or oval shape (e.g., Hinkle's pills). These are largely replaced by other dosage forms today.

plant parts or products Crude drugs that may be obtained from any part of various plants and used medicinally (e.g., ergot, digitalis, opium). Leaves, bark, fruit, roots, rhizomes, resin, and other parts may be used.

polycythemia (PŌL-ē-sī-THĔ-mē-ĕ) **vera** A condition characterized by increased numbers of red blood cells in the blood. Occasionally occurs as a premalignant disorder before the onset of leukemia. Common in individuals living at high altitudes for prolonged periods of time.

potentiation An effect that occurs when a drug increases or prolongs the action of another drug, the total effect being greater than the sum of the effects of each drug used alone.

powders Single-dose quantities of a drug or mixture of drugs in powdered form wrapped separately in powder papers (e.g., Seidlitz powder).

prescription An order for medication, therapy, or a therapeutic device given by a properly authorized person.

progesterone A hormone that prepares the uterus for reception of the ovum.

prophylactic (PRŌ-fĭ-LĂK-tĭk) An agent or device to prevent an undesired effect or disease.

prostaglandin inhibitors Agents that interfere with the effects of prostaglandins.

prostaglandins (PRŎS-tĕ-GLĂN-dĭn) Short-acting hormones that perform many functions in the body and exert their effect close to the site of production.

prothrombin A protein produced by the liver, necessary for normal blood clotting.

prothrombin time A measurement of the prothrombin level in the blood. Measurement is performed routinely to assess the effectiveness of anticoagulant therapy.

pruritus (prū-RĪ-tĕs) An itching sensation of the skin.

pseudoaddiction (SŪ-dō-ăd-DĬK-shŭn) Drug-seeking behaviors that may occur when a patient's pain is undertreated.

psychoactive (SĪ-kō-ĂK-tĭv) **drug** An agent possessing the ability to alter mood, behavior, or cognitive processes.

psychosis A severe mental disease in which the patient's contact with reality is diminished or lost.

PT Prothrombin time.

purpura (PŬR-pĕr-ĕ) Multiple small hemorrhagic areas in the skin or mucous membranes.

pyelitis (PĪ-ĕ-LĪ-tĭs) Inflammation of the pelvis of the kidney.

pyelonephritis (PĪ-ĕ-lō-nĕ-FRĪ-tĭs) Inflammation of the pelvis and glomerular tissues of the kidney.

Q

quinolones (KWĬN-ĕ-lōns) A group of synthetic antibiotics structurally related by having the same (quinolone) nucleus.

R

recombinant (rē-KŎM-bĭ-nĕnt) A cell or organism that has received genes from different parental strains.

Recommended Daily Allowance (RDA) Guidelines established by the U.S. Department of Agriculture listing the nutrients necessary for good health.

respiration The process of exchanging oxygen and carbon dioxide via the respiratory system.

rheumatoid arthritis A generalized connective tissue disease that inflames many joints.

rickets A condition caused by a deficiency of vitamin D. Calcium and phosphorus imbalances cause softening of the bones and characteristic deformations, such as bowed legs, rachitic "rosary" on the costochondral junctions, and so on.

ringworm A topical fungal infection of the skin, hair, or nails, often circular in appearance and spreading peripherally.

RNA A component of the cell nucleus or cytoplasm that carries genetic information and aids in the correct assembly of DNA and proteins.

S

schedules of controlled substances A classification system that categorizes drugs by their potential for abuse.

schizophrenia A type of psychosis in which the patient typically withdraws from reality, exhibiting unpredictable moods, disturbances in the stream of thought, and regressive tendencies to the point of deterioration, often with hallucinations and delusions.

scurvy A vitamin C deficiency characterized by weakness, gum hemorrhages, loosening of the teeth, and subcutaneous hemorrhages.

sedative An agent used to quiet the patient without inducing sleep.

seizure *See* Convulsion.

senility A term that relates to a variety of organic disorders, both physical and mental, that occur in old age.

selective serotonin reuptake (SĔR-ĕ-TŌ-nĭn rē-ŬP-tāk) **inhibitors (SSRIs)** Drugs that increase serotonin availability in the central nervous system, which is believed to produce an antidepressant effect.

shock A sudden drop in blood pressure as a result of an injury or blood loss.

side effect An unpredictable effect that is not related to the main action of the drug.

signa (Sig) The part of the prescription that gives directions to the patient.

solutions Aqueous liquid preparations containing one or more substances that are completely dissolved. Every solution has two parts: the *solute* (the dissolved substance) and the *solvent* (the substance, usually a liquid, in which the solute is dissolved).

spirits Alcoholic solutions of volatile substances. These are also known as essences or spirits (e.g., essence of peppermint, camphor spirit).

SSRI Selective serotonin reuptake inhibitor.

status asthmaticus A prolonged attack of asthma, poorly responsive to drug therapy and lasting as long as several days.

status epilepticus A rapid succession of epileptic seizures in which the patient does not regain consciousness between seizures.

stem cells Cells that are totipotent, or able to give rise to all the cells of the body.

steroid (STĬR-ŏyd) antagonists Diuretics that act by inhibiting aldosterone, an adrenal hormone that promotes the retention of sodium and the excretion of potassium.

Stevens-Johnson syndrome A severe, life-threatening allergic drug reaction. Excoriations of the skin, mucous membranes, and cornea and inflammation of the internal organs occur. Decreased blood pressure may bring about shock and death.

stimulant An agent that promotes or enhances the activity of a body organ or tissue.

stimulation An increase in the activity of cells produced by drugs.

subcutaneous (subQ) injection Insertion of a needle beneath the skin into the fat or connective tissue just underlying the dermis layer.

sublingual administration Placing medication under the patient's tongue, where it must be retained until it is dissolved or absorbed.

subscription The part of the prescription that gives directions to the pharmacist.

substance abuse The use or overuse of a chemical or substance in a way that leads to dependence and has adverse effects on the health and well-being of the user and others.

sulfonamides (sĕl-FŎN-ĕ-mīd) Antiinfective agents modeled after PABA; also known as "sulfa drugs."

suppositories Mixtures of drugs with some firm base such as cocoa butter, which can then be molded into shape for insertion into a body orifice. Rectal, vaginal, and urethral suppositories are the most common types (e.g., Furacin vaginal suppositories, Dulcolax suppositories), but nasal or otic suppositories may be made.

sympatholytic An agent that counteracts the effects of the sympathetic nervous system.

sympathomimetic (SĬM-pĕ-THŌ-mĭ-MĔT-ĭk) An agent that produces stimulating effects on the sympathetic nervous system.

synapse (SĬN-ăps) The connection between two or more neurons.

synergism (SĬN-ĕr-JĬSM) The joint action of agents in which their combined effect is more intense or longer in duration than the sum of their individual effects.

syrups Aqueous solutions of a sugar. These may or may not have medicinal substances added (e.g., simple syrup, ipecac syrup).

systemic effects General effects caused by a drug being absorbed into the blood and carried to one or more tissues in the body.

T

tablets Single-dose units made by compressing powdered drugs in a suitable mold (e.g., aspirin tablets). Special forms of tablets include *sublingual* tablets (to be held under the tongue until dissolved) and *enteric-coated* tablets (with a coating that prevents their absorption until they reach the intestinal tract).

tachycardia (TĂK-ē-KĂR-dē-ē) Increased heart rate.

terminal illness A disease expected to cause death within a short period of time.

testosterone The hormone responsible for development of the male reproductive tract and maintaining secondary sex characteristics.

tetany (TĔT-ĕ-nē) A condition caused by a decreased concentration of ionized calcium in the blood, leading to increased irritability of muscles and painful tonic muscle spasms.

tetracycline (TĔT-rĕ-SĪ-klēn) A broad-spectrum antibiotic.

therapeutic Pertaining to treatment of disease.

thiazide diuretics Diuretics that act partly by inhibiting carbonic anhydrase, partly by acting directly on the collecting tubules, and partly by promoting excretion of sodium, potassium, chloride, and bicarbonate along with water.

thrombolysis (thrŏm-BŎL-ĭ-sīs) The process of dissolving a blood clot.

thrombolytic (THRŎM-bŏ-LĬT-ĭk) **therapy** Drug therapy used to dissolved blood clots.

thrombophlebitis (THRŎM-bŏ-flĕ-BĪ-tĭs) Inflammation of the walls of a vein, with resultant clotting of blood at the site.

thrombus A blood clot in the heart or blood vessels that remains attached at the site of formation.

thrush *Candida albicans* infection of the oral mucous membranes, typically in the form of small, white macular spots.

tinctures Alcoholic or hydroalcoholic solutions prepared from drugs (e.g., iodine tincture, digitalis tincture).

tolerance Increasing resistance to the usual effects of an established dosage of a drug as a result of continued use.

toxicology The science that deals with poisons: their detection and the symptoms, diagnosis, and treatment of conditions caused by them.

toxin The poisonous substance released by microorganisms.

toxoid An altered form of toxin that may be injected to produce immunity to a specific disease or microorganism.

toxoplasmosis (TŎK-sō-plăz-MŌ-sĭs) A disease caused by infection with the protozoan *Toxoplasma*. May take the form of a respiratory infection, encephalomyelitis, or a dermatitis.

trachoma (trĕ-KŌ-mĕ) An inflammatory disease of the eye involving the conjunctiva and cornea, producing photophobia, pain, and excessive lacrimation. If not treated, it may lead to blindness through vascularization of the cornea.

tranquilizer (TRĂNG-kwĕ-LĬZ-ĕr) An agent used to calm anxiety or agitation during waking hours.

transgene A transplanted gene.

troches (TRŌ-kēs) Flat, round, or rectangular preparations that are held in the mouth until they dissolve; also called lozenges.

tumor An unnatural growth in the body.

U

ulcer A lesion through skin or mucous membrane resulting in loss of tissue, usually with inflammation.

ureter The tube that carries urine from the kidney to the bladder.

urethra The tube that carries urine from the bladder to the exterior of the body.

urticaria (ŬR-tĭ-KĔR-ē-ē) A condition in which pruritic wheals or welts appear on the skin, usually as a response to an allergic phenomenon; also known as hives.

V

vaccine Any preparation intended for use to produce active immunologic prevention of a disease.

vasoconstrictor (văs-ō-kŏn-STRĬK-tŏr) An agent that causes narrowing of the blood vessels.

vasodilator (văs-ō-DĬ-lā-tŏr) An agent that causes blood vessels to relax or increase in diameter.

vector A carrier of disease.

ventricle One of the lower chambers of the heart.

vertigo Dizziness.

virus A minute parasitic microorganism that is able to replicate only within a cell of a living plant or animal host.

vitamin An organic compound that cannot be synthesized in the human body, but is present in minute amounts in foodstuffs. It is required for normal growth, development, and well-being.

W

waters Saturated solutions of volatile oils (e.g., peppermint water, camphor water).

withdrawal A syndrome that occurs when a drug-dependent person discontinues the drug suddenly; characterized by anxiety, insomnia, irritability, and often physical illness that may be severe.

withdrawal symptoms Unpleasant or life-threatening symptoms that occur when an addict does not take the substance to which he or she is addicted.

Canadian Drug Information*

ALFRED J. RÉMILLARD, PHARMD, BCPP

INTERNATIONAL SYSTEM OF UNITS

In an attempt to standardize the large number of different units used worldwide and thus improve communication, the Système International d'Unités (International System of Units; SI) was recommended in 1954. In 1971, the mole (mol) was adopted as the standard for designating the amount of substance present, and the liter (L) was adopted as the standard for designating volume. The World Health Organization recommended the adoption of SI units in 1977. However, Canada had already implemented an equivalent system in 1971.

In therapeutics, the major change caused by adopting the SI was to express drug concentrations present in body fluids in molar units (e.g., mmol/L) rather than in mass units (e.g., mg/L). This allows a better comparison between the pharmacologic and pharmacodynamic effects of different drugs, since these properties are relative to the number of molecules (e.g., mmol) of drug present rather than to the number of mass units (e.g., mg).

DRUG SERUM CONCENTRATIONS

Many drugs have known therapeutic or toxic levels that are monitored in patients to ensure safety and efficacy. In Canada, clinical laboratories report these levels in SI units. Levels traditionally reported as milligrams per milliliter (mg/mL) can be converted to millimoles per liter (mmol/L) using the conversion factor (CF) for that specific drug:

$$CF = \frac{1000}{\text{molecular weight of the drug}}$$

To convert from micrograms per milliliter to SI units, the following equation is used:

$$\frac{mcg}{mL} \times CF = \frac{\mu mol}{L}$$

To convert from SI units to micrograms per milliliter, the following equation is used:

$$\frac{\mu mol}{L} \div CF = \frac{mcg}{mL}$$

From Lehne RA: *Pharmacology for nursing care,* ed 5, Philadelphia, 2004, WB Saunders, with permission.

Table A–1 lists some important drugs for which therapeutic or toxic levels have been established. For most of these drugs, the levels presented are trough (minimum) values, which are measured in blood samples drawn just prior to the next dose. For the aminoglycosides and vancomycin, two levels are listed: a trough level and a peak (maximum) level. Levels must remain between the peak and trough to ensure efficacy of these drugs and at the same time to minimize toxicity.

CANADIAN DRUG LEGISLATION

Two acts form the basis of the drug laws in Canada, the Food and Drug Act and the Controlled Drugs and Substance Act. The responsibility for administering these acts rests with the Therapeutic Products Directorate (TPD) at Health Canada.

The Food and Drug Act (1927), accompanied by the Food and Drug Regulations (1953, 1954, 1979), reviews the safety and efficacy of drugs before they are marketed, and the legislation determines whether the medicine is prescription or nonprescription. The Act controls the requirements for good manufacturing practices, labeling, distribution, and sale, including advertising of the drug.

PRESCRIPTION DRUGS (SCHEDULE F)

All drugs that require a prescription, except for narcotics and controlled substances, are listed in Schedule F of the Food and Drugs Regulations. Prescriptions for Schedule F medications may written (including facsimiles) or transmitted orally (i.e., telephone order directly to the pharmacist) by a medical practitioner, dentist, or veterinary surgeon. The prescription can be refilled as often as indicated by the physician. The symbol Pr must appear on all manufacturing labels. Individual provinces (or states in the United States) can legislate more restrictive control and require a prescription for a medication classified by the TPD as a nonprescription drug (e.g., digoxin).

The Controlled Drugs and Substance Act (1997) establishes the requirements for the control and sale of narcotics, controlled drugs, and substances of abuse in Canada. The Controlled Drugs and Substance Act lists eight schedules of controlled substances. Assignment to a schedule is based on potential for abuse and the ease with which illicit substances can be manufactured in illegal laboratories. The degree of control, the conditions of record keeping, and other regula-

Table **A-1** *Therapeutic Serum Drug Concentrations*

DRUGS	SI REFERENCE INTERVAL	SI UNIT	CONVERSION FACTOR	TRADITIONAL REFERENCE INTERVAL	TRADITIONAL REFERENCE UNIT
acetaminophen	13–40	μmol/L	66.15	0.2–0.6	mg/dL
acetylsalicylic acid	7.2–21.7	μmol/L	0.0724	100–300	mg/dL
amikacin*	—	—	—	15–25†; <8‡	mcg/mL
amitriptyline	430–9000§	mmol/L	3.605	120–250§	ng/mL
carbamazepine	17–42	μmol/L	4.233	4–10	mcg/mL
desipramine	430–750	nmol/L	3.754	115–200	ng/mL
digoxin	0.6–2.8	nmol/L	1.282	0.5–2.2	ng/mL
disopyramide	6–18	μmol/L	2.946	2–6	mcg/mL
gentamicin*	—	—	—	6–10†; <2‡	mcg/mL
imipramine	640–1070§	nmol/L	3.566	180–300§	ng/mL
lidocaine	4.5–21.5	μmol/L	4.267	1–5	mcg/mL
lithium	0.4–1.2	mmol/L	1.0	0.4–1.2	mEq/L
netilmicin*	—	—	—	6–10†; <2‡	mcg/mL
nortriptyline	190–570	nmol/L	3.797	50–150	ng/mL
phenobarbital	65–170	μmol/L	4.306	15–40	mcg/mL
phenytoin	40–80	μmol/L	3.964	10–20	mcg/mL
primidone	25–46	μmol/L	4.582	6–10	mcg/mL
procainamide	17–34§	μmol/L	4.249	4–8§	mcg/mL
quinidine	4.6–9.2	μmol/L	3.082	1.5–3	mcg/mL
theophylline	55–110	μmol/L	5.55	10–20	mcg/mL
tobramycin*	—	—	—	6–10†; <2‡	mcg/mL
valproic acid	300–700	μmol/L	6.934	50–100	mcg/mL
vancomycin*	—	—	—	25–40†; <10‡	mcg/mL

*Aminoglycosides (amikacin, gentamicin, netilmicin, tobramycin) and vancomycin are not reported in SI units because of the variability of their molecular weights.
†Peak drug level.
‡Trough drug level.
§Drug level reported as the total of the parent drug and its active metabolite.

tions depend on the specific schedule. For example, Schedule I, which includes the narcotic agents, requires written orders only and no repeat orders are allowed. Some provinces require prescriptions for certain narcotics, such as morphine, to be written on a triplicate prescription form with one copy to be sent to the practitioner's regulatory body. The symbol ◇ must appear on the labels of controlled products, while the letter N is printed on the label of all the narcotic agents. Schedules I through IV are defined below; Schedules V through VIII are not yet finalized.

- Schedule I: opium poppy and its derivatives (e.g., morphine, heroin); methadone; coca and its derivatives (e.g., cocaine)
- Schedule II: cannabis and its derivatives (e.g., marijuana, hashish)
- Schedule III: amphetamines, methylphenidate, lysergic acid diethylamide (LSD), methaqualone, psilocybin, mescaline
- Schedule IV: sedative-hypnotic agents (e.g., barbiturates, benzodiazepines); anabolic steroids

The Controlled Drugs and Substance Act also provides for the nonprescription sale of certain codeine preparations. The content must not exceed the equivalent of 8 mg codeine phosphate per solid dosage unit or 20 mg/30 mL of a liquid, and the preparation must also contain two additional non-narcotic medicinal ingredients (usually acetylsalicylic acid or acetaminophen and caffeine). These preparations may not be advertised or displayed and may be sold only by pharmacists. Some provinces restrict the amount that can be sold at any given time.

NONPRESCRIPTION MEDICATIONS

Currently there are three categories of nonprescription medications that govern their sale. Restricted Access Nonprescription Drugs are "kept behind the counter" and are available for sale directly from the pharmacist only. Examples include insulin, glucagon, ipecac, loperamide, and nitroglycerin. This restriction is to assure that patients are not self-diagnosing medically serious diseases such as diabetes mellitus or angina and to help ensure proper use of the medicines through appropriate counseling by the pharmacist. The second category, Pharmacy Only Nonprescription Drugs, are sold only through pharmacies and include most antihistamines and the low-dose ulcer medicines. It is expected that, if clients have questions, they could easily consult with the pharmacist. The third category includes nonprescription products that can be sold at any retail outlet. In general, these products are provided with adequate instruction to permit self-treatment. Examples are nicotine gum and patches, aspirin, ibuprofen, and some low-dose "cough and cold" preparations.

PROPOSED CHANGES TO NATIONAL DRUG SCHEDULES

As previously mentioned, individual provinces have enacted their own legislation controlling the sale of both prescription and nonprescription products. This has led to inconsistency and confusion for both the health care practitioner and the consumer. As a result, the National Association of Pharmacy Regulatory Authorities endorsed a proposal for a national drug scheduling model. This model will align the provincial drug schedules so that the conditions for the sale of drugs would be consistent across the country. The harmonized model includes all classes of medications—narcotics, controlled substances, prescription medications, and nonprescription medications—which are assigned to one of the following four categories:

- Schedule I: all prescription drugs, including narcotics and controlled substances
- Schedule II: Restricted Access Nonprescription Drugs (see Nonprescription Medications above)
- Schedule III: Pharmacy Only Nonprescription Drugs (see Nonprescription Medications above)
- Unscheduled Drugs: those drugs not assigned to the above categories, which can be sold at any retail outlet

The national drug schedule is in various stages of implementation across the provinces.

NEW DRUG DEVELOPMENT IN CANADA

The process for approving a new drug in Canada is very similar, if not identical, to the process in the United States. The same drug data that are required for approval by the Food and Drug Administration in the United States are required by the TPD in Canada. The principal difference between Canada and the United States is one of nomenclature: Once preclinical testing is completed, the manufacturer in Canada applies for a Preclinical New Drug Submission, versus an Investigational New Drug in the United States. At the end of clinical testing, the manufacturer in Canada seeks a New Drug Submission (NDS), versus a New Drug Application in the United States.

After all the information on a new drug has been submitted—including results of preclinical and clinical testing, method of manufacturing, packaging, labeling, and results of stability testing—the pharmaceutical company receives a Notice of Compliance (NOC) from the TPD, and the drug enters the market.

Although data collection for a new drug is thorough, there is no guarantee that all adverse reactions are known, especially when the drug is used concurrently with other drugs. Also, long-term effects are not fully appreciated. For these reasons, postmarketing surveillance plays a major role in monitoring new drugs. The Canadian Adverse Drug Reactions monitoring program has undergone extensive expansion in recent years. The manufacturer and all health care practitioners must immediately report any new clinical findings, unexpected adverse effects, or therapeutic failures to the TPD.

PATENT LAWS

Patent laws in Canada continue to evolve. In 1969, the Patent Act was changed to include compulsory licensing. This new provision allowed generic drug companies to manufacture and distribute patented drugs in Canada, provided that a minimal 4% royalty fee was paid to the patent holder. This system was introduced to help control drug prices. Unfortunately, the system caused a decline in revenue to "innovative" pharmaceutical companies, with a resultant decline in research on new drug development. After much debate, and retroactive to June 1987, the Patent Act was amended to give patent holders market exclusivity either (1) for 7 to 10 years or (2) until the 17-year patent (from date of filing) expires, whichever comes first. The Patent Act was then further amended to "make Canada's intellectual property legislation more in line with that of the major industrialized countries."

In response to provisions of the North American Free Trade Agreement (NAFTA) and the General Agreement on Tariffs and Trade (GATT), Bill C-91 was introduced in 1993. This bill (1) eliminated compulsory licensing and (2) extended patent protection on brand-name drugs to 20 years, thereby making Canadian patent laws consistent with those of the United States and other industrialized nations. Section 14 of Bill C-91 called for a parliamentary review of legislation in 1997. A special committee reviewed the impact of Bill C-91 on such factors as drug prices, drug research and development, and job creation. No changes to the legislation were made.

In order to respond to concerns arising from changes in the Patent Act, a Patented Medicine Prices Review Board was created. Its mandate is to (1) ensure that prices of patented medicines are not excessive and (2) report on the ratios of research and development expenditures relative to sales for individual patentees and for the pharmaceutical industry as a whole.

SOME IMPORTANT CANADIAN DRUG TRADE NAMES

For a list of common drug trade names used in Canada, see Table A–2.

REFERENCES

Bachynsky J: Nonprescription drugs in health care. In *Nonprescription drug reference for health professionals*, Ottawa, 1996, Canadian Pharmaceutical Association.

Evans WE, Schentag JJ, Jusko WJ (eds): *Applied pharmacokinetics: principles of therapeutic drug monitoring*, Spokane, WA, 1992, Applied Therapeutics, Inc.

Health protection and drug laws, Ottawa, 1988, Health and Welfare Canada/Canadian Publishing Center.

Health Protection Branch: *Information Newsletter* No. 798, 1991.

Johnson GE, Hannah KJ, Zerr SR: *Pharmacology and the nursing process*, ed 3, Philadelphia, 1992, WB Saunders.

Mailhot R: The Canadian drug regulatory process. *J Clin Pharmacol* 26:232, 1986.

McLeod DC: SI units in drug therapeutics. *Drug Intell Clin Pharm* 22:990, 1988.

Subcommittee of Metric Commission Canada, Sector 9.10: *SI manual in health care*, ed 2, Ottawa, 1982, Health and Welfare Canada.

Sullivan P: CMA to support increased patent protection for drugs but will attach strong qualifications. *CMAJ* 147:1669, 1992.

To the year 2000: the changing roles of nonprescription medicines and the practice of pharmacy, Ottawa, 1992, Nonprescription Drug Manufacturers Association of Canada.

Table A-2 | *Canadian Drug Names**

GENERIC NAME	TRADE NAME(S)
A	
5-aminosalicylic acid	Asacol, Mesasal, Novo-5 ASA, Pentasa, Salofalk
abacavir	Ziagen
abacavir-lamivudine-zidovudine	Trizivir
abciximab	ReoPro
acebutolol	Monitan, Rhotral, Sectral
acetaminophen	Abenol, Atasol, Panadol, Tempra, Tylenol
acetaminophen-chlorzoxazone	Acetazone, Parafon Forte
acetaminophen-methocarbamol	Methoxacet, Robaxacet
acetaminophen-oxycodone	Endocet, Oxycocet, Percocet
acetaminophen-pseudoephedrine	Dimetapp, Sinutab, Sudafed
acetaminophen-pseudoephedrine-triprolidine	Actifed Plus
acetaminophen-pyrilamine	Midol Extra Strength
acetazolamide	Diamox
acetylcysteine	Mucomyst, Parvolex
acetylsalicylic acid (ASA)	Asaphen, Aspirin, Entrophen, Novasen
acitretin	Soriatane
acyclovir	Zovirax
adapalene	Differin
adenosine	Adenocard
albuterol, *see* salbutamol	
aldesleukin	Proleukin
alendronate	Fosamax
alfacalcidol	One-Alpha
alfentanil	Alfenta
allopurinol	Zyloprim
alpha$_1$ proteinase inhibitor	Prolastin
alprazolam	Apo-Alpraz, Novo-Alprazol, Nu-Alpraz, Xanax
alprostadil	Caverject, Muse, Prostin VR
alteplase	Activase
amantadine	Edantadine, Symmetrel
amcinonide	Cyclocort
amikacin	Amikin
amiloride	Midamor
amiloride-hydrochlorothiazide	Apo-Amilzide, Moduret, Novamilor, Nu-Amilzide
aminobenzoate	Potaba
aminocaproic acid	Amicar
aminophylline	Phyllocontin
amiodarone	Cordarone
amitriptyline-perphenazine	Triavil
amlodipine	Norvasc
amobarbital	Amytal
amoxicillin	Amoxil, Apo-Amoxi, Nu-Amoxi
amoxicillin-clarithromycin-lansoprazole	HpPAC
amoxicillin-clavulanate	Apo-Amoxi-Clav, Clavulin
amphotericin B	Abelcet, AmBisome, Fungizone
ampicillin	Ampicin, Apo-Ampi, Nu-Ampi
anagrelide	Agrylin
anastrozole	Arimidex
antazoline-naphazoline	Albalon-A, Vasocon-A

Table A-2 | Canadian Drug Names*

GENERIC NAME	TRADE NAME(S)
antihemophilic factor	Kogenate, Re-Facto
apraclonidine	Iopidine
aprotinin	Trasylol
ASA-butalbital-caffeine	Fiorinal, Trianal
ASA-dipyridamole	Aggrenox
ASA-methocarbamol	Methoxasal, Robaxisal
ASA-oxycodone	Endodan, Oxycodan, Percodan
asparaginase	Kidrolase
atenolol	Apo-Atenol, Novo-Atenol, Nu-Atenol, Tenolin, Tenormin
atenolol-chlorthalidone	Tenoretic
atorvastatin	Lipitor
atovaquone	Mepron
atracurium	Tracrium
atropine	Atropisol
atropine-diphenoxylate	Lomotil
auranofin	Ridaura
aurothioglucose	Solganal
azatadine	Optimine
azathioprine	Imuran
azithromycin	Zithromax

B

bacampicillin	Penglobe
bacitracin	Baciguent, Bacitin
baclofen	Lioresal, Nu-Baclo
becaplermin	Regranex
beclomethasone	Gen-Beclo, Propaderm, Rivansa
benazepril	Lotensin
benserazide-levodopa	Prolopa
benzoyl peroxide	Acetoxyl, Benoxyl, Benzac, Oxyderm, PanOxyl
benztropine	Cogentin
beractant	Survanta
betahistine	Serc
betaine	Cystadane
betamethasone	Betaject, Celestone, Diprolene, Diprosone, Topilene
betaxolol	Betoptic
bethanechol	Duvoid, Myotonachol
bezafibrate	Bezalip
bicalutamide	Casodex
bimatoprost	Lumigan
biperiden	Akineton
bisacodyl	Dulcolax
bisoprolol	Monocor
bleomycin	Blenoxane
bosentan	Tracleer
bretylium	Bretylate
brimonidine	Alphagan
brinzolamide	Azopt
bromazepam	Lectopam
bromocriptine	Parlodel
brompheniramine	Dimetane
brompheniramine-phenylephrine	Dimetapp
budesonide	Entocort, Pulmicort, Rhinocort
bumetadine	Burinex
bupivacaine	Marcaine, Sensorcaine
bupropion	Wellbutrin SR, Zyban
buserelin	Suprefact
buspirone	BuSpar

Continued

Table **A-2** *Canadian Drug Names*—cont'd*

GENERIC NAME	TRADE NAME(S)
busulfan	Busulfex, Myleran
butorphanol	Stadol NS
C	
cadexomer	Iodosorb
caffeine-ergotamine	Cafergot
calcipotriol	Dovonex
calcitonin	Calcimar, Caltine, Miacalcin
calcitriol	Rocaltrol
candesartan	Atacand
candesartan-hydrochlorothiazide	Atacand Plus
cantharidin	Canthacur, Cantharone
capecitabine	Xeloda
capsaicin	Zostrix
captopril	Apo-Capto, Capoten
carbamazepine	Novo-Carbamaz, Tegretol
carbetocin	Duratocin
carbidopa-levodopa	Apo-Levocard, Novo-Levocarbidopa, Sinemet
carboplatin	Paraplatin
carmustine	BiCNU
carvedilol	Coreg
cefaclor	Ceclor
cefadroxil	Duricef
cefazolin	Ancef, Kefzol
cefepime	Maxipime
cefixime	Suprax
cefotaxime	Claforan
cefotetan	Cefotan
cefoxitin	Mefoxin
cefprozil	Cefzil
ceftazidime	Tazidime
ceftizoxime	Cefizox
ceftriaxone	Rocephin
cefuroxime	Ceftin, Kefurox, Zinacef
celecoxib	Celebrex
cephalexin	Apo-Cephalex, Novo-Lexin
cephalothin	Ceporacin, Keflin
cetirizine	Reactine
chlophedianol	Ulone
chloral hydrate, generic	—
chlorambucil	Leukeran
chloramphenicol	Chloromycetin, Pentamycetin
chlordiazepoxide-clidinium	Apo-Chlorax, Librax
chloroquine	Aralen
chlorpheniramine	Chlor-Tripolon
chlorpromazine	Largactil
chlorthalidone, generic	—
chlorthalidone-atenolol	Tenoretic
cholecalciferol	D-Vi-Sol, Os-Cal-D
cholestyramine	Novo-Cholamine, Questran
choline magnesium trisalicylate	Trilisate
choline salicylate	Teejel, Trilisate
ciclopirox	Loprox
cilastatin-imipenem	Primaxin
cilazapril	Inhibace
cilazapril-hydrochlorothiazide	Inhibace Plus
cimetidine	Novo-Cimetine, Nu-Cimet
ciprofloxacin	Ciloxan, Cipro

Table A-2 *Canadian Drug Names**

GENERIC NAME	TRADE NAME(S)
cisatracurium	Nimbex
cisplatin	Platinol
citalopram	Celexa
cladribine	Leustatin
clarithromycin	Biaxin
clarithromycin-amoxicillin-lansoprazole	HpPAC
clavulanate-amoxicillin	Apo-Amoxi-Clav, Clavulin
clidinium-chlordiazepoxide	Apo-Chlorax, Librax
clindamycin	Dalacin C
clobazam	Frisium
clobetasol	Derma-Sone, Dermovate
clodronate (bisphosphonate)	Bonefos, Ostac
clomiphene	Clomid, Serophene
clomipramine	Anafranil, Novo-Clopamine
clonazepam	Rivotril
clonidine	Catapres, Dixarit
clopidogrel	Plavix
clorazepate	Novo-Clopate
clotrimazole	Canesten, Clotrimaderm
cloxacillin	Apo-Cloxi, Novo-Cloxin, Nu-Cloxi, Tegopen
clozapine	Clozaril, Rhoxal-Clozapine
codeine, generic	—
colchicine, generic	—
colestipol	Colestid
cortisone	Cortone
cosyntropin	Cortrosyn, Synacthen Depot
cromolyn	Intal, Nalcrom, Opticrom, Rynacrom
cyanocobalamin	Bedoz
cyclobenzaprine	Flexeril, Novo-Cycloprine
cyclopentolate	Cyclogyl
cyclophosphamide	Cytoxan, Procytox
cyclosporine	Neoral, Sandimmune
cyproheptadine	Periactin
cyproterone	Androcur
cytarabine	Cytosar
D	
dacarbazine	DTIC
dactinomycin	Cosmegen
dalteparin	Fragmin
danaparoid	Orgaran
danazol	Cyclomen
dantrolene	Dantrium
darbepoetin	Aranesp
daunorubicin	Cerubidine
deferoxamine	Desferal
delavirdine	Rescriptor
demeclocycline	Declomycin
desipramine	Norpramin
desloratadine	Aerius
desmopressin	DDAVP, Octostim
desonide	Desocort
dexamethasone	Decadron, Dexasone, Maxidex
dexamphetamine	Dexedrine
dexbrompheniramine-pseudoephedrine	Drixoral, Drixtab
dexchlorpheniramine	Polaramine
dexrazoxane	Zinecard
dextromethorphan	Balminil, Benylin, Robitussin

Continued

Table A-2 | *Canadian Drug Names*—cont'd*

GENERIC NAME	TRADE NAME(S)
diazepam	Diazemuls, Valium
diazoxide	Hyperstat, Proglycem
diclofenac	Apo-Diclo, Diclotec, Novo-Difenac, Nu-Diclo, Vofenal, Voltaren
diclofenac-misoprostol	Arthrotec
dicyclomine	Bentylol, Lomine
didanosine	Videx
dienestrol	Ortho Dienestrol
diethylpropion	Tenuate
diethylstilbestrol	Honvol
digoxin	Lanoxin
digoxin immune Fab	Digibind
dihydroergotamine	Migranal
diltiazem	Apo-Diltiaz, Cardizem, Tiazac
dimenhydrinate	Gravol, Traveltabs
diphenhydramine	Allerdryl, Allernix, Benadryl, Nytol
diphenoxylate-atropine	Lomotil
dipivefrin	Propine
dipyridamole	Novo-Dipiradol, Persantine
dipyridamole-ASA	Aggrenox
disopyramide	Rythmodan
divalproex	Epival
dobutamine	Dobutrex
docetaxel	Taxotere
docusate calcium	Surfak
docusate sodium	Colace, Selax, Soflax
dolasetron	Anzemet
donepezil	Aricept
dopamine	Intropin
dornase alfa	Pulmozyme
doxacurium	Nuromax
doxazosin	Cardura
doxepin	Apo-Doxepin, Novo-Doxepin, Sinequan
doxorubicin	Adriamycin
doxycycline	Apo-Doxy, Doxycin, Novo-Doxylin, Vibra-Tabs
doxylamine-pyridoxine	Diclectin
dronabinol	Marinol
E	
econazole	Ecostatin
edrophonium	Enlon
efavirenz	Sustiva
emedestine	Emadine
enalapril	Vasotec
enalapril-hydrochlorothiazide	Vaseretic
enalaprilat	Vasotec IV
enoxaparin	Lovenox
entacapone	Comtan
epinephrine, generic	—
epoetin alfa	Eprex
epoprostenol	Flolan
eptifibatide	Integrilin
ergocalciferol	Drisdol, Ostoforte
ergoloid mesylates	Hydergine
ergotamine, generic	—
ergotamine-caffeine	Cafergot
erythromycin-sulfisoxazole	Pediazole
esmolol	Brevibloc
esomeprazole	Nexium

| Table A-2 | *Canadian Drug Names** |

GENERIC NAME	TRADE NAME(S)
estramustine	Emcyt
estropipate	Ogen
ethacrynic acid	Edecrin
ethambutol	Etibi
ethopropazine	Parsitan
ethosuximide	Zarontin
etidronate	Didronel
etodolac	Ultradol
etoposide	Vepesid
F	
famciclovir	Famvir
famotidine	Pepcid
felodipine	Plendil, Renedil
fenofibrate	Apo-Feno-Micro, Lipidil Micro
fenoprofen	Nalfon
fenoterol	Berotec
fenoterol-ipratropium	Duovent
fentanyl	Duragesic
ferrous fumarate	Palafer
ferrous sulfate	Fer-In-Sol, Slow-Fe
feverfew	Tanacet 125
fexofenadine	Allegra
filgrastim	Neupogen
finasteride	Propecia, Proscar
flecainide	Tambocor
floctafenine	Idarac
fluconazole	Diflucan
fludarabine	Fludara
fludrocortisone	Florinef
flumazenil	Anexate
flunarizine	Sibelium
fluocinolone	Fluoderm, Synalar
fluocinonide	Tiamol, Topsyn
fluorescein	Dioflur, Fluorescite
fluorometholone	Flarex
fluorouracil	Adrucil, Efudex
fluoxetine	Prozac
fluoxymesterone	Halotestin
flupenthixol	Fluanxol
fluphenazine	Modecate, Moditen
flurazepam	Dalmane
flurbiprofen	Ansaid, Froben, Ocufen
flutamide	Euflex
fluticasone	Flonase, Flovent
fluticasone-salmeterol	Advair Diskus
fluvastatin	Lescol
fluvoxamine	Luvox
follitropin	Puregon
fomepizole	Antizol
fondaparinus	Arixta
formoterol	Foradil, Oxeze
fosinopril	Monopril
fosphenytoin	Cerebyx
furosemide	Lasix
G	
gabapentin	Neurontin
gadodiamide	Omniscan

Continued

Table A-2 *Canadian Drug Names*—cont'd*

GENERIC NAME	TRADE NAME(S)
ganciclovir	Cytovene
ganirelix	Orgalutran
gemcitabine	Gemzar
gemfibrozil	Lopid
gentamicin	Alcomicin, Cidomycin, Garamycin
glatiramer	Copaxone
glicazide	Diamicron
glimepride	Amaryl
glyburide	Diabeta, Euglucon, Gen-Glybe
gonadorelin	Factrel, Lutrepulse
goserelin	Zoladex
granisetron	Kytril
griseofulvin	Fulvicin
H	
haloperidol	Haldol, Novo-Peridol, Peridol
heparin	Hepalean
homatropine, generic	—
hydralazine	Apresoline, Novo-Hylazin, Nu-Hydral
hydrochlorothiazide	Apo-Hydro, HydroDIURIL
hydrochlorothiazide-amiloride	Apo-Amilzide, Moduret, Novamilor, Nu-Amilzide
hydrochlorothiazide-candesartan	Atacand Plus
hydrochlorothiazide-cilazapril	Inhibace Plus
hydrochlorothiazide-enalapril	Vaseretic
hydrochlorothiazide-irbesartan	Avalide
hydrochlorothiazide-lisinopril	Prinzide, Zestoretic
hydrochlorothiazide-losartan	Hyzaar
hydrochlorothiazide-methyldopa	Apo-Methazide
hydrochlorothiazide-pindolol	Viskazide
hydrochlorothiazide-quinapril	Accuretic
hydrochlorothiazide-spironolactone	Aldactazide, Novo-Spirozine
hydrochlorothiazide-telmisartan	Micardis Plus
hydrochlorothiazide-triamterene	Apo-Triazide, Dyazide, Novo-Triamzide, Nu-Triazide
hydrochlorothiazide-valsartan	Diovan-HCT
hydrocodone	Hycodan
hydrocortisone	Cortate, Cortef, Hycort, Solu-Cortef
hydromorphone	Dilaudid, Hydromorph Contin
hydroquinone	Lustra, Solaquin, Ultraquin
hydroxurea	Hydrea
hydroxycobalamin, generic	—
hydroxyzine	Atarax
hyoscine	Buscopan
I	
ibuprofen	Advil, Motrin, Novo-Profen
idarubicin	Idamycin
idoxuridine	Herplex-D
ifosfamide	Ifex
imipenem-cilastatin	Primaxin
imipramine	Tofranil
imiquimod	Aldara
indapamide	Lozide
indinavir	Crixivan
indomethacin	Indocid, Novo-Methacin, Nu-Indo, Rhodacine
infliximab	Remicade
inosine	Imunovir
interferon alfa-2a	Roferon-A
interferon alfa-2b	Intron-A

Table A-2 *Canadian Drug Names**

GENERIC NAME	TRADE NAME(S)
interferon beta-1a	Anovex, Rebif
interferon beta-1b	Betaseron
iopromide	Ultravist
ipratropium	Apo-Ipravent, Atrovent, Novo-Ipramide
ipratropium-fenterol	Duovent
ipratropium-salbutamol	Combivent
irbesartan	Avapro
irbesartan-hydrochlorothiazide	Avalide
iron sorbitex	Jectofer
isoflurane, generic	—
isoniazid	Isotamine
isoniazid-rifampin-pyrazinamide	Rifater
isoproterenol, generic	—
isosorbide dinitrate	Apo-ISDN
isosorbide mononitrate	Imdur, Ismo
isotretinoin	Accutane, Isotrex
itraconazole	Sporanox
K	
ketamine	Ketalar
ketoconazole	Nizoral
ketoprofen	Apo-Keto, Novo-Keto, Orafen, Orudis, Oruvail, Rhodis, Rhovail
ketorolac	Acular, Toradol
ketotifen	Zaditen
L	
labetalol	Trandate
lamivudine	3TC, Heptovir
lamivudine-abacavir-zidovudine	Trizivir
lamivudine-zidovudine	Combivir
lamotrigine	Lamictal
lansoprazole	Prevacid
lansoprazole-amoxacillin-clarithromycin	HpPAC
latanoprost	Xalatan
leflunomide	Arava
lepirudin	Refludan
letrozole	Femara
leuprolide	Lupron
levamisole	Ergamisol
levarterenol, *see* norepinephrine	—
levobunolol	Betagan
levocabastine	Livostin
levodopa-benserazide	Prolopa
levodopa-carbidopa	Apo-Levocarb, Nu-Levocarb, Sinemet
levofloxacin	Levaquin
levomepromazine	Nozinan
ievonorgestrel	Norplant
levothyroxine	Eltroxin, Synthroid
lidocaine	Xylocaine, Xylocard
lincomycin	Lincocin
lindane	Hexit
liothyronine	Cytomel
lisinopril	Prinivil, Zestril
lisinopril-hydrochlorothiazide	Prinzide, Zestoretic
lithium carbonate	Carbolith, Duralith, Lithane
lodoxamide	Alomide
lomustine	CEENU

Continued

| Table A-2 | *Canadian Drug Names*—cont'd |

GENERIC NAME	TRADE NAME(S)
loperamide	Imodium
loratadine	Claritin
lorazepam	Ativan, Novo-Lorazem, Nu-Loraz
losartan	Cozaar
losartan-hydrochlorothiazide	Hyzaar
lovastatin	Mevacor
loxapine	Loxapac
l-tryptophan	Tryptan
M	
mazindol	Sanorex
mebendazole	Vermox
meclizine	Bonamine
medroxyprogesterone	Depo-Provera, Gen-Medroxy, Novo-Medrone, Provera
mefenamic acid	Ponstan
mefloquine	Lariam
meloxicam	Mobicox
melphalan	Alkeran
meperidine	Demerol
mepivacaine	Carbocaine
meprobamate-ASA-caffeine	282MEP
mercaptopurine	Purinethol
mesna	Uromitexan
metformin	Glucophage, Glycon
methacholine	Provocholine
methadone	Metadol
methazolamide, generic	—
methenamine	Mandelamine, Hip-Rex
methimazole	Tapazole
methocarbamol	Robaxin
methocarbamol-acetaminophen	Methoxacet, Robaxacet
methocarbamol-ASA	Methoxasal, Robaxisal
methotrexate	Rheumatrex
methotrimeprazine	Apo-Methoprazine, Novo-Meprazine, Nozinan
methoxamine	Vasoxyl
methoxsalen	Oxsoralen, Ultramop
methsuximide	Celontin
methyldopa	Novo-Medopa, Nu-Medopa
methyldopa-hydrochlorothiazide	Apo-Methazide
methylphenidate	Ritalin
methylprednisolone	Depo-Medrol, Medrol, Solu-Medrol
methysergide	Sansert
metoclopramide	Apo-Metoclop
metolazone	Zaroxolyn
metoprolol	Betaloc, Lopressor, Novo-Metoprol, Nu-Metop
metronidazole	Flagyl, Novo-Nidazol
metronidazole-nystatin	Flagystatin
miconazole	Micatin, Micozole, Monistat
midazolam	Versed
midodrine	Amatine
milrinone	Primacor
minocycline	Minocin
minoxidil	Apo-Gain, Loniten, Rogaine
mirtazapine	Remeron
misoprostol	Cytotec
misoprostol-diclofenac	Arthrotec
mitotane	Lysodren
moclobemide	Manerix
modafinil	Alertec

Table **A-2** | *Canadian Drug Names* *

GENERIC NAME	TRADE NAME(S)
montelukast	Singular
morphine	Kadian, M.O.S., MS Contin
mupirocin	Bactroban
muromonab-CD3	Orthoclone-OKT3
N	
nabilone	Cesamet
nabumetone	Relafen
nadolol	Apo-Nadol, Corgard
nadoparin	Fraxiparine
nafarelin	Synarel
nalidixic acid	Neggram
naloxone	Narcan
naltrexone	ReVia
nandrolone	Deca-Durabolin
naphazoline	Naphcon, Vasocon
naphazoline-antazoline	Albalon-A, Vasocon-A
naproxen	Anaprox, Apo-Napro, Naprosyn, Novo-Naprox, Nu-Naprox
naratriptan	Amerge
nedocromil	Alocril, Tilade
nefazodone	Serzone
nelfinavir	Viracept
neomycin, generic	—
neostigmine	Prostigmin
netilmicin	Netromycin
nevirapine	Viramune
nicotine	Habitrol, Nicoderm, Nicorette, Nicotrol
nicotinyl alcohol tartrate	Roniacol
nicoumalone	Sintrom
nifedipine	Adalat, Apo-Nifed, Novo-Nifedin, Nu-Nifed
nilutamide	Anandron
nimodipine	Nimotop
nitrazepam	Mogadon, Nitrazadon
nitrofurantoin	Macrodantin, Novo-Furantoin
nitroglycerin	Nitro-Dur, Nitrol, Nitrostat, Transderm-Nitro
nitroprusside	Nipride
norepinephrine	Levophed
norethindrone	Micronor, Norlutate
norfloxacin	Apo-Norflox, Noroxin
nylidrin	Arlidin
nystatin	Candistatin, Mycostatin, Nyaderm
nystatin-metronidazole	Flagystatin
O	
octreotide	Sandostatin
ofloxacin	Apo-Oflox, Floxin, Ocuflox
olanzepine	Zyprexa
olopatadine	Patanol
olsalazine	Dipentum
omeprazole	Losec
ondansetron	Zofran
orciprenaline, *see* metaproterenol	—
orlistat	Xenical
orphenadrine	Disipal, Norflex
oxaprozin	Daypro
oxazepam	Serax
oxcarbazepine	Trileptal

Continued

Table A-2 *Canadian Drug Names*—cont'd*

GENERIC NAME	TRADE NAME(S)
oxiconazole	Oxizole
oxprenolol	Slow-Trasicor, Trasicor
oxtriphylline	Choledyl
oxybutynin	Ditropan
oxycodone	OxyContin, Supeudol
oxycodone-acetaminophen	Endocet, Oxycocet, Percocet
oxycodone-ASA	Endodan, Oxycodan, Percodan
oxymetazoline, generic	—
oxymorphone	Numorphan
oxytocin, generic	—
P	
paclitaxel	Taxol
palivizumab	Synagis
pamidronate	Aredia
pancrelipase	Cotazym, Ultrase, Viokase
pancuronium, generic	—
pantoprazole	Pantoloc
papavarine, generic	—
paraldehyde, generic	—
paromomycin	Humatin
paroxetine	Paxil
penicillamine	Cuprimine
penicillin G	Bicillin
penicillin V	Apo-Pen-VK, Novo-Pen-VK, Nu-Pen-VK, Pen-Vee
pentamidine	Pentacarinat
pentazocine	Talwin
pentobarbital	Nembutal
pentoxifylline	Trental
pergolide	Permax
pericyazine	Neuleptil
perphenazine	Trilafon
perphenazine-amitriptyline	Triavil
pethidine, *see* meperidine	—
phenazopyridine	Phenazo, Pyridium
phenelzine	Nardil
phenobarbital, generic	—
phentermine	Ionamin
phentolamine	Rogitine
phenylephrine	Mydfrin, Neo-Synephrine
phenylpropanolamine	Coricidin
phenytoin	Dilantin
phytomenadione, generic	—
pilocarpine	Diocarpine, Isopto Carpine, Miocarpine, Pilopine, Salagen
pimozide	Orap
pinaverium	Dicetel
pindolol	Apo-Pindol, Novo-Pindol, Nu-Pindol, Visken
pindolol-hydrochlorothiazide	Viskazide
pioglitazone	Actos
piperacillin	Pipracil
piperacillin-tazobactam	Tazocin
piperazine	Entacyl
pipotiazine	Piportil-L4
piroxicam	Feldene, Novo-Pirocam, Nu-Pirox
pivampicillin	Pondocillin
pivmecillinam	Selexid
pizotifen	Sandomigran
podophyllum resin	Podofilm

Table A-2	*Canadian Drug Names**

GENERIC NAME	TRADE NAME(S)
polymyxin B	Polysporin
potassium	Apo-K, K-10, K-Dur, Slow-K
pralidoxime	Protopam
pramipexole	Miraprex
pravastatin	Apo-Pravachol, Pravachol
praziquantel	Biltricide
prazosin	Apo-Prazo, Minipress, Novo-Prazin, Nu-Prazo
prednisolone, generic	—
prednisone	Winpred
primaquine, generic	—
primidone	Mysoline
probenecid	Benemid, Benuryl
procainamide	Procan SR, Pronestyl
procaine	Novocain
procarbazine	Matulane
prochlorperazine	Nu-Prochlor, Stemetil
procyclidine	Procyclid
progesterone	Crinone, Prometrium
proguanil-atovaquone	Malarone
promazine, generic	—
promethazine	Phenergan
propafenone	Rythmol
propantheline	Propanthel
proparacaine	Alcaine
propofol	Diprivan
propoxyphene	Darvon-N
propranolol	Inderal
propylthiouracil	Propyl-Thyracil
protamine, generic	—
protirelin	Relefact TRH
protriptyline	Triptil
pseudoephedrine	Contact, Eltor
pseudoephedrine-acetaminophen	Sudafed
pseudoephedrine-triprolidine	Actifed
psyllium	Metamucil
pyrantel	Combantrin
pyrazinamide	Tebrazid
pyrazinamide-isoniazid-rifampin	Rifater
pyridostigmine	Mestinon
pyridoxine-doxylamine	Diclectin
pyrilamine-acetaminophen	Midol Extra Strength
pyrimethamine	Daraprim
pyrvinium pamoate	Vanquin
Q	
quetiapine	Seroquel
quinapril	Accupril
quinapril-hydrochlorothiazide	Accuretic
quinidine	Biquin Durules, Cardioquin, Quinidex
quinine, generic	—
R	
rabeprazole	Pariet
raloxifene	Evista
raltitrexed	Tomudex
ramipril	Altace
ranitidine	Novo-Ranidine, Nu-Ranit, Zantac
remifentanil	Ultiva

Continued

Table A-2 | *Canadian Drug Names*—cont'd

GENERIC NAME	TRADE NAME(S)
repaglinide	Gluconorm
reteplase	Retavase
Rh$_o$(D) immune globulin	Win-Rho
ribavirin	Virazole
ribavarin–interferon alfa-2b	Rebetron
ribavarin–peg-interferon alfa-2b	Pegetron
rifabutin	Mycobutin
rifampin	Rifadin, Rofact
rifampin-isoniazid-pyrazinamide	Rifater
riluzole	Riluter
rimexolone	Vexol
risedronate	Actonel
risperidone	Risperdal
ritonavir	Norvir
ritonavir-lopinavir	Kaletra
rivastigmine	Rituxan
rizatriptan	Maxalt
rocuronium	Zemuron
ropinirole	Requip
ropivacaine	Naropin
rosiglitazone	Avandia
S	
salbutamol (albuterol)	Apo-Salvent, Novo-Salmol, Ventolin
salbutamol-ipratropium	Combivent
salmeterol	Serevent
salmeterol-fluticasone	Advair Diskus
saquinavir	Fortovase, Invirase
scopolamine	Transderm V
selegiline	Eldepryl
sennosides	Senokot, X-Prep
sertraline	Zoloft
sevelamer	Renagel
sevoflurane	Sevorane
sibutramine	Meridia
sildenafil	Viagra
silver sulfadiazine	Dermazin, Flamazine
simethicone	Mylanta, Ovol
simvastatin	Zocor
sirolimus	Rapamune
somatostatin	Stilamin
somatrem	Protropin
somatropin	Humatrope, Nutropin, Saizen, Serostin
sotalol	Apo-Sotalol, Novo-Sotalol, Sotacor
spiramycin	Rovamycine
spironolactone	Aldactone, Novo-Spiroton
spironolactone-hydrochlorothiazide	Aldactazide, Novo-Spirozine
stavudine	Zerit
sterculia	Normacol
streptomycin, generic	—
streptozocin	Zanosar
succinylcholine	Quelcin
sucralfate	Sulcrate
sufentanil	Sufenta
sulfacetamide	Cetamide, Sulamyd
sulfadiazine-trimethoprim	Coptin
sulfamethoxazole-trimethoprim	Apo-Sulfatrim, Novo-Trimel, Nu-Cotrimox, Septra
sulfasalazine	Salazopyrin, S.A.S.

Table A-2   *Canadian Drug Names**

GENERIC NAME	TRADE NAME(S)
sulfisoxazole-erythromycin	Pediazole
sulindac	Apo-Sulin, Novo-Sundac
sumatriptan	Imitrex
T	
tacrolimus	Prograf, Protopic
tamoxifen	Apo-Tamox, Nolvadex, Tamofen
tamsulosin	Flomax
tazarotene	Tazorac
tazobactam-piperacillin	Tazocin
telmisartan	Micardis
telmisartan-hydrochlorothiazide	Micardis Plus
temazepam	Restoril
temozolomide	Temodal
tenecteplase	TNKase
teniposide	Vumon
terazosin	Hytrin
terbinafine	Lamisil
terbutaline	Bricanyl
terconazole	Terazol
testosterone	Andriol, Delatestryl
tetrabenazine	Nitoman
tetracaine	Ametop
tetracycline	Apo-Tetra, Novo-Tetra, Nu-Tetra
theophylline	Apo-Theo LA, Novo-Theophyl, Quibron, Theo-Dur, Uniphyl
thioguanine	Lanvis
thiopental	Pentothal
thioproperazine	Majeptil
thiothixene	Navane
tiaprofenic acid	Surgam
ticarcillin-clavulanate	Timentin
ticlopidine	Ticlid
timolol	Apo-Timol, Novo-Timol, Timoptic
tirofiban	Aggrastat
tobramycin	Nebcin, Tobrex
tolbutamide, generic	—
tolmetin	Tolectin
tolnaftate	Zeasorb
tolterodine	Detrol, Unidet
topiramate	Topamax
topotecan	Hycamtin
trandolapril	Mavik
trandolapril-verapamil	Tarka
tranexamic acid	Cyclokapron
tranylcypromine	Parnate
trastuzumab	Herceptin
travoprost	Travatan
trazodone	Desyrel, Trazorel
tretinoin	Renova, Retin-A, Stieva-A, Vesanoid, Vitamin A Acid
tretinoin-erythromycin	Stievamycin
triamcinolone	Aristocort
triamterene-hydrochlorothiazide	Apo-Triazide, Dyazide, Novo-Triamzide, Nu-Triazide
triazolam	Apo-Triazo, Halcion
trifluridine	Viroptic
trihexyphenidyl	Apo-Trihex
trimebutine	Modulon
trimeprazine	Panectyl
trimethoprim	Proloprim

Continued

Table **A-2** *Canadian Drug Names*—cont'd*

GENERIC NAME	TRADE NAME(S)
trimethoprim-sulfadiazine	Coptin
trimethoprim-sulfamethoxazole	Apo-Sulfatrim, Bactrim, Novo-Trimel, Nu-Cotrimox, Septra
trimipramine	Apo-Trimip, Nu-Tripramine, Rhotrimine, Surmontil
triprolidine-pseudoephedrine	Actifed
tropicamide	Diotrope, Mydriacyl
U	
ursodiol	Urso
V	
valacyclovir	Valtrex
valganciclovir	Valcyte
valproic acid	Depakene
valrubicin	Valtaxin
valsartan	Diovan
valsartan-hydrochlorothiazide	Diovan-HCT
vancomycin	Vancocin
vasopressin	Pressyn
vecuronium	Norcuron
venlafaxine	Effexor
verapamil	Apo-Verap, Chronovera, Isoptin, Novo-Veramil, Nu-Verap
verapamil-trandolapril	Tarka
vigabatrin	Sabril
vinblastine, generic	—
vincristine, generic	—
vinorelbine	Navelbine
W	
warfarin	Coumadin
X	
xylometazoline	Decongest
Y	
yohimbine	Yocon
Z	
zafirlukast	Accolate
zalcitabine	Hivid
zaleplon	Starnoc
zanamivir	Relenza
zidovudine	Novo-AZT, Retrovir
zidovudine-abacavir-lamivudine	Trizivir
zidovudine-lamivudine	Combivir
zolmitriptan	Zomig
zopiclone	Imovane, Rhovane
zuclopenthixol	Clopixol, Clopixol-Acuphase

*This table contains common trade names used in Canada, many of which are the same as those used in the United States. Trade names that are formed by simply adding a manufacturer's prefix to a generic name are not included; examples of such names are Apo-Flurazepam (flurazepam), Novo-Digoxin (digoxin), PMS-Isoniazid (isoniazid), and Syn-Diltiazem (diltiazem).
From Evolve Learning Resources to Accompany Lehne RA: *Pharmacology for nursing care,* ed 5, Philadelphia, 2004, WB Saunders (available at *http://evolve.elsevier.com/Lehne/*).

Answers to Exercises and Review Questions

Chapter 1
(p. 1)
A.
1. **XXXV**
2. **LXXXIX**
3. **LXXII**
4. **LV**
5. **CI**
6. **XCII**
7. **CXXXV**
8. **MDLXXX**
9. **CCCXLI**
10. **DCCXXIX**

B.
1. **1211**
2. **720**
3. **166**
4. **529**
5. **3006**
6. **800**
7. **56**
8. **75**
9. **2673**
10. **61**

Chapter 2
(p. 3)
A.
1. $1\frac{1}{2}$
2. $1\frac{2}{5}$
3. 2
4. 3
5. $1\frac{5}{6}$
6. $3\frac{1}{8}$
7. $15\frac{2}{5}$
8. $7\frac{1}{3}$
9. $8\frac{2}{3}$
10. $4\frac{1}{10}$

B.
1. $\frac{5}{3}$
2. $\frac{9}{2}$
3. $\frac{703}{7}$
4. $\frac{73}{8}$
5. $\frac{54}{5}$
6. $\frac{34}{5}$
7. $\frac{17}{8}$
8. $\frac{69}{4}$
9. $\frac{965}{12}$
10. $\frac{441}{4}$

(p. 4)
1. $\frac{5}{20}$
2. $\frac{18}{39}$
3. $\frac{24}{60}$
4. $\frac{14}{36}$
5. $\frac{40}{32}$
6. $\frac{24}{51}$
7. $\frac{49}{63}$
8. $\frac{18}{16}$
9. $\frac{18}{21}$
10. $\frac{21}{10}$

(p. 4)
1. $\frac{7}{12}$ **and** $\frac{6}{12}$
2. $\frac{18}{21}$ **and** $\frac{14}{21}$
3. $\frac{3}{9}$ **and** $\frac{2}{9}$
4. $\frac{8}{20}$ **and** $\frac{8}{20}$
5. $\frac{3}{24}$ **and** $\frac{8}{24}$
6. $\frac{15}{60}$, $\frac{12}{60}$, $\frac{10}{60}$
7. $\frac{8}{12}$, $\frac{6}{12}$, $\frac{9}{12}$
8. $\frac{18}{24}$, $\frac{20}{24}$, $\frac{21}{24}$
9. $\frac{80}{90}$, $\frac{81}{90}$, $\frac{30}{90}$
10. $\frac{20}{75}$, $\frac{45}{75}$, $\frac{12}{75}$
11. $\frac{16}{12}$, $\frac{6}{12}$, $\frac{3}{12}$
12. $\frac{18}{30}$, $\frac{20}{30}$, $\frac{12}{30}$

(pp. 4–5)
1. $1\frac{7}{36}$
2. $1\frac{2}{3}$
3. $6\frac{11}{24}$
4. $18\frac{1}{3}$
5. $1\frac{5}{12}$
6. $11\frac{1}{5}$
7. $5\frac{7}{12}$
8. $6\frac{5}{6}$
9. $37\frac{33}{66}$
10. $10\frac{1}{8}$

(p. 5)
1. $\frac{5}{18}$
2. $\frac{1}{21}$
3. $\frac{5}{8}$
4. $1\frac{3}{7}$
5. $1\frac{3}{8}$
6. $3\frac{1}{5}$
7. $3\frac{1}{3}$
8. $14\frac{5}{6}$
9. $3\frac{1}{12}$
10. $3\frac{1}{6}$

(pp. 5–6)
1. $\frac{1}{12}$
2. $\frac{35}{72}$

3. 4
4. $1\frac{17}{75}$
5. $14\frac{1}{6}$
6. 33
7. 4
8. 20
9. $\frac{2}{27}$
10. $\frac{1}{25}$

(p. 6)
1. $\frac{24}{35}$
2. $\frac{1}{4}$
3. $\frac{7}{9}$
4. $\frac{1}{6}$
5. 6
6. $1\frac{1}{8}$
7. 2
8. $\frac{7}{8}$
9. $1\frac{1}{5}$
10. $\frac{41}{100}$

(p. 6)
1. $\frac{1}{3}$
2. $\frac{5}{7}$
3. $\frac{1}{500}$
4. $\frac{1}{9}$
5. $\frac{42}{83}$
6. $\frac{2}{17}$
7. $\frac{1}{8}$
8. $\frac{1}{11}$
9. $\frac{1}{75}$
10. $\frac{4}{9}$

Chapter 3
(p. 7)
A.
1. **Three one-hundredths**
2. **Eighty-nine one-thousandths**
3. **Twenty-three and five tenths**
4. **Five and twenty-one one-hundredths**
5. **Twenty-nine ten-thousandths**
6. **Two hundred and nine one-hundredths**
7. **Thirty-seven and two hundred eighty-two one-thousandths**
8. **Four thousand two hundred fifty-six and three hundred fifty-three one-thousandths**
9. **Two hundred fifty-six and one one-thousandth**
10. **Eight ten-thousandths**

B.
1. 0.004
2. 0.26
3. 5.000003
4. 0.07
5. 3.1
6. 0.088
7. 233.000057
8. 2.3
9. 8.04
10. 25.003

(p. 8)
1. 10.898
2. 49.59
3. 12.42
4. 6.53
5. 302.76
6. 1.783
7. 6.09
8. 7.045
9. 77.68
10. 2.47

(p. 8)
1. 0.646
2. 0.04
3. 41.28
4. 728.697
5. 0.018
6. 3.22
7. 4.7
8. 34.5
9. 2.837
10. 105.71

(p. 8)
1. 3.2
2. 0.011
3. 0.0945
4. 140
5. 0.8907
6. 120
7. 0.00009
8. 99.446
9. 120
10. 11.24508

(p. 9)
1. 60.000
2. 2.338
3. 133.461
4. 6.195
5. 20.000
6. 3.650
7. 20.000
8. 8.456
9. 3.435
10. 0.085

(p. 9)

A.
1. 0.8
2. 0.166

3. 0.22
4. 0.866
5. 4.4
6. 7.125
7. 0.703
8. 0.6754
9. 4.718
10. 2.611

B.
1. $^{28}/_{100}$ **reduced to** $^{7}/_{25}$
2. $5^{7}/_{100}$
3. $^{22}/_{10,000}$ **reduced to** $^{11}/_{5000}$
4. $1^{28}/_{100}$ **reduced to** $1^{7}/_{25}$
5. $3^{4}/_{100}$ **reduced to** $3^{1}/_{25}$
6. $^{575}/_{1000}$ **reduced to** $^{23}/_{40}$
7. $^{76}/_{100}$ **reduced to** $^{19}/_{25}$
8. $^{15,325}/_{100,000}$ **reduced to** $^{613}/_{4000}$
9. $6^{9}/_{100}$
10. $^{1}/_{100}$

Chapter 4
(p. 10)

	Fraction	Decimal	Percent
1.	—	0.25	23%
2.	$1^{25}/_{100}$	—	125%
3.	¾	0.75	—
4.	—	0.125	12.5%
5.	$^{14}/_{25}$	—	56%
6.	—	0.006	0.6%
7.	$^{3}/_{50}$	0.06	—
8.	¾	—	75%
9.	⅕	0.2	—
10.	$^{3}/_{25}$	0.12	—
11.	$^{1}/_{20}$	—	5%
12.	$^{18}/_{25}$	0.72	—

(pp. 10–11)
1. 18
2. 4.2
3. 0.75
4. 216
5. 13.4
6. 0.02
7. 37.5
8. 6
9. 1.20
10. 50.544
11. 137.5
12. 3.237

(p. 11)
1. 10%
2. 40%
3. 17.6%
4. 31.2%
5. 60%
6. 56.2%
7. 17.6%
8. 200%
9. 400%
10. 20%
11. 20%
12. 200%

Chapter 5
(p. 12)
1. 4
2. 400
3. 20
4. 10
5. 5000
6. 48
7. 3
8. 5
9. 36
10. 48
11. 90
12. 14
13. 28
14. 1.04
15. 25

Chapter 6
(pp. 13–14)
1. 68° F
2. 140° F
3. 215.6° F
4. 95° F
5. 104° F
6. 38.3° C
7. 21.1° C
8. 48.8° C
9. 40° C
10. 36° C

Chapter 7
(p. 15)
1. 1 gm
2. 0.5 gm
3. 2 L
4. 1.5 gm
5. 100 mL
6. 0.75 gm
7. 1000 gm
8. 5000 mL
9. 0.004 gm
10. 0.1 kg
11. 250 mL
12. 6 mg
13. 0.25 gm
14. 2500 mL
15. 50 mg

(p. 16)

A.
1. 2 teaspoons
2. 16 ounces
3. 4.5 kg
4. 2 ounces
5. 10 kg
6. 90 gm
7. 12 teaspoons
8. 1 fluid ounce
9. 18 teaspoons
10. 154 pounds

B.
1. **500 mL**
2. **4 cc**
3. **15 mg**
4. **100 mg**
5. **1 pint**
6. **15 mL**
7. **13.6 kg**
8. **6 teaspoons**
9. **1.5 gm**
10. **60 gm**
11. **75 mL**
12. **2½ ounces**
13. **1000 mg**
14. **2 teaspoons**
15. **1/2 ounce**
16. **2500 mL**
17. **1 ounce**
18. **6.6 pounds**
19. **75 kg**
20. **1½ quarts**

Chapter 8
(pp. 17–19)
1. **6 mg**
2. **3 mL**
3. **100 mg**
4. **0.6 mL**
5. **6 mg**
6. **48 mg**
7. **100,000 units**
8. **0.3 mL**
9. **1 mL**
10. **2 mg**
11. **33 mg**
12. **0.6 mL**
13. **3 mg**
14. **1.3 mL**
15. a. **3.0 mL**
    b. **2.0 mL**
    c. **2.5 mL**
    d. **7.5 mL**
16. **0.8 m² = 100 mg/day**
17. **On the chart, this is 0.9 m²;**
    125 × 0.9 = 112.5 mg/day

Chapter 9
(p. 21)
1. a. **0.2 mL**
    b. **0.6 mL**
    c. **1.2 mL**
2. **100,000 units**
3. **500,000 units**
4. **250,000 units**
5. **3.3 mL**
6. **4 mL**
7. **2 mL**
8. a. **1.5 mL**
    b. **0.6 mL**
    c. **0.5 mL**
9. a. **0.5 mL**
    b. **0.75 mL**
    c. **1.0 mL**
10. **0.15 mL**

Chapter 11
(p. 26)
1. **a**
2. **a**
3. **d**
4. **d**
5. **d**

Chapter 12
(p. 28)
1. **b**
2. **c**
3. **c**
4. **d**
5. **d**

Chapter 13
(p. 31)
1. **d**
2. **d**
3. **c**
4. **c**
5. **d**
6. **a**
7. **d**
8. **b**
9. **b**
10. **c**

Chapter 14
(pp. 39–40)
1. **b**
2. **c**
3. **a**
4. **d**
5. **c**
6. **c**
7. **b**
8. **a**
9. **c**
10. **a**

Chapter 15
(p. 47)
1. **c**
2. **c**
3. **d**
4. **b**
5. **c**
6. **d**
7. **c**
8. **b**
9. **b**
10. **c**

Chapter 16
(p. 64)
1. **a**
2. **c**
3. **c**
4. **c**
5. **d**
6. **c**
7. **c**
8. **a**

9. **b**
10. **d**

Chapter 17
(pp. 69–70)
1. **d**
2. **b**
3. **a**
4. **d**
5. **c**
6. **a**
7. **a**
8. **b**
9. **c**
10. **d**

Chapter 18
(pp. 78–79)
1. **d**
2. **a**
3. **b**
4. **d**
5. **b**
6. **c**
7. **a**
8. **c**
9. **d**
10. **c**

Chapter 19
(p. 86)
1. **b**
2. **d**
3. **b**
4. **d**
5. **a**
6. **d**
7. **a**
8. **c**
9. **d**
10. **d**

Chapter 20
(p. 100)
1. **c**
2. **a**
3. **c**
4. **a**
5. **d**
6. **d**
7. **c**
8. **b**
9. **d**
10. **b**

Chapter 21
(p. 113)
1. **a**
2. **d**
3. **d**
4. **c**
5. **d**
6. **a**
7. **d**

8. d
9. a
10. c

Chapter 22
(pp. 120–121)

1. c
2. b
3. c
4. d
5. c
6. d
7. d
8. a
9. b
10. a

Chapter 23
(pp. 129–130)

1. b
2. c
3. d
4. b
5. a
6. b
7. d
8. d
9. b
10. b

Chapter 24
(p. 135)

1. b
2. d
3. a
4. c
5. c
6. b
7. c
8. a
9. c
10. c

Chapter 25
(pp. 142–143)

1. b
2. a
3. c
4. b
5. c
6. d
7. c
8. a
9. a
10. d

Chapter 26
(pp. 152–153)

1. d
2. c
3. b
4. c
5. b

6. d
7. c
8. b
9. b
10. a

Chapter 27
(pp. 166–167)

1. a
2. b
3. a
4. a
5. b
6. c
7. c
8. d
9. a
10. d

Chapter 28
(p. 175)

1. a
2. c
3. c
4. c
5. d
6. a
7. b
8. d
9. c
10. b

Chapter 29
(p. 185)

1. b
2. c
3. c
4. a
5. c
6. b
7. a
8. c
9. d
10. d

Chapter 30
(p. 193)

1. b
2. c
3. c
4. b
5. d
6. c
7. c
8. b
9. a
10. a

Chapter 31
(p. 198)

1. a
2. c
3. c

4. d
5. a
6. b
7. c
8. a
9. c
10. d

Chapter 32
(pp. 206–207)

1. b
2. c
3. c
4. c
5. a
6. c
7. b
8. a
9. a
10. d

Chapter 33
(p. 215)

1. d
2. b
3. d
4. c
5. b
6. d
7. b
8. c
9. a
10. c

Chapter 34
(p. 220)

1. c
2. d
3. a
4. b
5. c
6. d
7. d
8. b
9. d
10. d

Chapter 35
(pp. 227–228)

1. b
2. b
3. c
4. a
5. c
6. b
7. d
8. a
9. c
10. c

Disorders Index

Therapeutic Index

In this index, drugs are listed by prescribing category. It is an informational index only and should not be considered to be comprehensive or complete. Page numbers followed by t denote tables.

General Index

Page numbers followed by t denote tables.